'Reiter has recruited an all-star line-up of leading practitioners in couples' work. From case conceptualizations to clear case examples, they illustrate a wide range of theoretical orientations and practices that offer clear maps and guidelines for working with couples. Beginning therapists and seasoned clinicians will find this invaluable resource a must have for their library.'

Jim Duvall, *Co-Director, JST Institute and Editor,*
Journal of Systemic Therapies

'Dr. Reiter and his co-authors brilliantly showcase 11 marriage and family therapy theories in action through a captivating clinical case centered on intricate systemic relational challenges. With engaging mock transcripts of initial sessions, each chapter masterfully dissects the case, conceptualizing problem formation and resolution within each model. An invaluable resource, offering marriage and family therapists an illuminating guide to witness theories come alive in real-world practice!'

Lori Pantaleao, Ph.D., LMFT, LMHC, CAP, CTP,
Assistant Professor and Director of Master's in Couple and Family
Therapy Program, Nova Southeastern University, Fort Lauderdale, FL

T0299773

Case Conceptualization in Couple Therapy

This textbook provides undergraduate and graduate students with a comprehensive and in-depth exploration of the primary models of couples counseling, allowing them to compare and contrast each theory alongside a single case.

Designed to be the core text for couple therapy courses, the book begins by introducing the field as well as presenting Carissa and Steve, a couple whom readers will follow as each model is applied to their case. The chapters focus on 11 different theoretical models such as Bowen family systems theory, emotionally focused couple therapy, the Gottman method, solution-focused couples counseling, narrative couple therapy, and more, with expert therapists writing on each of these unique models. Each chapter addresses the history of the model, the conceptualization of problem formation, diversity considerations, and the conceptualization of problem resolution. With session transcripts throughout, this book allows training therapists to easily compare, contrast, and apply the most prevalent models in couples counseling.

This textbook is a core text for graduate marriage and family therapy, mental health counseling, clinical psychology, and social work students. The book is also useful for practicing professionals who want to explore how to apply a specific model of counseling to couples.

Michael D. Reiter, Ph.D., is an LMFT, an AAMFT Approved Supervisor, a therapist with 30 years' experience, and a full-time faculty member for over 20 years. He currently teaches and supervises at Capella University, Minneapolis.

Case Conceptualization in Couple Therapy

Comparing and Contrasting Theories

Edited by Michael D. Reiter

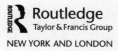

Routledge
Taylor & Francis Group

NEW YORK AND LONDON

Designed cover image: © J. Michael Fernandez

First published 2025
by Routledge
605 Third Avenue, New York, NY 10158

and by Routledge
4 Park Square, Milton Park, Abingdon, Oxon, OX14 4RN

Routledge is an imprint of the Taylor & Francis Group, an informa business

ISBN: 9781032438429 (hbk)
ISBN: 9781032438412 (pbk)
ISBN: 9781003369097 (ebk)

DOI: 10.4324/9781003369097

Typeset in Times New Roman
by Newgen Publishing UK

This book is dedicated to my wife, Yukari.

Thank you for going on this journey of life with me.

Contents

Editor

Michael D. Reiter, Ph.D., LMFT, has been a practicing family therapist for the past 30 years. He earned his M.S. and Ed.S. in Counselor Education from the University of Florida with specializations in Marriage and Family Therapy and Mental Health Counseling and a Ph.D. in Family Therapy from Nova Southeastern University. Michael is a licensed marriage and family therapist in the State of Florida and an Approved Supervisor through the American Association of Marriage and Family Therapy (AAMFT). He is also a State Approved Supervisor for both marriage and family therapy and mental health counseling. For 23 years he was a faculty member at Nova Southeastern University, teaching in the Divisions of Social and Behavioral Sciences, Clinical Psychology, Mental Health Counseling, and the Department of Family Therapy. He is currently a faculty member at Capella University, Minneapolis. Michael has been heavily engaged in scholarship, having written 14 books, including *Succeeding in Your Practicum and Internship* (2024), *Family Therapy: The Basics* (2023), *A Therapist's Guide to Writing in Psychotherapy* (2023), *Therapeutic Interviewing* (2nd ed., 2022), *The Craft of Family Therapy* (2nd ed.) (co-written with Salvador Minuchin; 2021), *Systems Theories for Psychotherapists* (2019), *Family Therapy: An Introduction to Process, Practice, & Theory* (2018), and *Case Conceptualization in Family Therapy* (2014). His books have been translated into Spanish, Polish, Chinese, Italian, and Korean.

Contributing Authors

Carl Bagnini, LCSW, BCD (Board Certified Diplomate in Clinical Social Work), was a senior faculty member and National Program Chair of the Child, Couple and Family Psychotherapy Program at the International Psychotherapy Institute in Washington, D.C. Carl is also a faculty member and Supervisor of the Derner Post Graduate Programs in Psychoanalysis, Psychotherapy and Couple Therapy at Adelphi University, New York. He is the author of *Keeping Couples in Treatment: Working from Surface to Depth* (2012) and has written or co-written many book chapters and papers. Carl is a guest presenter in the United States and internationally on Object Relations topics. He has a private practice in Port Washington, New York.

Christopher Burnett, Psy.D., is an Associate Professor of Human Relationship Systems at Nova Southeastern University in Fort Lauderdale, Florida. He has been with the university since 1993 and has been involved with Bowen family systems theory for over 40 years. He utilizes the human relationship systems principles embedded in Bowen family systems theory in both his clinical practice as well as his organizational consulting business.

Gene Combs, Co-Director of Evanston Family Therapy Center, is internationally recognized for his contributions to narrative therapy theory and training. With his partner-in-all-things Jill Freedman, he has co-authored more than 30 journal articles and book chapters and three books. Now retired from his position as Clinical Associate Professor at the University of Chicago, he is increasingly upset with what professional psychiatry has become over the 45 years since he was certified to practice it. He believes it is important to see people and the world in more complex and less pathologizing ways than does the DSM-based and big-pharma-influenced model that has become standard.

Norman B. Epstein, Ph.D., is Professor Emeritus in the Department of Family Science, School of Public Health, at the University of Maryland, College Park, and a licensed clinical psychologist. He is a Fellow of the American Psychological Association, Fellow of the Association for Behavioral and Cognitive Therapies, Professional Member of the American Association for Marriage and Family Therapy, Founding Fellow of the Academy of Cognitive Therapy, and Diplomate of the Society of Assessment Psychology. He is a pioneer in the development of cognitive-behavioral therapy with couples and families.

Jill Freedman, MSW, is Co-Director of the Evanston Family Therapy Center in the United States and an international faculty member of Dulwich Centre in Adelaide, Australia. She is co-author of three books with Gene Combs: *Symbol, Story and Ceremony: Using Metaphor in Individual and Family Therapy* (1990), *Narrative Therapy: The Social Construction of Preferred Realities* (1996), and *Narrative Therapy with Couples… and a Whole Lot More!* (2002). She is co-author with David Denborough and Cheryl White of *Strengthening Resistance: The Use of Narrative Practices in Working with Genocide Survivors* (2018). She teaches internationally, has a therapy and supervision practice, and consults to non-profit agencies and schools.

James L. Furrow, Ph.D., is a recognized leader and contributor to the practice of emotionally focused therapy (EFT) with couples and families. His works include: *Emotionally Focused Family Therapy: Restoring Connection and Promoting Resilience* (2019) and *Becoming an Emotionally Focused Therapist: The Workbook* (2022). He teaches in the Couple and Family Therapy Program, Seattle University, Seattle, Washington.

Nicholas Lee is an Assistant Professor of Counseling Psychology in the Department of Counseling Psychology, Social Psychology, and Counseling at Ball State University. He is a licensed psychologist and Health Service Provider in Psychology in Indiana. He is a certified emotionally focused couple therapist.

Wade Luquet, Ph.D., LCSW, is Professor of Social Work at Gwynedd Mercy University in suburban Philadelphia. He is the author of *Short-Term Couples Therapy: The Imago Model in Action* (1996) and co-editor of *Healing in the Relational Paradigm: The Imago Relationship Therapy Casebook* (1998) and *Imago Relationship Therapy: Perspectives on Theory* (2005). He maintains a private practice in North Wales, Pennsylvania.

Vagdevi Meunier, Psy.D., is a licensed clinical psychologist and a Clinical Assistant Professor in the Clinical Psychology Doctoral Program at the University of Texas in Austin. She has a private clinical and consulting practice in Austin where she specializes in couples and family therapy, couples' workshops, training and supervision, and organizational consultation. Vagdevi is the founder and Executive Director of The Center for Relationships, a wellness center that specializes in counseling, outreach, education, and research based on relationship science. She has also been a certified Gottman couples therapist and a certified Gottman workshop leader since 2006.

Hannah S. Myung, Ph.D., is an Assistant Professor in the Department of Psychology at the University of Utah Asia Campus and a licensed psychologist in California.

Patricia A. Robey, Ed.D., LPC, NCC, is a Full Professor in Psychology and Counseling at Governors State University in Illinois. She is a licensed professional counselor, a nationally certified counselor, and coach. Dr. Robey is a senior faculty member of William Glasser International and the Glasser Institute for Choice Theory in the United States. She is the author of numerous articles and contributions to professional textbooks and is the lead editor and contributing author to *Contemporary Issues in Couples Counseling: A Choice Theory and Reality Therapy Approach* (2012).

Kayleigh Sabo, M.S., Ph.D. Candidate, is a licensed marriage and family therapist in the State of Florida. She is currently working on her Ph.D. dissertation in Couple and Family Therapy. Kayleigh has published six articles, co-authored three book chapters, and co-authored *Succeeding in Your Practicum and Internship: Tips, Tools, and Tales from Interns and Supervisors* (2024).

Jon Sperry, Ph.D., is an Associate Professor of Clinical Mental Health Counseling at Lynn University, Boca Raton, Florida. He teaches, writes, and researches case conceptualization, and conducts workshops on it worldwide. Sperry holds a Diplomate in Adlerian Psychotherapy and is currently the co-editor of the *Journal of Individual Psychology*.

Len Sperry, M.D., Ph.D., is a Professor Emeritus at Florida Atlantic University and Clinical Professor at the Medical College of Wisconsin. His 1,100+ publications include *Highly Effective Therapy: Effecting Deep Change in Counseling and Psychotherapy* (2nd ed., 2022).

Preface

In 2014, I wrote *Case Conceptualization in Family Therapy* (published by Pearson). That book was based on showing *The Gloria Tapes*, those most famous psychotherapy sessions where the client, Gloria, worked with Carl Rogers, Fritz Perls, and Albert Ellis. After viewing them in class, my students were able to better compare and contrast how various models understood why people have difficulties and what to do with them. In the book, I created a case family. Then I presented nine different family therapy models, highlighting the theory of problem formation and the theory of problem resolution along with a focus on diversity conceptualization. Each chapter ended with a transcript of what a first session using that model might look like. Each chapter was co-written with a colleague who was a content expert in that model. Over the years since that book was published, thousands of students have used the book to help them learn the primary models of family therapy and, most importantly, be able to apply them. Knowing the concepts of the model is useful when taking an exam. However, the application of the model is crucial for actual engagement with clients.

This book, *Case Conceptualization in Couple Therapy*, is the natural follow-up to that original book. I took what made the first book a success, the use of a standard case and a focus on case conceptualization, and implemented that in the design of this book. I was fortunate to bring on board some leading U.S. experts on couple therapy to write the various chapters. I provided them with the case (the Hogarths, whom you will meet in Chapter 2) and asked them to organize the chapter as such:

1 History of the Model
2 Conceptualization of Problem Formation
3 Conceptualizing Diversity
4 The Role of the Therapist
5 Conceptualization of Problem Resolution
6 Case Transcript

The hope of this book is that you will have a solid understanding of each of the models as well as the ability to compare and contrast them with one another. However, I recognize that the chapters of this book alone are not sufficient for you to be fully knowledgeable and functional in that model. Learning any model of therapy takes time. Yet, after reading this book, you should have leanings as to which model(s) makes the most sense for you. Once you do, please explore them more; read from the founders, watch sessions from that model, and begin to incorporate these ideas into your practice.

This book could definitely not have come to fruition without the contributions of the various chapter authors. I want to thank them all again: Carl Bagnini, Christopher Burnett, Gene Combs,

Norman Epstein, Jill Freedman, James L. Furrow, Nicholas Lee, Wade Luquet, Vagdevi Meunier, Hannah Myung, Patricia Robey, Kayleigh Sabo, Jon Sperry, and Len Sperry. I also want to thank Brye Moss for her help in the transcript development for the Bowen couple therapy chapter (Chapter 5) and Yukari Tomozawa for genogram development. Julia Giordano, of Routledge, helped see this project through fruition.

1   An Introduction to Couple Therapy

Michael D. Reiter

When clients seek therapeutic services, they do so in a variety of configurations, whether it be as an individual, couple, family, or other relational connection. Although therapists may apply a single model across these formats, each format poses unique challenges. This book provides an introduction to major theoretical models for working with couples, aiming to establish a comprehensive understanding of these models for conceptualizing therapeutic approaches. This chapter offers an overview of couples, couple therapy, and case conceptualizations, contextualizing the specific theoretical case conceptualizations that will be presented throughout this book.

Understanding Couples

Couples may be one of the most difficult populations to work with as many times, couples will come to the first session and say some variation of the following: "Things are terrible between us. If it doesn't work with you, we are going to end the relationship." The good news is that they are finally working on improving their relationship with a trained professional. The bad news is that they have likely waited a long time and may have built up much resentment, anger, and negative patterns of interactions.

A **couple** is a unit, composing a subsystem of two larger systems, each partner's family of origin. As a unit, they are connected in a myriad of ways. The subjective closeness of the couple is referred to as **"we-ness"** and is an important factor in their satisfaction with the relationship (Cruwys et al., 2023). Couples who use a "we" orientation rather than an "I" orientation tend to have more positive therapeutic outcomes (D'Arrigo-Patrick et al., 2020). Many people in couples, however, tend to operate more from an "I" orientation, exemplified by a disagreement on whether they want/need therapy (Doss et al., 2004).

Couples come to therapy for a variety of reasons. Gurman (2010) explained, "Generally, couples seek therapy because of threats to the security and stability of their relationships with the most significant attachment figures of adult life" (p. 3). Many times, they will come stating that they are having "communication issues" (Beckerman & Shepherd, 2002) as well as a deficit in emotional affection (Doss et al., 2004). One of the main reasons that couples come to therapy is a concern that their partner does not understand them, especially around areas that lead to conflict (Crenshaw et al., 2019). To further confound this situation, greater levels of stress result in lower levels of empathic accuracy for members of a couple (Crenshaw et al., 2019). That is, as the relationship becomes more difficult, each member has a tougher time being able to appreciate and understand the internal experience of their partner.

Not all couple issues are at the same level. Some are minor while others are severe. Beckerman and Shepherd (2002) found that high-conflict areas for couples included those around sex and making major decisions. Moderate-conflict areas included money, in-laws, and religion. For whatever reason the couple seeks therapy, they likely present their reasons for doing so in terms of

DOI: 10.4324/9781003369097-1

blaming their partner. Many couples come to therapy where one or both partners blame and accuse the other of wrongdoing (Smoliak et al., 2022). Couple distress is also predicated on blaming one another, withdrawal strategies, and aggression (Parnell et al., 2018).

In the United Kingdom, couples who go to therapy tend to be White, 25–54 years old, and present with interpersonal issues (Duncan et al., 2020). Only about one-quarter of couples present with a concern about mental health problems, demonstrating that they are more concerned about interpersonal rather than psychological problems. In heterosexual couples, the female tends to be the first to perceive a relationship problem and is likely the person to reach out for therapeutic help (Parnell et al., 2018). These researchers found that males tend to fear being judged and feel a sense of failure in considering going to couple therapy. Men are more reluctant than women to pursue couple therapy (Spiker et al., 2019). When men have more positive attitudes about couple therapy, they are more likely to seek it out and participate.

As explained, couples do not come to therapy at the first sign of trouble in their relationship. Usually, they wait quite a long time before seeking therapeutic assistance. They likely experienced a gradual reduction in their marital satisfaction and an increased desire for relationship dissolution (Owen et al., 2018). There are numerous reasons why couples do not seek therapeutic services, reflecting general significant barriers to accessing mental health services (Salivar et al., 2020). These include direct (money) and indirect (time off work, childcare, and transportation) costs. Further, there still exists a stigma that some people experience when thinking about seeking out therapy.

Couple therapy continues to gain recognition throughout the world based on three main factors (Lebow & Snyder, 2022). First, couples experience distress throughout their relationship. Second, this distress impacts the emotional and physical well-being of the partners in the couple (as well as any children they may have). Last, people entering a couple relationship these days expect more from it. At one point in time, the dominant discourse was that the members of the couple had to hold an acceptance of marital disharmony since they had said in their vows, "For better or for worse." Modern couples are less likely to accept unhappiness in the relationship or even expect that the relationship must progress to marriage or be monogamous.

Telehealth and Couple Therapy

Traditionally, couple therapy occurred between three people who sat in the therapist's office for one hour per week for weekly sessions. The Covid-19 pandemic turned this typical format on its head and most couple therapists began providing services through videoconferencing technology. The therapist might have been in a room of their house while the partners of the couple were on the other end of a computer or smartphone via the camera, which allowed them to be in their home environment (or anywhere else they wanted to be during the session). Further, the members of the couple could be in different locations at the same time, with one partner at home and the other in their car during their lunch break from work. We will not talk much in this book about teletherapy, although it is likely to continue to be a significant means of providing therapeutic services to couples (Lebow & Snyder, 2022; Wrape & McGinn, 2018).

One of the reasons for teletherapy is that potentially more clients will access services. This may be to avoid the potential stigma of going to therapy (i.e., being seen in the therapist's office), transportation issues, or childcare issues. Teletherapy has the potential to provide underserved populations with more access to mental healthcare. However, for higher-risk issues (such as intimate partner violence, infidelity, divorce, or other self-harm issues), in-person therapy may be more appropriate (Salivar et al., 2020).

While there are many advantages to conducting couple sessions via telehealth, there are also some unique concerns (Wrape & McGinn, 2018). These include having the process interrupted by normal occurrences in the house, missing out on various non-verbal cues, difficulties in joining the couple, and safety. For instance, if things begin to escalate between the partners, it is more difficult for the therapist to intervene and de-escalate the situation. Lord (2022) suggested that, when engaging couples via telehealth, it is extremely important to lay the foundation at the beginning of therapy to ensure clear professional boundaries and safety issues. Further, assessing safety is important throughout the course of the therapy process.

Models of Couple Therapy

Few therapists are trained in couple therapy during their graduate degree (Doherty, 2002). Most likely, someone getting a degree in family therapy will be required to take a course in couple therapy. Other professions are likely not to have a couple therapy class, perhaps covering this topic for a class session or two in some courses. Thus, most therapists learn how to do couple therapy after they have gotten their academic qualification, learning on the job.

Gurman (2010) explained,

> Couple therapy, traditionally referred to as "marital therapy" … refers to a varied set of psychotherapeutic interventions, techniques, methods, strategies, and perspectives intended to help intimate relationship partners reduce important (and usually recurrent) aspects of relationship distress and enhance relationship satisfaction.
>
> (Gurman, 2010, p. 1)

Couple therapy helps to improve communication for couples and provides them with a space to come to a resolution about the status of their relationship (Beckerman & Shepherd, 2002).

Lebow and Snyder (2022) stated, "By definition, couple therapies focus on the couple dyad and, for the most part, on the aggregate subjective balance of couple distress versus well-being" (p. 14).

Contemporary couple therapy models tend to be predicated on general systems theory, cybernetics, and family development theory (Gurman, 2008). Other influencing factors include psychodynamic, humanistic, and cognitive and social learning theories as well as feminism, multiculturalism, and postmodernism. Recently, couple therapy has been informed by relationship science as well as neuroscience (Lebow & Snyder, 2022). Wittenborn and Holtrop (2022) stated,

> Couple and family interventions are based on the well-established science that close relationships play a role in the development and maintenance of mental and behavioral disorders and health conditions and that relationship dynamics can be altered or harnessed to improve symptoms.
>
> (Wittenborn & Holtrop, 2022, p. 20)

Gurman and Fraenkel (2002) broke down the history of couple therapy into four phases. Phase I is called **Atheoretical marriage counseling formation** and lasted from 1930 to 1963. In the early 1930s, three different major marriage counseling institutes were developed. Marriage counseling was in many ways a side project of professionals such as doctors, religious leaders, and social workers. They worked with couples who were not having severe issues but rather were seeking pre-marital counseling or guidance about typical married life.

Phase II of couple therapy is the **Psychoanalytic experimentation**, which lasted from 1931 to 1966. As can be seen, there is an overlap in years between phases I and II. This is because there were two different paths being taken simultaneously by two different groups of professionals. Phase II was led by those clinicians who operated from a psychoanalytic perspective. These individuals, all of whom were psychiatrists, strayed from the fundamentalist psychoanalytic practice by at first seeing one partner in analysis after their partner's therapy ended. They then engaged in a concurrent treatment where the analyst worked with both partners but not at the same time. What was happening was a shift of thought where the therapist was becoming more central in the therapy process. They were still conceptualizing cases primarily from an individualistic perspective, but the ground was fertile for conjoint therapy.

Phase III of couple therapy is **Family therapy incorporation**, which lasted from 1963 to 1985. Family therapy was born in the late 1950s and early 1960s. The notion of conjoint therapy, where multiple members of the family were seen at the same time was an innovation at this time. Further, there was a move away from conceptualizing the problem as being inherent in one person (deemed the identified patient) to the processes and interactions that occur between people.

The last phase of couple therapy, Phase IV, is called **Refinement, extension, diversification, and integration**, which began in 1986 and continues to the present. Theories and models of couple therapy emerged, all with a robust research base. The three most significant models included behavioral marital therapy, emotionally focused couple therapy, and insight-oriented marital therapy. During this time there was also a reemergence of psychodynamic (psychoanalytic) couple therapy. Gurman and Fraenkel (2002) hypothesized that psychoanalytic couple therapy had this reemergence due to a push for integration, where both intrapsychic and interpersonal aspects of functioning and distress came more prominently to the forefront. The diversification in the field arose from viewing the couple as a subsystem of larger systems such as social and political contexts. Areas such as feminism, postmodernism, and multiculturalism helped inform therapists about how couples organized and functioned.

At the end of the 20th century, couple therapy had several key trends (Johnson & Lebow, 2000). First, couple therapy was recognized as the treatment of choice for clients who were coming in with couple distress. Second, the science of relationships was taking off, providing a framework for couple functioning and intervention. Third, more researchers were conducting studies that were showing the effectiveness of couple therapy. Fourth, psychotherapy had a greater recognition of the role of gender in relationships. Fifth, there was a growing appreciation of the diversity of ways that people come together and enter couples and/or families. Sixth, emotion was becoming a more important component in psychotherapy. Seventh, postmodernism was influencing the field, holding that there is no inherently defined truth or meaning. Eighth, domestic violence (interpersonal violence) was becoming more widely recognized as an issue, moving from a private to a more public matter. Last, integration across models was becoming more prevalent.

Couple therapy is distinct from individual and family therapy. For instance, while some couple therapists might meet, perhaps for a one-time session, individually with each partner, most couple therapists will refer one or both partners to a different therapist for individual therapy (Lebow & Snyder, 2022). Further, couple therapy attempts to understand the client system (the couple) within the various contexts in which they live. This brings in factors of diversity where oppression, marginalization, and privilege are relevant. Lebow and Snyder explained,

> Understanding couples in the context of culture, race, ethnicity, gender, sexual orientation, and other aspects of social location that afford persons greater or less privilege (and greater or lesser experiences of marginalization and oppression) has become an essential aspect of couple therapy.
>
> (Lebow & Snyder, 2022, p. 8)

Given all of this, this is not a book about the generalities of doing couple therapy; rather, it focuses on the various theoretical models you might use. However, there are some generalities of practice that cut across models. By utilizing one of the models in this book, you will have a structure and plan that you can use in your couple sessions. This should provide you with a map and guideline that will assist you and your clients in making changes that are useful and lead to clients achieving their goals.

While the various models of couple therapy have many similarities, they also have distinct differences. These include how they define the important elements of a successful relationship, who should come to sessions, and the role of the therapist (Lebow & Snyder, 2022) as well as what they target in terms of change processes along with their primary techniques. Most couple therapy sessions are conjoint sessions—both parties are in the therapy room at the same time. However, practitioners from various models may differ on whether they have spontaneously or as a fixed component of their therapeutic process individual interviews. Usually, these individual sessions are for assessment purposes or to provide a safe space for the partners where they might talk about, among other things, intimate partner violence, substance abuse, infidelity, or a desire to leave the relationship. Regardless of theoretical model, most couple therapy lasts between 3 and 12 months (Lebow & Snyder, 2022).

Effectiveness of Couple Therapy

Research demonstrates that couple therapy is quite effective (Carr, 2019; Gurman, 2011; Johnson & Lebow, 2000; Klann et al., 2011; Lebow et al., 2012; Lebow & Snyder, 2022; Roesler, 2020; Snyder et al., 2006; Stratton et al., 2015). However, when exploring typical practice settings, the gains for couples are not as large as in a research setting (Halford et al., 2016). One reason for this is that research-efficacy trials tend to mainly include couples who are seeking to enhance their relationship while practice-effectiveness trials contain a greater mix of couples wanting to enhance their relationship and those who are trying to determine whether to stay in the relationship.

The overarching good news is that approximately 70 percent of couples have significant positive change when engaging in couple therapy (Lebow et al., 2012). This change can happen in one or more areas of a couple's relationship. While couple therapy helps to improve overall relationship satisfaction (Petch et al., 2014), it is also effective in treating a couple's sexual relationship, aspects of physical aggression, substance abuse, mental health issues, and infidelity issues (Snyder et al., 2006). Not only is couple therapy effective in reducing distress between the partners, but it helps to reduce psychiatric symptoms in individual members (Lundblad & Hansson, 2005), particularly depression (Roesler, 2020). Couple therapy is useful for relational distress as well as to treat individual problems (Halford & Pepping, 2019). Thus, therapists should consider the use of couple therapy when relationship issues are the presenting problem, but also potentially when a person reports a psychological disorder.

To help in leading to these therapy benefits, therapists need to have and operate from a model of therapy. Doss et al. (2022) explained,

> There is strong support for therapists to utilize well-established couple therapy approaches in their work with dissatisfied couples. While the evidence base is still thin, the available evidence suggests that the well-established approaches to couple therapy are effective for couples from diverse racial and socio-economic backgrounds.
>
> (Doss et al., 2022, p. 299)

Several factors help boost the positive impact of couple therapy. Couples who come for multiple sessions are better able to achieve their goals versus those who only attend one or two sessions (Hampson et al., 1999). Further, members of couples who seek therapy tend to state that they find that therapists are the most helpful aspect of couple therapy (Eldridge et al., 2022). Hampson et al. (1999) found that couples without children had better outcomes than those who did have children. In their study, remarried couples without children did the best in treatment.

As explained, in general, couple therapy is effective. There are specific things that couple therapists do that may be more useful than other techniques. For instance, the most helpful intervention in the perception of therapists and clients was a communication-directed intervention (Vansteenwegen, 1998). These included asking a partner to explain themselves in greater depth, preventing partners from interrupting one another, having partners communicate via I-statements, etc. The lowest-rated intervention was reassurances, which may be because this intervention may focus on just one partner in the couple rather than the relationship. Vansteenwegen (1998) also found that directive interventions were perceived as more helpful than non-directive interventions. Eldridge et al. (2022) explained,

> Clients' reports confirm that the following three principles of change are viewed by them as particularly helpful: (a) altering the view of the problems to be more objective, dyadic, and contextualized, (b) eliciting emotion-based, avoided, private behavior, and (c) increasing constructive communication.
>
> (Eldridge et al., 2022, p. 293)

Couples do not always come to therapy with the same goals. One partner may want to mend the relationship while the other wants out. They both may want to stay in the relationship, but one may want more closeness while the other wants more separation. Couple therapists need to help partners to become more aligned so that their goals match. Couples who have aligned goals begin therapy in quite a different place from those whose goals are mismatched (Smith et al., 2020). When couples entering therapy are misaligned in their goals, they experience lower levels of sexual satisfaction and lower commitment. Most couple therapists attempt, throughout treatment, to help the couple develop shared mutual goals, increasing the within-couple-alliance. While many clients come to therapy for couple therapy and find it useful, others do not.

D'Aniello et al. (2021) found that, specifically for female partners, a lack of positive interactions between partners was associated with therapy discontinuation. Owen et al. (2018) found that once couple therapy started, relationship satisfaction stopped decreasing and leveled off. However, these researchers noted that relationship satisfaction tended to not increase over time.

While couple therapy is quite useful and effective for many couples, it is not a panacea. Couples will drop out or perhaps experience an increase in their interpersonal distress. For instance, Roesler (2020) found that of couples receiving counseling in Germany, approximately half prematurely discontinued therapy or had increased symptoms. One potential reason for this is that couples come to therapy when stress, tension, and conflict are at their peak and one or both members of the couple are contemplating relationship dissolution.

Case Conceptualization

Psychotherapists need a way to understand what to do when they are working with clients. This happens when they develop a **case conceptualization** (also sometimes referred to as a case formulation). A clear and thorough case conceptualization is the key to effective treatment. As Sperry (2019) explains, "Clinically useful and valuable case conceptualizations provide therapists with a coherent treatment strategy for planning and focusing treatment interventions to increase the likelihood of effecting change" (p. 24). Instead of going into a therapy session not knowing how to understand why the client is having difficulty or what your potential pathways to change are, case conceptualizations provide a road map that therapists can navigate to help get clients to their goals. Case conceptualizations can be model-specific or integrative. In this book, the authors present a model-specific case conceptualization. For integrative conceptualizations, therapists tend to have a foundational model and then build around that by integrating concepts and techniques from other approaches.

This book will discuss case conceptualization by focusing on problem formation and problem resolution (Reiter, 2014). These conceptualizations have multiple components to them. For instance, Eells (2022) described case formulation as having both content and process aspects. The content includes all the information that describes and explains the difficulties the client is currently experiencing. The process aspect is how the therapist elicits this information. Eells defined **case formulation** as follows: "Psychotherapy case formulation is a process of developing a hypothesis about the causes, precipitants, and maintaining influences of a person's psychological, interpersonal, and behavioral problems, as well as a plan to address these problems" (p. 2). Thus, the content of the formulation is the understanding of problem formation while the process is the therapist's conceptualization of problem resolution.

While there are different definitions of case conceptualization, they all focus on allowing the therapist to understand the client's presenting problem and provide a pathway for change. For instance, Sperry and Sperry (2020) defined case conceptualization "as a method and clinical strategy for obtaining and organizing information about a client, understanding and explaining the client's situation and maladaptive patterns, guiding and focusing treatment, anticipating challenges and roadblocks, and preparing for successful termination" (pp. 3–4). Again, whichever therapeutic model you use to develop your case conceptualization, you are doing so to gain a guide that will lead you to an understanding of the client and to make informed clinical decisions.

A clinically useful case conceptualization includes an explanatory power (describing an understanding of problem formation) as well as a predictive power (anticipating potential obstacles) that guide the treatment process (Sperry & Sperry, 2020). That is, therapists should be able to come to an understanding of what is bringing the client into therapy and what they might do in therapy to help move the client toward change. Each of the models that is presented in this book provides both the explanatory and predictive power of a good case conceptualization. They help you to see where the problems are located in the couple's relationship and what tools and pathways to use and take to help the couple have a more satisfactory relationship.

Sperry and Sperry (2020) explained that there are four components of case conceptualizations: diagnostic formulation, clinical formulation, cultural formulation, and treatment formulation. The **diagnostic formulation** provides an understanding of the client's presenting situation. This component answers the "what" question—"What happened?" The **clinical formulation** provides an understanding of the client's pattern. It answers the "why" question—"Why did this happen?" The **cultural formulation** provides an understanding of how cultural and social factors weigh in on the client's situation and functioning. It answers the "what role" question—"What role does culture play in the situation?" Last, the **treatment formulation** provides a plan of how to get the client to achieve the treatment goals. It answers the "how" question—"How does the client change?"

Why is having a case conceptualization important? Case conceptualizations are a competency that therapists need to understand and work with clients more effectively (Sperry & Sperry, 2020). And not all therapists are equally competent in this skill. More experienced therapists tend to produce higher-quality case formulations (Eells et al., 2005), which results in their treatment plans being better connected to the client's presenting problems and their case formulations being more consistent from case to case.

Common Factors

This first chapter ends by talking about the **common factors of psychotherapy** since all the models that will be presented are effective in leading to positive changes for the couple. Over the course of psychotherapy's history, there has sometimes been a model war, where two models are put against one another to see which is better (more effective at alleviating the client's distress). What has been found is that one model is not more effective than another (Lambert & Bergin, 1994; Miller et al., 1997). However, having a model is extremely important.

There are several models of common factors in psychotherapy (see Lambert, 1992; Miller et al., 1997; Sprenkle et al., 2009). Perhaps the most popular of these was put forth by Michael Lambert. In exploring Lambert's meta-analysis of psychotherapy outcome research, there are four common factors: extratherapeutic factors; therapeutic relationship; hope, expectancy, and placebo; and model factors.

Extratherapeutic factors are aspects of the client that lead to change. These account for 40 percent of positive client change (Lambert, 1992). Clients come to therapy with preexisting strengths, resources, and resiliencies. A client's sense of humor, positive viewpoint, or various experiences that they have may all be protective and growth-producing elements. These factors can lead clients to change outside of therapy while also being potential areas of exploration during the therapeutic process.

Therapeutic relationship factors focus on the importance of the therapeutic alliance. All models of therapy function through the connection between therapist and client. For some models, this relationship is described more prominently while for others it is more covert. A positive therapeutic relationship accounts for 30 percent of positive change for clients (Lambert, 1992). Developing and maintaining a strong therapeutic alliance with each member of the couple, while holding the couple as the unit of treatment, is key in couple therapy. The establishment of an early therapeutic alliance is a significant predictor of positive progress in therapy for couples (Tilden et al., 2021). Aponte (2016) explained, "The first task of couple therapy is to gain the trust and partnership of the clients, the foundation of the therapeutic relationship" (p. 11). Alliance occurs through both verbal and non-verbal (i.e., posture synchrony and movement mirroring) means (Kykyri et al., 2019). This is important since clients have expressed that their therapist being warm, empathic, and non-judgmental was integral in positive change (Madden & Timulak, 2022). The converse is also applicable, as clients find change hampered when the therapist is patronizing, unfriendly, and a poor listener.

Hope, expectancy, and placebo factors account for 15 percent of positive change (Lambert, 1992). The more that clients believe that therapy will be helpful, the more they increase their motivation to make changes in their lives. Further, the more the therapist believes and expects change to happen for the client, the more the client will believe that positive change can happen for them.

Model factors focus on the specific techniques that each theory of therapy utilizes. These factors account for 15 percent of positive change for clients. Each theory has its own techniques. Proper use of the techniques leads to beneficial changes for people. The bulk of this book will focus on model factors; however, each model, in its own way, incorporates aspects from the other factors—highlighting client competence, the therapeutic relationship, and the belief in a positive outcome.

We can also look at **therapist effects**, which is the amount of variance of outcomes that is based upon the therapist. Willis et al. (2021) found that the therapist accounted for 9.4 percent of the variance in couple dropouts. Therapists are differentially effective between each other and between clients. That is, the same therapist will be effective with some clients, somewhat helpful with others, and ineffective with the rest (Miller & Hubble, 2016). This is why it is important for us as therapists to obtain feedback from clients of what they find useful in our engagement with them and what they do not find useful so that we can tailor our approach to that particular client.

Sprenkle et al. (2009) promoted four common factors specific to therapists who engage in couple or family therapy. The first is that these therapists can conceptualize problems in relational terms. Rather than viewing one person as the identified problem, couple therapists can conceptualize the problem as interpersonal. The more that therapists can create an equal sense of understanding between themselves and each member of the couple, the greater the therapeutic alliance and the increased probability for positive change (Madden & Timulak, 2022). Partners in a couple may disagree with one another about the etiology of the problem, with one viewing it as more couple-related and the other as more individualistic. The more the partners view the problem differently, with one seeing it as relational and the other as an individual issue, the greater the discrepancies in the therapeutic alliance (Wu et al., 2020). However, throughout treatment, their discrepancy is likely to diminish. The second relational common factor is the ability to disrupt dysfunctional relational patterns. These patterns are the ways in which the couple has been engaging one another. The third relational common factor is expanding the direct treatment system, where the therapist can work with more than one individual. The fourth relational common factor is expanding the therapeutic alliance where the therapist can develop a therapeutic relationship with multiple people simultaneously.

Understanding the various common factors is quite useful for positive therapeutic outcomes for our clients. Snyder et al. (2006) stated, "Couple therapists should be trained in common factors and mechanisms of change that potentially undergird most forms of successful treatment" (p. 338). A further common factor is being able to accept client feedback. Those couples who were prompted to provide the therapist with feedback to track their progress showed statistically significant improvement over those couples who did not provide feedback (Reese et al., 2010). Anker et al. (2009) also found that couples who provided feedback to their therapist had a moderate to large effect size of improved results compared to couples who received treatment as usual. This effect was preset at post-treatment and follow-up.

In this book, you will have the opportunity to explore 11 different models for couple therapy. Each model is potentially useful for you (and ultimately for your couple clients). The trick is to find a model that fits you and will fit your clients. The more you believe that your use of that model will be useful for the couple, the more the couple will believe the therapy will be useful for them—thus, your increased expectancy of positive change helps promote the client's sense of hope and expectancy of change. I encourage you to explore how each of the models addresses each of the common factors.

Competencies

We have explored how couple therapists should have a clear understanding of case conceptualization and common factors. This is so they can efficiently put into practice the pathways to positive change. However, we also discussed how therapists are differentially effective. Some therapists are better in providing a therapeutic context than others. Those who are more effective have a greater grasp of the varying competencies needed when engaging in couple therapy. Halford and Pepping (2019) provided several competencies specific to couple therapists.

The first couple therapist competency is the development of a couple-based formulation. You need to be able to take all the information present and put it together as a whole so that you can make an assessment and then appropriate interventions. That is what this book is designed to do, provide you with a conceptualization of the theory of problem formation (the content of a case formulation) along with a guide for the theory of problem resolution (the process of therapy).

When engaging in couple therapy, the therapist is working with two individuals. Thus, building a couple-based therapeutic alliance is a core competency. Sometimes things go awry in couple therapy when one partner believes the therapist has completely taken the other partner's side. The therapist needs to be able to connect with both individuals while also connecting with them as a couple. This is the development of a positive working relationship where the couple experiences the therapist working for them in their movement toward their goals.

Invariably, the partners of a couple will have conflict within the therapy room. Sometimes this may be extreme through cursing and yelling at each other or potentially through intimidation and physical attack. At other times the partners may be civil with one another, but will not agree with one another on a decision to be made, what they think happened, or the goal of therapy. This is why managing couple conflict in session can is considered a core competency in couple therapy. This competency is enacted when the therapist shifts partners from complaining about one another to enacting conflict resolution skills.

The last competency for couple therapy that Halford and Pepping (2019) put forth is fostering intimacy, communication, and security. Inevitably, couples that come to therapy will bring up communication difficulties as one of the primary reasons they are seeking therapy. Depending on the approach, a portion of therapy will be focused on helping partners to express themselves and to receive these expressions more effectively from each other. This may come in the form of skills training, having the couple engage in activities to increase intimacy, and working on interactions centered on positive engagement with one another.

Another competency of couple therapy includes helping partners take responsibility for their actions (Smoliak et al., 2022). This is sometimes difficult as people (primarily males) tend to deny responsibility, usually by attributing fault to something outside of themselves, which many times is their partner. Partners may also deny responsibility through justification, trying to explain why they couldn't do anything but what they did or did not do. Smoliak et al. explained, "Supporting partners in moving beyond the blame cycle and fostering mutual responsibility for couple distress is a key aspect of couple therapy" (p. 360).

Hopefully, you engage in all these competencies. However, there are some common mistakes that couple therapists tend to make. Some are made more by beginning therapists while others are made by more experienced therapists. Doherty (2002) discussed several mistakes that beginners to couple therapy tend to make. Perhaps the most common of these is a lack of structure for sessions. When this happens, sessions become a free-for-all with interrupting, yelling, accusations, and little growth and change. The second mistake is not having a plan for change. Here, therapists do not actively push for each member of the couple to make some type of change in their day-to-day relationship. The third common mistake of couple therapy is giving up. This usually happens when the therapist is feeling overwhelmed.

Doherty (2002) also explained that experienced couple therapists tend to make two primary mistakes. First, they may think that all couples are equal. This discounts the context in which the couple relates to each other and larger systems. First marriage, remarriage, not being married, open relationships, same-sex relationships, with or without children, interracial, intercultural, interfaith, being an older or younger couple, etc., all impact that couple's dynamics. The second mistake that Doherty believes experienced couple therapists might make is not standing by marriage. This mistake is quite debatable as other therapists might hold that trying to keep a very unhappy couple together can be problematic.

These are not the only mistakes couple therapists might make. Weeks et al. (2005) listed several generic mistakes including:

- Failing to acknowledge that mistakes exist
- Failing to use theory when intervening
- Failing to use a chosen theory or theories correctly
- Failing to discard a theory when it is not applicable
- Failing to act when action is clearly warranted
- Failing to restrain oneself from intervening when it is not time

(Weeks et al., 2005, p. 2)

These authors explain a few more specific mistakes of couple therapists. The first is not winning the battle for structure, where the therapist is supposed to determine the ground rules and provide the structure for therapy. Second, the therapist may lose neutrality and ally with one member of the couple. Third, they believe mistakes happen when the therapist overemphasizes the past or the present. Rather, they hold that there should be a balance where the therapist can easily move back and forth between these time frames to help contextualize the couple's situation. A fourth common mistake is the therapist not engaging in careful listening, where they are listening with the third ear and hearing the overt communication as well as the unsaid processes. This includes a recognition that one or both people will overemphasize, underemphasize, or fail to bring up concerns. A fifth mistake happens around conflict. This might occur if the therapist tries to avoid at all costs the couple having a conflict or allows a chaotic session to occur by letting conflict happen for too long.

Mistakes might be avoided by thinking about what you could do and not do when working with a couple. Weeks and Treat (2001, pp. 4–8) provided a list of don'ts for the couple therapist. These included:

- Don't take sides.
- Don't intervene too quickly.
- Don't answer questions from the couple until ready.
- Don't proceed until the problem(s) and goal(s) have been clarified.
- Don't discuss problems abstractly and non-concretely.
- Don't discount problems, even small problems.
- Don't allow differences to escalate.
- Don't assume the partners in the couple will perceive the problem in the same way.
- Don't unbalance the system.
- Don't make premature interpretations.
- Don't get hooked in the past.
- Don't get hooked on the partners' theories or explanations.
- Don't allow the couple to tell stories.
- Don't allow emotion to take charge of the session.
- Don't allow the couple to take charge of the session.

Most of these are applicable regardless of the theoretic model, while others may be interpreted differently based on one's theoretical orientation.

These are just a few of the common mistakes that couple therapists might make. There are, unfortunately, many more. I hope that this book will help prevent these common couple therapy mistakes. The more that you can situate yourself based on theory, the greater the likelihood that you will effectively engage the couple and lead to positive therapeutic change.

Structure of the Book

The underpinning of this book is designed so you can see how the various models presented engage in case conceptualization. To better enact that, I created a couple that is an amalgamation of many of the couples I have seen over the course of my career. The couple is presented to you in Chapter 2. In the succeeding chapters, each chapter author will cover the following areas, all while applying their model to the case so that you can more easily compare and contrast the models:

- History of the Model
- Conceptualization of Problem Formation
- Conceptualization of Diversity
- The Role of the Therapist
- Conceptualization of Problem Resolution
- Case Transcript

It is hoped that this consistent format across chapters will help you understand each model and how they uniquely conceptualize why a couple is having difficulties and what they would do with the couple, particularly in a first session.

References

Anker, M. G., Duncan, B. L., & Sparks, J. A. (2009). Using client feedback to improve couple therapy outcomes: A randomized clinical trial in a naturalistic setting. *Journal of Consulting and Clinical Psychology, 77*(4), 693–704. DOI: 10.1037/a0016062

Aponte, H. J. (2016). Joining: From the perspective of the use of self. In G. R. Weeks, S. T. Fife, & C. M. Peterson (Eds.), *Techniques for the couple therapist: Essential interventions from the experts* (pp. 11–14). Routledge.

Beckerman, N. L., & Shepherd, L. (2002). Couple therapy: Identification of conflict areas. *Family Therapy, 29*(2), 77–87.

Carr, A. (2019). Couple therapy, family therapy and systemic interventions for adult-focused problems: The current evidence base. *Journal of Family Therapy, 41*(4), 492–536. DOI: 10.1111/1467-6427.12225

Crenshaw, A. O., Leo, K., & Baucom, B. R. W. (2019). The effect of stress on empathic accuracy in romantic couple. *Journal of Family Psychology, 33*(3), 327–337. DOI: 10.1037/fam0000508

Cruwys, T., South, E. I., Halford, W. K., Murray, J. A., & Fladerer, M. P. (2023). Measuring "we-ness" in couple relationships: A social identity approach. *Family Process, 62*(2), 795–817. DOI: 10.1111/famp.12811

D'Aniello, C., Anderson, S. R., & Tambling, R. R. (2021). Psychotherapeutic processes associated with couple therapy discontinuance: An observational analysis using the rapid marital interaction coding system. *Journal of Marital and Family Therapy, 47*(4), 891–908. DOI: 10.1111/jmft.12482

D'Arrigo-Patrick, E., Samman, S. K., & Knudson-Martin, C. (2020). Moving from "I" to "We": A grounded theory analysis of couple therapy with liver patients and their partners. *Family Process, 59*(4), 1517–1529. DOI: 10.1111/famp.12528

Doherty, W. J. (2002). Bad couple therapy: How to avoid it. *Psychotherapy Networker, 26*(6).

Doss, B. D., Roddy, M. K., Wiebe, S. A., & Johnson, S. M. (2022). A review of the research during 2010–2019 on evidence-based treatments for couple relationship distress. *Journal of Marital and Family Therapy, 48*(1), 283–306. DOI: 10.1111/jmft.12552

Doss, B. D., Simpson, L. E., & Christensen, A. (2004). Why do couple seek marital therapy? *Professional Psychology: Research and Practice, 35*(6), 608–614. DOI: 10.1037/0735-7028.35.6.608

Duncan, C., Ryan, G. S., Moller, N. P., & Davies, R. (2020). Who attends couple counseling in the UK and why? *Journal of Sex & Marital Therapy, 46*(2), 177–186. DOI: 10.1080/0092623x.2019.1654584

Eells, T. D. (2022). History and current status of psychotherapy case formulation. In T. D. Eells (Ed.), *Handbook of psychotherapy case formulation* (3rd ed., pp. 1–35). Guilford.

Eells, T. D., Lombart, K. G., Kendjelic, E. M., Turner, L. C., & Lucas, C. P. (2005). The quality of psychotherapy case formulations: A comparison of expert, experienced, and novice cognitive-behavioral and psychodynamic therapists. *Journal of Consulting and Clinical Psychology, 73*(4), 579–589. DOI: 10.1-37/0022-006X.73.4.579

Eldridge, K., Mason, J., & Christensen, A. (2022). Client perceptions of the most and least helpful aspects of couple therapy. *Journal of Couple & Relationship Therapy, 21*(3), 277–303. DOI: 10.1080/15332691.2021.1925611

Gurman, A. S. (2008). A framework for the comparative study of couple therapy: History, models, and applications. In A. S. Gurman (Ed.), *Clinical handbook of couple therapy* (4th ed., pp. 1–30). Guiford.

Gurman, A. S. (2010). The evolving clinical practice of couple therapy. In A. S. Gurman (Ed.), *Clinical casebook of couple therapy* (pp. 1–20). Guilford.

Gurman, A. S. (2011). Couple therapy research and the practice of couple therapy: Can we talk? *Family Process, 50*(3), 280–292.

Gurman, A. S., & Fraenkel, P. (2002). The history of couple therapy: A millennial review. *Family Process, 41*(2), 199–260.

Halford, W. K., & Pepping, C. A. (2019). What every therapist needs to know about couple therapy. *Behaviour Change, 36*(3), 121–142. DOI: 10.1017/bec.2019.12

Halford, W. K., Pepping, C. A., & Petch, J. (2016). The gap between couple therapy research efficacy and practice effectiveness. *Journal of Marital and Family Therapy, 42*(1), 32–44.

Hampson, R. B., Prince, C. C., & Beavers, W. R. (1999). Marital therapy: Qualities of couple who fare better or worse in treatment. *Journal of Marital and Family Therapy, 25*(4), 411–424.

Johnson, S., & Lebow, J. (2000). The "coming of age" of couple therapy: A decade review. *Journal of Marital and Family Therapy, 26*(1), 23–38.

Klann, N., Hahlweg, K., Baucom, D. H., & Kroeger, C. (2011). The effectiveness of couple therapy in Germany: A replication study. *Journal of Marital and Family Therapy, 37*(2), 200–208. DOI: 10.1111/j.1752-0606.2009.00164x

Kykyri, V-L., Tourunen, A., Nyman-Salonen, P., Kurri, K., Wahlström, J., Kaartinen, J., Penttonen, M., & Seikkula, J. (2019). Alliance formations in couple therapy—A Multi-modal and multi-method study. *Journal of Couple and Relationship Therapy, 18*(3), 189–222. DOI: 10.1080/15332691.2018.1551166

Lambert, M. J. (1992). Psychotherapy outcome research: Implications for integrative and eclectic therapists. In J. C. Norcross & M. R. Goldfried (Eds.), *Handbook of psychotherapy integration* (pp. 94–129). Basic Books.

Lambert, M. J., & Bergin, A. E. (1994). The effectiveness of psychotherapy. In A. E. Bergin & S. L. Garfield (Eds.), *Handbook of psychotherapy and behavior change* (4th ed., pp. 143–189). Wiley.

Lebow, J. L., Chambers, A. L., Christensen, A., & Johnson, S. M. (2012). Research on the treatment of couple distress. *Journal of Marital and Family Therapy, 38*(1), 145–168. DOI: 10.1111/j.1752-0606.2011.00249

Lebow, J., & Snyder, D. K. (2022). Couple therapy in the 2020s: Current status and emerging developments. *Family Process, 61*(4), 1359–1385. DOI: 10.1111/famp.12824

Lord, S. A. (2022). COVID couple therapy: Telehealth and somatic action techniques. *Australian and New Zealand Journal of Family Therapy, 43*(2), 197–209. DOI: 10.1002/anzf.1487

Lundblad, A-M., & Hansson, K. (2005). Outcomes in couple therapy: Reduced psychiatric symptoms and improved sense of coherence. *Nordic Journal of Psychiatry, 59*(5), 374–380. DOI: 10.1080/08039480500319795

Madden, L., & Timulak, L. (2022). It takes three to tango: Clients' experiences of couple therapy-A meta-analysis of qualitative research studies. *Counseling Psychology Quarterly*. DOI: 10.1080/09515070.2022.2151978

Miller, S. D., Duncan, B. L., & Hubble, M. A. (1997). *Escape from Babel: Toward a unifying language for psychotherapy practice*. Norton.

Miller, S. D., & Hubble, M. A. (2016). The road to mastery: Three steps for improving performance as a couple therapist. In G. R. Weeks, S. T. Fife & C. M. Peterson (Eds.), *Techniques for the couple therapist: Essential interventions from the experts* (pp. 15–18). Routledge.

Owen, J., Rhoades, G. K., Stanley, S. M., Markman, H. J., & Allen, E. S. (2018). Treatment-as-usual for couple: Trajectories before and after beginning couple therapy. *Family Process, 58*(2), 273–286. DOI: 10.1111/famp.12390

Parnell, K. J., Scheel, M. J., Davis, C. K., & Black, W. W. (2018). An investigation of couple' help-seeking: A multiple case study. *Contemporary Family Therapy, 40*, 110–117. DOI: 10.1007/s10591-017-9427-9

Petch, J., Lee, J., Huntingdon, B., & Murray, J. (2014). Couple counselling outcomes in an Australian not for profit: Evidence for the effectiveness of couple counselling conducted within routine practice. *Australian & New Zealand Journal of Family Therapy, 35*(4), 445–461. DOI: 10.1002/anzf.1074

Reese, R. J., Toland, M. D., Slone, M. C., & Norsworthy, L. A. (2010). Effect of client feedback on couple psychotherapy outcomes. *Psychotherapy Theory, Research, Practice, & Training, 47*(4), 616–630. DOI: 10.1037/a0021182

Reiter, M. D. (2014). *Case conceptualization in family therapy*. Pearson.

Roesler, C. (2020). Effectiveness of couple therapy in practice settings and identification of potential predictors for different outcomes: Results of a German Nationwide naturalistic study. *Family Process, 59*(2), 390–408.

Salivar, Em. J. G., Rothman, K., Roddy, M. K., & Doss, B. D. (2020). Relative cost effectiveness of in-person and internet interventions for relationship distress. *Family Process, 59*(1), 66–80. DOI: 10.1111/famp.12414

Smith, A. D., Quirk, K., Pinsof, W., & Goldstein, J. (2020). It's a match? The influence of goal matching in couple therapy. *Journal of Couple & Relationship Therapy, 19*(2), 95–114. DOI: 10.1080/15332691.2019.1667935

Smoliak, O., Rice, C., Knudson-Martin, C., Briscoe, C., LeCouteur, A., LaMarre, A., Tseliou, E., Addison, M., Myers, M., Velikonja, L., & Vesely, L. (2022). Denials of responsibility in couple therapy. *Journal of Couple & Relationship Therapy, 21*(4), 344–365. DOI: 10.1080/15332691.2021.1967248

Snyder, D. K., Castellani, A. M., & Whisman, M. A. (2006). Current status and future directions in couple therapy. *Annual Review of Psychology, 57*, 317–344. DOI: 10.1146/annurev.psych.56.091103.080154

Sperry, L. (2019). Assessment and case conceptualization with couple and families. In L. Sperry (Ed.), *Couple and family assessment: Contemporary and cutting-edge strategies* (3rd ed., pp. 20–32). Routledge.

Sperry, L., & Sperry, J. (2020). *Case conceptualization: Mastering this competency with ease and confidence* (2nd ed.). Routledge.

Spiker, D. A., Hammer, J. H., & Parnell, K. J. (2019). Men in unhappy relationships: Perceptions of couple therapy. *Journal of Social and Personal Relationships, 36*(7), 2015–2035. DOI: 10.1177/0265407518775537

Sprenkle, D. H., Davis, S. D., & Lebow, J. L. (2009). *Common factors in couple and family therapy*. Guilford.

Stratton, P., Silver, E., Nasimento, N., McDonnell, L., Powell, G., & Nowotny, E. (2015). Couple and family therapy outcome research in the previous decade: What does the evidence tell us? *Contemporary Family Therapy, 37*(1), 1–12. DOI: 10.1007/s10591-014-9314-6

Tilden, T., Johnson, S. U., Hoffart, A., Zahl-Olsen, R., Wampold, B. E., Ulvenes, P., & Håland, A. T. (2021). Alliance predicting progress in couple therapy. *Psychotherapy, 58*(3), 391–400. DOI: 10.1037/pst0000355

Vansteenwegen, A. (1998). Helpfulness of therapist verbal interventions in couple therapy. *Sexual and Marital Therapy, 13*(1), 15–20. DOI: 10.1080/02674659808406540

Weeks, G. R., Odell, M., & Methven, S. (2005). *If only I had known...: Avoiding common mistakes in couple therapy*. W. W. Norton & Company.

Weeks, G. R., & Treat, S. R. (2001). *Couple in treatment: Techniques and approaches for effective practice* (2nd ed.). Brunner-Routledge.

Willis, K. L., Miller, R. B., Anderson, S. R., Bradford, A. B., Johnson, L. N., & Yorgason, J. B. (2021). Therapist effects on dropout in couple therapy. *Journal of Marital and Family Therapy, 47*(1), 104–119. DOI: 10.1111/jmft.12473

Wittenborn, A. K., & Holtrop, K. (2022). Introduction to the special issue on the efficacy and effectiveness of couple and family interventions: Evidence base update 2010–2019. *Journal of Marital and Family Therapy, 48*(1), 5–22. DOI: 10.1111/jmft.12576

Wrape, E. R., & McGinn, M. M. (2018). Clinical and ethical considerations or delivering couple and family therapy via telehealth. *Journal of Marital and Family Therapy, 45*(2), 296–308. DOI: 10.1111/jmft.12319

Wu, Q., McWey, L. M., & Ledermann, T. (2020). Clients' attributions of the presenting problem and the therapeutic alliance in couple therapy: Systemic versus intrapersonal perspectives. *Journal of Marital and Family Therapy, 46*(4), 661–673. DOI: 10.1111/jmft.12432

2 The Case

Steve and Carissa Hogarth

Michael D. Reiter

The Couple's History[1]

Steve and Carissa Hogarth have been married for five years. The first two to three years were quite happy. Steve is a 29-year-old White cisgender male while Carissa is a 28-year-old Black cisgender female. They met seven years ago at the University of Florida when Steve was a senior and Carissa a junior. They had both been out at a club, somehow found themselves talking with one another, and by the end of the night were in Steve's bed.

Their relationship got off to quite a rapid start, with Carissa spending most nights at Steve's apartment as she lived with two female roommates while Steve lived alone in a one-bedroom flat. This was the third relationship for Carissa who had never previously dated a White guy. Both prior boyfriends were Black. Steve had never dated a Black female. Carissa was his fourth serious relationship. Two previous girlfriends were White, and one was Hispanic. While being in an interracial relationship was new to both, they were excited about being in it and seemed to get along well.

Neither Steve nor Carissa saw anything wrong or deviant in the relationship but this relationship was happening in the South. While no one in Gainesville, Florida, showed outright disdain for the relationship, each would occasionally see someone staring at them while they held hands. Their friends would privately ask them what it was like to be in an interracial relationship, but they felt supported by their friends. Where each was concerned was when they were going to tell their families.

Carissa was the first to tell her parents she was in a relationship with a White guy. She waited four months until she knew that the relationship was serious. Carissa came from Bushnell, Florida, a small town about an hour south of the university. She couldn't remember anyone from her hometown being in an interracial relationship. She had seen some interracial couples on television, especially Black football players marrying White females. She couldn't recall ever seeing a Black female with a White male. On a trip home, she told her parents she was dating, describing Steve, his personality, and his life ambitions. She then said, "There's one big thing that you should know. He's White." She could see a bit of shock on her parents' faces, but not disdain. They asked if he treated her well, and when she said yes, they let her know that was the most important thing to them.

Steve's experience telling his parents was a bit more difficult. His parents had been divorced for about 20 years. The first person he told was his mother, who seemed fine with the situation. Her advice was not to listen to anyone else if they had an issue with it and that he should do what made him happy. Steve held off for several more months before telling his father, as he knew that his father had some prejudicial attitudes. When he told his father, he received the response he expected. His father told him that there would be too many issues and that it wouldn't last.

Upon graduation, Steve took a job at a large national company headquartered in Orlando, Florida. He had another offer for a company located in Charlotte, North Carolina, but took the

DOI: 10.4324/9781003369097-2

Orlando job because it was closer to Carissa who was entering her senior year of college. They saw each other almost every weekend as the drive from Orlando to Gainesville was less than two hours. Since Bushnell, Carissa's hometown, was right in the middle of the two cities, they would meet there a lot. This provided Steve with a chance to really get to know Carissa's parents, whom he came to really appreciate. They seemed to accept him into their family. For Christmas that year, Steve took Carissa down to Miami to celebrate the holidays with his family, particularly his mother. While there wasn't the same connection that Steve had with Carissa's family, Carissa and Steve's mother got along fine. Steve took Carissa to meet his father for a few hours and everyone felt the tension.

One year after Steve moved to Orlando, Carissa followed him there and they moved in together. Carissa graduated from the University of Florida with a degree in accounting. She then applied and was accepted into the Master's of Accounting Program at the University of Central Florida. She also picked up a job as an accounting clerk. Moving in together went well and the couple began to get into a smooth rhythm with one another. Carissa, who tended to be easygoing, made friends at school and work. Steve had made a few friends at his job and would hang with them on the weekends playing disc golf, softball, or watching football. At first, Carissa was fine with Steve hanging with his friends on the weekends as she had a lot of homework. This routine would eventually be problematic once she graduated and no longer had schoolwork to occupy her weekends.

During the celebration dinner for Carissa's graduation from her Master's program, Steve proposed to her. Carissa accepted and they began planning their wedding. They decided to have the ceremony in Orlando as it was almost in the middle of where their families lived. They were both quite happy on their wedding day and enjoyed their honeymoon, a cruise out of Port Canaveral, Florida, to the Caribbean. At the wedding itself, there was not much interaction between Steve and Carissa's families. The mothers spent some time talking with one another, but Steve's father did not say anything to anyone in Carissa's family.

The first couple of years of marriage went by in a routine. Steve and Carissa worked hard during the week and spent time together at night cooking and eating together, exercising, and watching television shows together. On the weekends, Steve would spend time with his friends, and he and Carissa would go to a lot of parties their various friends would hold. Carissa would occasionally make comments to Steve that she would like to spend more time with him on the weekends, but things did not really change.

Two years into marriage, Steve and Carissa began to observe many of their couple friends having children. This started to reduce their weekend get-togethers as the other couples were caring for their children. They then had an open conversation about starting a family. Carissa explained that she really wanted to become a mother and thought she was ready. Steve said that he was okay with having a child or not having one, but since Carissa was so passionate about having a child they would start to try.

Steve's History

Steve is the second of three children. He has a sister, Vanessa, who is five years older. Patrick, his brother, is two years younger. Steve and his siblings were born and raised in Miami, Florida. Steve's parents, Ethan and Melanie, married when Ethan was 26 and Melanie was 24. They met through mutual friends who thought that they would make a good pair. They dated for nine months and were engaged for seven. Within six months of being married, Melanie was pregnant. They viewed themselves as a typical couple.

Ethan had gone to university and earned a degree in political science with the hope of getting into law school. However, his grades were mediocre, and he did not do well on the Law School

Admission Test (LSAT). Ethan had never been a good standardized test taker and found that the prep work he did for the LSAT was not sufficient. Out of university, he got a job as a paralegal in a big law firm in Miami. Ethan was disappointed in himself for not living up to his potential. His parents were expecting him to become a lawyer, and Ethan felt that he was letting down not only himself but his parents. Ethan's older brother, Edward, was a very good student who had completed medical school and was doing quite well in his career. Throughout his whole childhood, Ethan felt like he could never live up to his brother's standards.

Ethan met Melanie on a blind date set up by his best friend and best friend's girlfriend as Melanie was a good friend to her. They seemed to get along well, and Ethan pursued the relationship. Melanie had just completed her degree in elementary education and was starting her career as a teacher. Within two years they were married and had their first child, Vanessa, one year later. Based on their finances, Melanie continued to teach as they needed the dual income to pay rent, bills, and student loans. Ethan felt bad that he was not making enough money to support the two of them so that Melanie did not have to work. He compared himself to his brother, Edward, whose wife was able to stay home to look after the children and the household.

Melanie actually wanted to continue to work and was not aware of Ethan's guilt as he never talked with her about it. She enjoyed feeling productive and loved being in the classroom, working primarily with 3rd graders. She was content with her job and loved being a mother. She had always wanted a large family and she and Ethan kept trying for another child, but they had some difficulties as she had two full-term miscarriages. The couple kept trying although the hope, anticipation, and then fear around the pregnancies brought tension into the relationship. Ethan told Melanie that they didn't need to keep trying and that he was fine with only having Vanessa. Melanie started to experience depression, thinking there was something wrong with her body. When she became pregnant for the third time, she took an extended leave of absence from her school so that she could focus on not straining herself physically or emotionally.

The pregnancy went well, and Steve was eventually born. They named him after Melanie's grandfather, whom she was close with. Vanessa was happy that she had a baby brother and tried to be involved in his caretaking, asking to help pick out which outfits he would wear that day, reading to him, and helping with baths. Melanie's mood improved and she and Ethan found a routine where Ethan would go to work from 9 to 5 while Melanie took care of both children.

A little over one year later, Melanie was pregnant again. When Patrick was born, Ethan told Melanie that he did not want any more children. She tried for perhaps two weeks to talk to him more about this, to see if he might change his mind as she did want more children. Ethan was steadfast in his decision. One day he came home and told Melanie that he had gotten a vasectomy. She was quite upset as he did this without consulting with her first, and now she would not have any more children. Melanie then put her energies into raising her children.

Over time, Steve could feel the discord between his parents. They would frequently have verbal arguments with one another in front of the children. He could also hear them yell at each other through their bedroom door. When Steve was 10 years old his father moved out and his parents eventually divorced. Two years later his father remarried Patricia, who had been divorced for a couple of years and had two teenage sons, Charlie and Dean. Steve has never been close with his stepbrothers but has nothing against them. He didn't see his father that often as his father had moved an hour away from where they lived.

From an early age, Steve knew that there were certain expectations that he and his siblings had to live by. These included doing well in school, not getting into trouble, and getting along with family members. He had a better relationship with his younger brother, but appreciated that his sister tried occasionally to include him in activities. However, as she got into her teen years, she spent more and more time with her friends and away from her family. Steve never got into trouble at school, but he was not as naturally good a student as Vanessa. Patrick was more social than he was and the two had some friends that they shared, playing baseball or basketball together with the group of friends.

Vanessa eventually went off to college in pursuit of becoming a pharmacist. Steve entered high school having a core group of friends and doing fairly well in school. He was in advanced classes but knew that he wasn't one of the smartest in his class. He did not spend a lot of time studying and knew that there was a hint of disappointment from his parents as his sister had been in the top five percent of her graduating class. When Steve did graduate, he was in the top 10 percent, had a mediocre score in the SAT Reasoning Test, and wasn't quite sure what he wanted to do for a career. He was accepted to the University of Florida through early admission, where he had to start during the summer and prove himself in those classes. Steve was able to focus and succeed in the classes and was matriculated into the College of Business. He knew that his parents would have preferred him to have a pathway to professional schools, such as medicine or law, but he didn't have an interest in those careers.

Carissa's History

Carissa is one of two siblings. She has an older sister, Lori, who is two years older than her. Carissa was born and raised in Bushnell, Florida, a very small town of about 2,000 people in North-Central Florida. Carissa's parents, Earl and Natalie, met in middle school and began dating when they were sophomores in high school. They had bonded as they were two of the few Black students in the school, which was primarily White. Natalie never really experienced any outright prejudice or discrimination. However, Earl had a few scuffles during his middle- and high-school career, primarily with other boys in his class.

After graduating from high school, Natalie got a job at the elementary school. Earl found employment at a fast-food restaurant. At 20 years old, Earl asked Natalie to marry him. They married at the courthouse and had a small reception at his parents' house. They had saved up enough to buy a small house with a small plot of land, but money was always tight. Within a year, Lori was born. Fortunately, the birth occurred over the summer so Natalie did not have to take any time off from work. When the school year started, Natalie's mother, Abigail, looked after Lori. Two years later, Carissa was born.

Lori and Carissa were quite close growing up. While they had occasional sibling spats, they were mainly each other's best friends. They were very close with their mother and grandmother. When Carissa was 10 years old, her father moved out of the house for two weeks. Years later she was to learn that he had cheated on her mother. However, it seemed that after the two-week separation her parents were able to reconcile. They are currently still married.

Lori was an average student. Their parents pushed them to do their schoolwork but were not overbearing on education. After graduating from high school, Lori moved to Gainesville to attend Santa Fe College to earn a degree in nursing. Carissa was a better student than her sister, especially in mathematics. She was accepted into the University of Florida and moved to Gainesville. After her freshman year, she moved in with Lori who had gotten a job as a nursing assistant at the local hospital. Carissa received several scholarships to help pay for school as her parents could not help much financially. After her freshman year, she obtained a job at the mall to help cover some of her expenses.

Carissa enjoyed her time at the university. She joined several clubs including a dance club, a math club, and Zeta Phi Beta, a primarily Black sorority. She made many friends, including a strong core group. Carissa did well in her accounting major and eventually graduated with a 3.6 grade point average (gpa).

The Couple's Current Problem

Steve and Carissa have made an appointment for couples therapy as they frequently argue with one another. This way of being has been steadily increasing over the last two years. They are primarily arguing over the potential of Carissa becoming pregnant. They have been actively trying for three years, with no successful results. The couple has gone to fertility doctors who could not pinpoint what the difficulties were. They have tried various methods of conception including in-vitro fertilization. Steve is at the point where he is wanting to stop trying as it is taking both a financial and emotional toll on their relationship. Carissa has a strong desire to be a mother, and more significantly, a biological mother.

The longer that Carissa went without getting pregnant the greater the tension within the couple's relationship. They would find that they sniped at each other more often about what seemed like inconsequential items. For instance, here is a recent exchange between the two:

Carissa: What's that smell?
Steve: What smell?
Carissa: That! It's so pungent. You scooped the cat litter, right?
Steve: Not yet today.
Carissa: Why not? I've told you that that's your responsibility. It's not going to scoop itself.
Steve: I've been doing it.
Carissa: Clearly not enough. When are you doing it?
Steve: Before I go to sleep.
Carissa: It needs to be done more than that! In the morning. In the evening. Maybe even the afternoon.
Steve: If you want it done so often, then you scoop it. I do it before bed.
Carissa: You want our house to smell like cat shit? What's wrong with you?

The couple has not yet had an open conversation about their growing tension. Carissa is wondering whether she made a mistake in marrying Steve. She has contemplated divorce, thinking that it would be easier to do it now before they have a child. Steve thinks he is being a good husband and that the only problem they have is that Carissa is becoming more out of control. Carissa has spent more time at her family's home, spending weekends away from Steve. When her mother asks her what is going on, she has explained that she doesn't sense the passion from Steve that was there at the beginning of their relationship. Her mother recommended that they try to work things out.

After one fight where Carissa yelled at Steve for going golfing with his friends, he yelled back that she needed to go to therapy. This enraged her and they both shouted at one another for a long while. At the end of this encounter, they both agreed that they would give couples therapy a try since neither is happy with how things currently are in their relationship.

Note

1 Chapter authors used this chapter as the jumping off point to apply their models. However, they may add or change some information for explanatory purposes.

3 Object Relations Couple Therapy

Carl Bagnini and Michael D. Reiter

History of the Model

Object relations couple therapy is a form of psychoanalytic therapy that is influenced by multiple factors. Out of the varying forms of psychoanalytic therapy, it is perhaps the one most applicable to couples (Scharff & Scharff, 1997). The roots of the model can be seen in the work of British Independent analysts such as Michael Balint, Ronald Fairbairn, Harry Guntrip, and Donald Winnicott. Several other influential analysts include Melanie Klein and Henry Dicks as well as Otto Kernberg, Heinz Kohut, and Margaret Mahler (Siegel, 2022). However, out of all these individuals, perhaps the two most influential contributors are Melanie Klein and Ronald Fairbairn, sometimes viewed as the mother and father of object relations couple therapy (Ludlam, 2022). While the British object relations therapy played a significant part in its worldwide usage (Scharff & Scharff, 1995), the American school of object relations also significantly impacted how people utilize the model in working with couples (Siegel, 2022). This chapter presents an amalgam of these various influences, knowing that depending on time, location, and context, object relations therapy may take on a somewhat different shape.

Object relations, like all models of therapy, initially had roots in psychoanalysis, which was the first and most influential model of psychotherapy. Freudian psychoanalysis was born in the late 19th century and was revolutionary for being perhaps the first talk therapy approach. Object relations theory was developed as a counter to the limitation of Freudian theory, with the child–parent relationship being expanded to explore a relational context (Siegel, 2022). Rather than stemming from the Freudian focus on drives (such as sexual and aggressive drives) as the basis for human motivation, object relations theorists focused on the infant's needs. Object relations therapists tend to concentrate on the context of relationships—especially early attachment relationships to significant caregivers—where the object provides security for the infant.

It is this attachment relationship that is primary for object relations theorists, as this is the context for the developing sense of relatedness that the infant builds. This context provides space for the child to experience meaning, since their primary need is to be in a relationship. In this model, "An 'object' is a person, place, thing, fantasy, idea, or memory that is invested with strong emotion" (Applegate, 1990, p. 87). The person's relationship with the object plays a significant role in the development of their psyche.

Object relations couple therapy is an integration between individual psychodynamic theory and a systemic formulation of couples (Scharff & de Varela, 2005). The first person to explicitly apply object relations theory to married couples was Dicks (1967), who worked at the Tavistock Clinic. He held that people tend to seek out partners whose personality unconsciously meets their own split-off aspects of self. Ronald Fairbairn, perhaps the most significant contributor to object relations couple therapy, shifted psychoanalytic thinking away from the drive-centered modality

DOI: 10.4324/9781003369097-3

of Freud to a more cybernetic perspective in which there is an integration of a psychic structure of dynamically related internal parts with general systems theory (Scharff & de Varela, 2005).

Object relations couple therapy can be viewed as a systems theory since it conceptualizes individuals as being organized on the basis of their experiences with a group of people—namely, their primary caregivers—and that it is these relationships that are internalized. The theory explores how these internal and external connections function to either create secure attachments and functioning or more insecure attachments and difficulties later in life. Solomon and Lynn (2002) explained, "Object-relations theory provides both a normative model of healthy and adaptive functioning and a way of understanding small, repetitive attachment failures that cause disruptions in normal growth and development" (p. 389).

Object relations theory views infants as competent in the beginning stages of life. They are born with an unformed self, which, over their life span, will be enriched by their experiences and will become their total personality (Scharff & Scharff, 1995). The self is composed of three parts: an **ego**, which is the executive mechanism; the **internal objects**; and **object relations**, which is the connection between the objects and parts of the ego. This last component of the self is also called **internal object relationships** and tends to maintain itself throughout the person's life but is modifiable.

While Freud focused on inner drives, object relations theorists pay attention to people's needs. Scharff and Scharff (1997) described object relations theory thus:

> an individual psychology drawn from study of the relationship between patient and therapist, object relations theory holds that the motivating factor in growth and development of the human infant is the need to be in a relationship with a mothering person.
>
> (Scharff & Scharff, 1997, p. 141)

That is, from birth, the infant is object seeking, trying to develop a relationship with another person (Ludlam, 2022).

When the infant reaches out in their search for connection, the object can be accepting or rejecting. Accepting objects (e.g., mother or father) help lead the infant to secure attachments and positive psychological growth. When a parent is sensitive to an infant's signals and needs, the infant develops trust and confidence in the caregiver, increased self-confidence, awareness of others, and open communication occurs between parent and child (Solomon & Lynn, 2002). However, when the infant's attempts to seek love from the object are rejected, they receive confusing messages that can be quite traumatic (Ludlam, 2022). This usually results in anxiety that plays out in what is known as separation anxiety.

The infant handles the situation of rejection by the object by splitting off the object and repressing it in the unconscious (Ludlam, 2022). Here, we can see the connection between what happens outside and what happens inside where there is an external object and an internal object. The **external object** is the actual significant other with whom the person is in a relationship (Scharff & Scharff, 1995). For a baby, this is usually the mother or father. It can also be a sibling, grandparent, or any other significant caregiver. The external object then becomes a part of the person and is known as the **internal object**. Scharff and Scharff (1995) stated, "An internal object is a piece of psychic structure that formed from the person's experience with the important caretaking person in earlier life, captured in the personality as the trace of that earlier relationship" (p. 5).

This process is significant since it shapes the person's personality and becomes a primary operating system for the person in their later relationships with other people. Siegel (2020) further explained this dynamic:

Relationships between an individual and his/her earlier loved objects create a meaning template that informs how future objects' behavior and intentions are interpreted. Beliefs about the self in relation to others are also held in memories that surface in reenactments of certain dynamics.

(Siegel, 2020, p. 12)

The earlier in life that the defenses get imprinted, the more they become entrenched (Solomon & Lynn, 2002).

Conceptualization of Problem Formation

Object relations theory goes back to birth. As mentioned, infants attempt to develop attachments with a significant care person, many times the mother or a mothering figure (Scharff & Scharff, 1997). The term "mother" is used in much of object relations literature but does not actually have to refer to the biological mother. When used, it refers to a primary caregiver of the child.

All people have needs. In this case, it is the caregiver's role to be able to address the needs of their infant. When the caregiver can keep the infant and their needs in mind, they have engaged in an emotional and cognitive process called **containment** (Scharff & Scharff, 1995). However, regardless of how well the caregiver engages in nurturing, the infant's needs cannot be met without the caregiver causing some type of discomfort. When this happens, the infant will develop a level of frustration.

Frustration that persists and increases leads to the infant viewing the caretaker as rejecting. Scharff and Scharff (1997) described what happens during this process:

To cope with the pain, the infant takes in (introjects) the experience of the mother as a rejecting object and rejects that image inside the self by splitting it off from the image of the ideal mother and pushing it out of consciousness (repressing it). This is called the rejected object.

(Scharff & Scharff, 1997, p. 142)

While the infant is trying to cope with the various frustrations in their needs being met by their primary caretaker, they are developing personality patterns. In healthy individuals, these patterns evolve as the person moves through the normal developmental stages (e.g., childhood, adolescence, young adult, etc.). For those who experience a rejecting caregiver, the person becomes stuck and is unable to deal with the various requirements of their life. It is these early interactions with one's parents that determine a person's defensive structures that tend to persist for the whole of their lives (Solomon & Lynn, 2002).

A series of splits then happens to the person's consciousness (self) which leads to three selves: a central self, a craving self, and a rejecting self (Ludlam, 2022; Scharff & Scharff, 1997). The **central self** attaches to an **ideal internal object**, leading to a sense of satisfaction and security. The **craving self** attaches to an **exciting internal object** but is unsatisfied and experiences a sense of longing. The **rejecting self** attaches to a **rejecting internal object,** leading to a sense of anger. These objects relate to one another within the individual's psyche, leading to the notion that within each individual, there is a dynamic internal object relations (Scharff & Scharff, 1997).

So far, we have discussed what happens for an individual, especially in their early history. Yet, people have a need to be in relationships. People will resultantly engage others in ways to get fulfillment of their needs throughout their life. Intimate relationships provide people with a space where they can experience commitment, devotion, intimacy, and physicality (Scharff & Scharff, 1997). Relationships are potentially containing for the partners as they can work through their object relationships while also engaging in development (Morgan, 2016). In romantic relationships, being connected allows each member of the couple to explore self and other. The repressed parts of the self may seek out a spouse who is accepting. When becoming a couple, each member seeks out from the other person those parts that have been previously split because of frustration with past need satisfaction.

Members of a couple unconsciously reenact various dynamics from their early relationships within the current relationship. This may take the form of recreating previous patterns of engagement, such as trying to be close to the other or withdrawing from the other as a form of protection. These unresolved childhood issues rise up in the couple relationship where their unmet needs or attachment insecurities as infants and children come to the surface. The conflicts that happen in couples usually happen because of the dynamics between the partners' internalized object representations and projections onto each other. This leads to misunderstandings, as each person is engaging the other through perceptions that have been shaped by their internalized experiences.

Positive internal object relationships provide a foundation for healthy romantic relationships. Conversely, a lack of preparation for adult intimate relationships eventually leads to attitudes and behaviors derived from child-based neglect and shame-based super-ego constructs that threaten well-being and prevent flexibility in dealing with differences between self and other. Arrests in developmental achievement are traceable to absent or insufficient nurturing supplies and are fueled by a partner's prior exposure to neglect, abandonment, or traumatic situations.

One way of conceptualizing couples on the brink of relationship dissolution through an object relations lens is that, after falling in love, the couple was not capable of "elevating" in love. The early romantic or exciting aspects of an early attraction may yield an idealized attachment that provides an illusion of a "forever" needed connection. In time, partners notice that change in one or both is occurring, for which personality structures are insufficiently mature for negotiation of needs. The result is often that only one partner can be receiving while the other is giving. Hence, mutuality is a lacking couple developmental requirement and the result is reduced or chronically absent emotional intimacy, increasing depressive anxieties, and/or open conflict about unmet needs or minutiae.

Basic Object Relations Concepts

A One and Two Body Theory of Projective Identification (regarding couples):
"A projection is to a perception, what projective identification is to an influence!" (Bagnini, teaching notes).

Projective identification occurs when one partner unknowingly encourages the other partner to relate to them in a way that permits an emotionally charged theme from their past to reoccur in the present (Siegel, 2020). It is an intrapsychic and interpersonal defense mechanism which gets another person to act out the internalized self or object image (Slipp, 2014). Siegel (2020) explained, "In that moment, there is a blurring of past and present, as beliefs, expectations, and emotions from earlier experiences infiltrate the here-and-now" (p. 13). For the couple, the members unwittingly take on roles that reflect one or the other's early interpersonal negative experiences. For instance, one partner may take on the role of the critical parent while the other takes on the role of the demeaned child. The therapist working with the Hogarths will need to determine how much of their relational patterns are based on each of their early histories where they are bringing those longings into the marriage. When this happens, conflict is likely to follow.

People will always experience conflict or failure. Many people can handle this, even though they may experience some level of sadness, disappointment, or fear when they try to deal with the situation. However, those who had early object rejection will likely engage in projective identification, which distorts their understanding of self and other (Siegel, 2020). That is, people engage in a repetition of their early childhood interpersonal experience in the present, usually with the person they love and are closest to (Solomon & Lynn, 2002). This leads to both members feeling shame and blame. Carissa's frequent pushes to get Steve to engage more with her or Steve's withdrawal and avoidance of conflict may be windows into each of their pasts. They are currently each feeling discomfort—Carissa experiences the view of herself (by Steve and perhaps by herself) as overbearing, and Steve experiences the view of himself (by Carissa and perhaps by himself) as not good enough. The question for the object relations therapist is where these ways of being originated. Some questions the therapist might ask themself include: What was the relationship like between Carissa and her caregivers? How secure did she feel in her relationship with her mother? How secure did she feel with her grandmother, Abigail, who played a significant parenting role since both of Carissa's parents worked? Although Lori, Carissa's sister, is older, it seems Carissa was a better student. Might she have felt pushed by someone to do better and might that experience be playing out in her relationship with Steve where she is pushing him to do more? What role did Steve's parents' conflict with one another have on his sense of security? Since Steve knew from an early age that there were expectations of him (and his siblings), might he have chosen Carissa as his wife to maintain him in a lower position of hierarchy where he doesn't live up to expectations, which encourages the other person to be more overbearing?

When asking oneself these questions, an object relations therapist can also remember that projective identification follows a developmental line within a range of adaptive to maladaptive aspects. Each person carries a psychic structure that guides perception and behavior toward another. Using a psychoanalytic lens gives one an interpersonal–interpsychic vantage point from which to comprehend the projective process. Mental constructs or precepts predetermine what will transpire between self and other. It is important to recognize that, for a couple, both members are involved in this process. Middelberg (2001) explained "that the second partner is not a passive recipient of projections but is actively engaged in a mutual projection process and must have a valency or hook for the projection" (p. 343).

From a **one-body perspective**, we do not need an external object for projective identification. In the subject, there are internal images lodged in the psyche that embody object relations. Perceptions, often infused with unmetabolized affects and mental images, are identified with. From a one-body perspective, we live in a solipsistic world, as there is no objective certainty about an outside world. The individual has a core that is enduring and not merely subject to outside tampering.

In a **two-body perspective**, the process of projective identification is identical, but we include the reactions of the external other. Unwanted and longed-for percepts (objects of perception) seek out another who might take them in and identify with them, behaving according to the unconscious matching or valence between the two unconscious minds and their actions. The object does not have to identify with the subject, and the projections of one may not result in a reciprocal accommodation.

For example, in a marriage, one partner may project worthlessness while the other feels worthy. If the partners are sufficiently integrated individuals, the projected unwanted part is not successful in promoting a collusion in the other; thus, a blurring of boundaries does not occur. In another situation, a couple that is poorly differentiated may collude in a basic assumption of contempt. The partners trade the projective material in which one partner feels contemptuous and hostile, but the other holds the guilt for being unlovable. In this dance, the projective identifications divide the couple into a doer and a done to. The projections can also become reversed. The unlovable partner may project a standard of sacrifice that the contemptuous partner identifies with; both partners then feel unlovable and contemptuous. Each partner carries an aspect of what is split off by the other. One partner may fire up the contempt while the other cools it down. In **malignant projective processes**, there is a valence, or absorption, that is sustained due to unconscious negative or idealized elements in each partner's prior object relations. The idea that love will be sufficient to manage significant primitive distortions is overrated and generally short-lived.

Let's apply this to our treatment couple. Steve and Carissa likely believed that, when they got married, they would be experiencing bliss for the rest of their lives. In five short years, that fantasy bubble has been popped. Through their projective identifications, Carissa has stepped into the position of blamer while Steve takes on a victim stance.

So far, we have been talking about projective identification. The complementary process to projective identification is **introjective identification** (Scharff & Scharff, 1995). Here, "a person takes in the projections of the other to solve an internal problem and then acts in identification with those parts" (p. 133). For projective identification to occur fully, introjective identification has to occur as well. This happens when one person has an internal experience of splitting a painful part of an internal object relationship and puts it into another person. However, the other person must take in that part, which happens without them knowing it. Object relations couple therapy is useful in bringing this unconscious process to the surface. In this way, the dynamic of projective identification/introjective identification can be seen as unconscious communication between the couple.

The processes of projective identification and introjective identification shift the therapist's view of the couple dynamic of blaming one person to seeing that what is happening to them is a joint process (this excludes certain aspects such as domestic violence). Carissa takes in Steve's push for connection to someone who sets and holds high expectations of others. This puts Carissa into a position above him and unbalances the relationship. Steve does not feel he can live up to her standards. Steve takes in Carissa's unconscious push for him to be fully committed and connected as her father wasn't (at times).

Counter to projective identification is **disidentification**. These two processes both involve past relational dynamics from early childhood playing a role in the current interpersonal relationship between the couple. However, whereas projective identification leads to a reenactment of the past unresolved themes, disidentification entails the person trying not to repeat the negative aspects of the past (Siegel, 2022). Rather, they try to evade and not engage in the situation when treated in a way that brings up the past trauma.

Earlier, we mentioned that it is inevitable for people to experience frustrations in their life. This is the case even when, in infancy, parents do their best to meet our needs. Those who function healthily can usually handle these frustrations fairly well. Those with intense early childhood rejections from their objects will likely begin to spiral when their past memories and/or internal representations seep into their awareness (Siegel, 2022). This will lead them to experience **emotional flooding**. Siegel explained, "When an individual experiences flooding, similar situations from the past are triggered along with the emotions that were stored in the memory" (p. 155). During the early part of their relationship, Steve and Carissa were in a honeymoon period—this period happened even before they got married; they were excited about the relationship and hopeful of what it could bring to their lives. Unfortunately for them, like with all couples, the honeymoon eventually ends. Based on each of their projective identifications and introjective identifications, they find themselves stuck in a consistent pattern of conflict. Both are likely to experience emotional flooding where their past internalized rejecting experiences with significant care people are now coming forth and influencing the unconscious push-and-pull they are having with one another.

Applying Theory to Practice

Let's talk more about how the object relations theory manifests in an object relations therapist's conceptualization of our treatment couple. First, it is important to note that people choose partners for an intimate relationship for many reasons. Consciously, it may be for attractiveness, family background, similar interests, and so on. However, it is the unconscious fit that determines the quality of the relationship, which is predicated on the way that object relations are gratified between the couple (Dicks, 1967). In some ways, this can be viewed as the couple developing a joint personality as parts of the ego and parts of the object connect them in a dynamic internal and dynamic external system.

Being involved in a couple provides an opportunity for projection and introjection to occur. During coupling, one partner is likely to discover parts of themselves in the other. However, those parts cannot stay in the partner. If so, the individual will remain impoverished. One of the functions of couplehood is to allow a reemergence of lost parts of the self. This happens when the object relations are acknowledged, allowing them to shift from being repressed.

Couplehood specifically is an experiment in relationship intimacy. Relatedness is motivated by unconscious and conscious processes. Couples do not ordinarily view serious intimate relationships in this way, but our experience indicates that they are complex and multi-faceted. Spending time with a couple in therapy reveals patterns of relating that the couple had little awareness of or never considered important. It is important for us, as therapists, to track varieties of couple relationships to identify the areas of couple experience that we need to address.

Needs

Rather than the Freudian view of the id and the push for the pleasure principle, object relations therapists believe that each person has a need to be cared about and a desire to care about someone else. The couple relationship is the medium in which adults can care about each other in a mutually satisfying manner. However, as they lose the goodwill they have toward one another and are not able to learn new ways of relating, they find themselves losing their sense of intimacy (Siegel, 1992). The longer that Steve and Carissa experience difficulties in their marriage, the more they hold to their rigid ways of relating to one another. At this point in their marriage, they are unaware of what they have each brought with them from their family-of-origin. They likely are taking a very limited view of what the problem is—and who the problem is. For each, it is the other. For Steve, Carissa is too overbearing and inflexible. For Carissa, Steve is too unemotional and disconnected. These views are quite partial, viewing only one person and not the mutual ways that they impact each other. However, even that is a partial view, as it doesn't take into consideration how each person was and still is impacted by their early internal object relationships, and how that plays a role in the interpersonal dynamics of their marriage through projective identification and introjective identification.

For couplehood to work, which is often—although not always—what two individuals expect when entering into a romantic relationship, two personalities have to blend in an emotionally satisfying way over time. What makes it difficult to accomplish and sustain emotional satisfaction over time is that the developmental trajectories of each partner have separate and distinct emotional/experiential origins that challenge the adaptability of each partner. Solomon and Lynn (2002) explained that "Two people will not form a relationship unless the partnership appears to preserve an internal structure that for each of them recapitulates experiences that are familiar and, in fact, are object relationships" (p. 390). We can use the succotash metaphor to describe an intimate partnership in which lima beans and corn are distinct flavors but are transformed into a third position or flavor called succotash when blended. Partners stuck in one flavor do not easily give up distinctness (knowledge as fact) for a surprising alternative.

Internalized prior relationships produce a mixture of frustrations, satisfactions, and good experiences metabolized for use along with bad, unsorted, hot triggers signaling unresolved conflicts and disturbances. The essential ingredients for relative success in coupling are giving and receiving, giving patience and forgiveness, and tolerating and embracing differences. Most important is the capacity to be curious about self and other when times are difficult. **Curiosity** is the single most important psychological tool a couple can have, even when adult love exists on a reasonably compatible level. Curiosity about a capacity for change in oneself and to accept change in others is what allows the couple to evolve. In the beginning of their relationship, Steve and Carissa found that they contained many of these ingredients for a successful relationship. They were curious about the other person, were interested in their likes and dislikes, and provided space and understanding around each other's worldviews. Over the last couple of years, perhaps spurred on by the difficulties in Carissa getting pregnant, they have put aside their sense of curiosity. Instead of leaning into their joint frustrations, the process of trying to get Carissa pregnant has led each to become a silo, isolated from the other. Inquiries are not about what is going on for the other person, but how they need to conform to the other's wants. For the object relations therapist, curiosity happens by wanting to explore the internalized prior relationships. For instance, it would be interesting to explore what was going on for Steve internally since his parents experienced significant conflict when they were having difficulties conceiving a child and were trying to figure out whether they would have more children.

Unfortunately, the expectations for couplehood are becoming increasingly risky. We live in an age of "selfies" and are flooded by technologically-driven narcissistic motives—the thought process is often "It's all about me." Coupling is centered on what the other can do for me, and what is the least I have to sacrifice or suffer to be invested in the partner. Solomon and Lynn (2002) described this concept as such:

> Marital problems often begin because most people unconsciously look for a match to their own early object-relations patterns, unconsciously hoping that what went wrong in the past will be healed with a new partner, who is expected to represent an improvement over the original caretaker.

(Solomon & Lynn, 2002, p. 392)

As an infant, the child looks to the parent to fulfill needs and provide security and esteem. This power shifts to the partner in an adult intimate relationship. Siegel (2022) stated, "When the new object fails to provide these functions or unconditional love, there is typically a strong emotional reaction—either a shutdown/implosion, or heightened emotions/explosion" (p. 159). Each person loses the desire to understand the other better. Further, they likely also lose the push to understand themselves better. The importance of *soul* in relating—courage, compassion, and contemplation (seeking the truth)—is, according to Edmundson (2018), too little appreciated.

This very brief reference to modern attitudes toward coupling takes us to a few time-tested observations about types of couples encountered in treatment. There are ordinary dynamics in intimate relations that oscillate within every couple—there is the wish for autonomy–separateness and the wish for togetherness–connection. Each couple that enters our office brings variations of their prior and current relationship successes and failures, and the partners' degrees of success or failure are atmospherically felt. The successes they experience tend to be tied to their previous family-of-origin experiences around positive caring. Solomon and Lynn (2002) explained, "The bonds of love in adults are an accumulation of the loving attachments developed early in life" (p. 402). On the one hand, Carissa's parents seem to have had a more loving relationship than Steve's. While there was an affair and a brief separation, they were not very openly conflictual as a couple. Steve, on the other hand, experienced the tension surrounding his parents' contentious marriage. This may lead him to shy away from conflict in relationships. Each of their early experiences of nurturing and need rejection play some role in the organization of their current coupling.

Schemas

In this section, we will talk about a few different organizing schemas for how two people may come together to form a couple. The first schema, by Mendelsohn (2014), suggests five types of couple that might be seen in therapy: parasitic, symbiotic, narcissistic, sibling, and oedipal. **Parasitic couples** occur when one part of a person's psyche is connected to and dependent on the other person. This leads to a malignant projective identification. Change is difficult in parasitic couples since both people operate based on the dependency. Similarly, the **symbiotic couple** is aware that they are separate people but strive for indivisibility. This couple develops a strong boundary between themselves and outsiders, leading to an "us against the rest of the world" mentality. This couple would likely initiate therapy when their fantasy of oneness has been shaken, either by people in their relational field (e.g., children, parents) or when a rupture has occurred (perhaps due to an affair or other such event). The **narcissistic couple** needs the other person to support their own self-esteem. Their connection is primarily for this purpose, where they seek a perfect mate. The **sibling couple** tend to have a relationship similar to that of siblings where a form of rivalry happens between them. Members either tend to have childhoods where they experienced much love and attention, or childhoods where they experienced one or more siblings receiving much more love and affection than they got. Last, the **oedipal couple** contains one or more members who choose the partner based on their resemblance to an important parental figure. These couples experience triangulation, either with an actual person or a fantasized person. Steve and Carissa likely equate to the oedipal couple, as Carissa probably resembles Steve's mother where he felt strong expectations put on him. Carissa may have unconsciously chosen Steve based on his ability to connect yet be somewhat disconnected—perhaps, in some ways, similar to her father.

Based on Melanie Klein's ideas, we can also view couples as being one of two types: paranoid/schizoid and depressed. The **paranoid/schizoid couple** tends to have mutual distrust and suspicion, emotional distance and detachment, pushes for independence over intimacy, has trust issues, and limited emotional connection. With the **depressed couple**, they are able to move away from splitting and integrate both positive and negative aspects of self and other. These couples tend to engage in idealization and devaluation, fear loss and abandonment, experience guilt and self-blame, demonstrate insecurity and lack of trust, have difficulty managing ambivalence, have strained communication and emotional expression, and exhibit intense emotional turmoil and dysregulation. The Hogarths fall more into the depressed couple type. There are ways that they can connect to the other person, yet there is some sense of insecurity and difficulty in communication.

Next, we present an adhesive mental organization for couple types. We want to point out that this is not standard object relations terminology, but has been an efficient theoretical construct to help make distinctions in how different couples come together and function.

Elmer's Glue: These couples comprise neurotic partners that move from rationalizations and intellectualizations to guilt and remorse. They are capable of ambivalence and insight and do not rigidly *stick* to defenses—there is some capacity for fluidity and movement between the depressed and paranoid/schizoid positions in sessions and over time. With these couples, the therapist would help them to mourn losses and recover lost objects for working on and through the current and deeper issues that were unconscious prior to treatment. For these couples, transferences are accessible and can be modified.

Crazy Glue: These couples are volatile, disorganized, affectively over-stimulated, loosely structured in survival mode, primitive and moody. They are prone to persecutory fears and rejection anxieties. They have psychosomatic complaints and part-object transferences that utilize the therapist to supply proxy functions, such as soothing, calming, joining, and being a bearer of suffering and painful psychic events.

Epoxy Glue: These couples display rigid defenses, concrete beliefs, insulated relational engage-ment, and tend to be antagonistic in relation to the therapist. Transferences to the therapist are not forthcoming. The inside stays mostly inside, and the border between self and other remains rigid. For example, this would be the couple that presents one partner as totally crushed, miserable, and bereft and the other as happy, unruffled, and perhaps a bit puzzled. Steve and Carissa would fall mostly into this type of couple.

Splitting

Some couples are part-object related; their individual fears range from exploitation to neglect so they have to control their objects. Libidinal pursuits are put aside accordingly, and unacknowledged projective identifications entice the partner whose desires for connection may temporarily assuage both partners' deeper catastrophic worries. The fears and longings are split in an unconscious collusion. One partner with abandonment anxiety is pressed into the role of caregiver and solicitor of the other's dependency. The other partner is fearful of needing and yet losing the solicitous one's seeming devotion, secretly harboring exploitation anxieties. The price of being given to is very high. This may result in **splitting**, which is an unconscious defense mechanism where individuals compartmentalize conflicting aspects of themselves or their partners into "all-good" or "all-bad" representations (Middelberg, 2001). This may seem to be problematic, but is actually viewed by object relations theorists as being a normal defense mechanism in early childhood (Siegel, 2022). Splitting is the outcome in a long-term relationship when the solicitous partner seeks connection but does not find it through admiration and doing for the other. The other enjoys yet fears becoming overwhelmed by the partner's unexpressed neediness. A struggle ensues, splitting the two part-ners' unmet libidinal needs into a "doer–done to" role exchange. Anti-libidinal motives strain the couple's ability to stay in contact with one another.

People may also engage in a dyadic splitting where they adopt an "all-or-nothing" view of their partner and/or the relationship (Siegel, 2022). Many times, this is as an "all-bad" position where a filter is developed so that the partner can only take in information that confirms the devalued pos-ition. This increases the pessimism that overwhelms the system, preventing people from having effective understanding of or engagement with one another. This can currently be seen in the Hogarths' marriage. There has been a dyadic splitting where each is primarily viewing the other as "all-bad." What once was fine is now taboo. For instance, Steve had for years gotten together with his friends to play sports or hang out. As the marriage has continued to fracture, these behaviors are now being seen as problematic and endemic to a view of Steve as not caring about or being present in the relationship.

Working with the Hogarths involves a review of any and all models of couple relations that each partner heard about and experienced from birth onwards. The therapist would want to understand the internal object relations and real-world aspects that carry into the marriage issues or tensions, which include prior generational influences on both sides. The transmission of intergenerational or current relational anxieties, traumatic losses, and family separations and conflicts would be of interest in determining the couple's holding capacities under conditions of interpersonal or indi-vidual prior or current life stress. Carissa's mother had the experience of infidelity, and although the couple recovered, more details are needed, as the affair's effects on the children would help to determine interpersonal processes. Further, themes such as trust—in males especially—would be an important consideration.

Another familial dynamic that likely had an impact on Steve and Carissa's relationship is Steve's father's opinions on their relationship. Steve's father was holding and expressing racist attitudes and anxieties regarding Steve's future in being with and marrying a Black woman; these were present from the beginning when Steve disclosed being with Carissa. Racist attitudes and a complete disregard for Steve's need for support and pleasure in his new marriage were then clearly displayed by his father's snubbing of Carissa's family at the wedding. This emotional cut-off likely continued throughout the marriage. Steve's mother did not intervene on the new couple's behalf at the wedding, so the post-divorce attitude toward having supportive unity appears missing within the parental pair. In therapy, a greater examination of Steve's childhood before and since the age of 10 (when Steve's parents divorced) would help to provide insight into his possible internal object relationships and projective identifications in the present.

It would be just as important to explore Steve's childhood and life after his parents' divorce. Divorce usually doesn't occur suddenly, as marriage problems may be brewing for months or years. These marital difficulties influence a young child's confidence, lead to confusion, increase triangulation or oedipal anxieties, and increase parent–child conflict or inner turmoil regarding parental unity or schism in child-rearing practices. The object relations therapist would want to explore the impact that Steve's parents' divorce had on his psyche. What internal object relationships had he developed? In what ways is he engaging in projective identification with Carissa? With a biracial couple, it would be important to ask about Carissa's experiences with White individuals (particularly males), the effects of these experiences on her well-being, and her family's experiences and attitudes regarding racial and racist culture.

Conceptualizing Diversity

While traditionally focused on intrapsychic dynamics, object relations therapy has evolved to acknowledge the importance of diversity and cultural factors in shaping object relations. Originally, much of the view of the family was based on a White, Western middle-class family (Applegate, 1990). However, over the last several decades, the importance of culture has increasingly had a significant impact on therapists' understandings. Cultural influences shape individuals' internalized objects, influencing their relationships, attachment styles, and emotional experiences. People are influenced by cultural norms, values, and familial structures. Clients may internalize culturally specific objects, affecting their relational patterns. Object relations therapy involves exploring clients' family and cultural narratives to understand the intergenerational transmission of cultural objects, values, and relational patterns. Every culture makes various assumptions about individual and family development. These cultural discourses find their way to people through family experience, and the family takes them in and interprets them in unique ways. In essence, the family has their own culture within the wider lens of the greater societal culture.

Object relations theory integrates an intersectional lens to understand how multiple aspects of identity (e.g., race, ethnicity, sexual orientation) converge to shape clients' object relations. These intersecting identities influence clients' internalized objects and relational experiences. Bucci (2002) stated that "the nature of the inner structures in adaptive and pathological forms and the nature of the symbolizing process will vary across diverse cultures; it is necessary to identify these differences to treat patients effectively" (p. 219).

Object relations therapy holds a humanistic position that is equally focused on male and female development (Scharff & Scharff, 1995). It is a nonauthoritarian approach that values people regardless of factors such as age, gender, sex, sexual orientation, or race. For instance, object relations therapy is especially applicable to those in a same-sex relationship who may experience discrimination or hostility from the social environment because of their sexual orientation (Sussal, 1999). There is a good fit for gay and lesbian couples and object relations therapy because of the notion of developing a therapeutic holding environment where clients are provided with safety by a caregiver (the therapist). For children of color who grow up in the United States, their object relations are more complex, as they have to develop a bicultural identity where they experience their ethnic subculture within the larger culture of the White majority (Applegate, 1990). For minority parents, the therapist can help them affirm and value their ethnic heritage, which can promote positive ethnic self-representations in their children.

Given the importance of the self of the therapist in the object relations therapeutic process, the therapist will need to acknowledge their own cultural biases and how these might impact transference and countertransference processes. Being culturally sensitive allows therapists to recognize how their own cultural experiences might influence their understanding of clients' object relations. When there are cultural differences between the therapist and the couple, the therapist needs to explore them so that they become understood. However, this is also the case when there is a similarity of culture between therapist and client so that these similarities don't get taken for granted.

The Role of the Therapist

A lot of the therapeutic work in object relations couple therapy comes by working with the partners to help them understand the impact of their early childhood experiences on their internal representations, and how those are playing a part in their current relationship. To do this, the therapist's first role is to create a safe therapeutic environment (Siegel, 2022). They can do this by taking on the role of a participant/observer (Siegel, 2020), holding a curious stance as to how the members of the couple interpret and relate to one another.

In therapy, the clients are likely to bring up complaints about the other or have a perspective that differs from their partner. Those with difficulty in regulating their emotions may quickly become detached from the process, defensive, attacking, or in denial. The therapist needs to be able to regulate the process between the couple so that they can take control and prevent an escalation. Siegel (2022) referred to this role as that of a referee, where the therapist prevents partners from making attacks and counterattacks.

Another role of the therapist is to bring forth insight for the members of the couple so that they can understand how their emotions and the current relational situation are related to their earlier childhood longings and object rejections (Siegel, 2020). "This often involves understanding the systemic sequence, the meaning that has been attributed to events, and emotional responses that may not have been fully acknowledged" (Siegel, 2022, p. 156). Here, the therapist can move beyond being a referee to the role of a detective and interpreter. They try to dig deep to find the emotionally laden aspects of relationships rather than the he-said/she-said of an event. The therapist helps to bring forth each person's voice as they explore their repressed pain. To do so, the therapist needs to be comfortable addressing difficult emotions. Many object relations couple therapists go to their own therapy or engage in supervision so that they can enhance their emotional balance (Siegel, 2022).

The object relations therapist is not manualized, but rather interacts based on open communication wherein the therapist doesn't try to go for a quick fix or structure the conversation (Bagnini, 2011). This happens by creating a context of safety that allows the clients to relate to the therapist in ways that help bring forth their previous object relations. Object relations therapists observe and respond to relational connections, disconnections, and ambivalences toward self and others. They work from inside the couple system to outside, noticing defenses, aggression, detachment, frustrations, self-protection, conscious and unconscious wishes and desires, and psychosomatic body language that suggests moods and modes of dealing with anxieties.

The role of the object relations therapist consists of paying attention to unconscious process, maintaining a position of managing anxieties (psychological containment), and remaining essentially non-directive. This is done by initially and mostly refraining from offering advice, and directing couple behavior away from their usual mode of communicating their distress (Morgan, 2016). The general attitude is not to do too much in order to pay attention to unconscious material, including the clients' dreams and associations that come into the session and feelings about the therapist's behavior when interacting with each partner.

The therapist observes and remains attentive to how the couple utilizes the therapist in two ways. First, to promote empathic understanding of the couple's levels of distress and suffering without taking sides. Second, the therapist traces the function of and puts words to survival defenses and anxieties that cause breakdowns. This may involve naming regressive pulls away from couple creativity and collaboration.

The therapist's tool kit is comprised of identifying individual and couple object relations and their unconscious impact on relating. The aim is to become useful to partners by being perceived and responded to as the sought-after maternal good object that was absent in the past or as the bad or rejecting object that over-gratified or seduced the partner as a child in an incestuous triangle.

When seeing the Hogarths in an initial object relations assessment and during ongoing treatment, the therapist would access unconscious defenses, anxieties, or hidden object relations issues enacted in the marriage. These internalized object relations are historicized and unresolved and are serious preconditions for causing pathological relating, ambiguities, conflicts, and estrangement in the couple.

Conceptualization of Problem Resolution

There is not a set of prescribed tools and techniques for object relations couple therapy. Rather, therapy is based on an attitude by the therapist that sets the frame of the sessions to allow a deep therapeutic relationship (Scharff & Scharff, 1995). The therapist engages in active listening— they listen for the conscious and unconscious organizational patterns of the individuals and the couple as a whole. This is one way in which object relations therapy is different from some other approaches that are more actively interventive.

The Therapeutic Frame

At the beginning of object relations therapy, the therapist is primarily concerned with setting the frame of therapy, maintaining a neutral position, and developing a therapeutic space for the intrapersonal and interpersonal processes to occur (Scharff & Scharff, 1995). As therapy progresses, other techniques come into play, such as the therapist's use of self, the use of transference and countertransference, the incorporation of dreams and fantasy, interpretations (of defenses, anxieties, and object relations), working through, and then termination.

The frame of therapy in problem resolution has multiple levels (Scharff & Scharff, 1995). On an administrative level, the therapist sets the frame by organizing the parameters of therapy, such as who should come, the time, frequency, duration of sessions, and the cost. The **therapeutic frame** consists of what is to be talked about and the interpersonal process between client and therapist. Attempts by the client to modify the frame are seen as reenactments of the client's inner object world.

Object relations couple therapy holds that it is the relationship between therapist and clients that is the center of the work (Scharff & Scharff, 1995). The therapist understands they must be aware of and explore each individual's object relationships, the couple's relationship with one another, and the relationship between the clients and the therapist. Each of these areas provides fodder for exploration of the internal and interpersonal worlds of the client.

When a couple comes to therapy, the therapist observes their dynamics, as that is the vehicle for understanding each person's internal object relationships and how they manifest in the current relationship (Solomon & Lynn, 2002). The couple's relationship is viewed developmentally, as processes differ depending on whether the couple is new, has recently had children, or has been together for many decades. Whichever stage the couple is in, the object relations therapist helps the couple to address the couple stage of development they are in (Scharff & de Varela, 2005).

The object relations couple therapist also helps each member of the couple to realize that the concerns which are present for them in the relationship are connected to their early in-life connections (and disconnections) that have solidified into dysfunctional patterns (Solomon & Lynn, 2002). There is therefore an inevitable moving back and forth and connection of the there-and-then and the here-and-now. Scharff and Scharff (1995) described this process in therapy as a core affective exchange, which can occur between the couple or between one or both members of the couple and the therapist. A **core affective exchange** is when internal object relationships become present in the therapy room and are reflected upon and understood to gain insight into the members' projective/introjective identification processes. During these times of intense exchange of feelings, the therapist asks the members to remember old experiences that are reminiscent of the current difficult situation.

Additionally, as in many other forms of couple therapy (or any therapy for that matter), the therapist's ability to be empathetic is quite important. While empathy is not the change agent in object relations couple therapy, its use helps the couple to communicate, especially their under-lying wounds, as well as to reclaim their projections and accept those qualities they have previously disavowed (Solomon & Lynn, 2002). In essence, the therapist gets a living history where the client's early history is connected to what is currently happening in the therapy room (Scharff & Scharff, 1995). This usually happens when clients are highly emotional in the interpersonal process.

This living history helps bring forth early attempts for need fulfillment and the splitting of parts of the self that happened for the internal object relationships. This happens for both members of the couple. Solomon and Lynn (2002) explained, "If therapy is to be successful, the goal is to help each reclaim split-off parts and, without shame, recognize the defenses used to hide these split-off aspects of self" (p. 402). Thus, symptom relief is not the primary goal of therapy. Rather, an explor-ation of the projective identification and introjective identification helps people to see how their history and their current experience intertwine.

Clinically, a therapist's core perspective on the projective process specifically depends on what point of view they hold about the role of projection in shaping the client's world. Therapists keep in mind that ideas about interpreting the transference depend on one's view of projection and projective identification. Therapists also study the role of client identifications with their primary objects that find their way into the transference with the therapist. The **transference** (discussed in more detail later in the chapter) is the means whereby the therapist is pressured to take on the primary emotional experiences of the child portion of the client's original family environment. The therapist will feel treated like they are the subject portion of the client's injured self, while the client either (a) takes on the parental object of neglect, aggression, or absence or (b) will feel obligated to be the source of repair, at first idealized, to become the rescuer. Later, unfortunately, the therapist is hated, feared and longed for, and unavailable, confirming the client's inferiority, neediness, and inability to be loved.

The object relations couple therapist listens for flexible, flat, or charged verbal accounts of the couple's circumstances and monitors projections that range from narcissistic to flexible relating. They make note of interactional patterns that support their compatibility or stir tensions and conflicts. The problem within the couple's intimacy boundary is depicted by variations of fight–flight, closeness–distance, and togetherness–separateness dimensions that can be observed in the setting. The boundaries are immediately influenced as the therapist takes notice and adjusts the way the couple enters a potential dialogue. When projective material is negotiable and a couple can mourn lost objects and take back hurtful and malevolent projections, the couple progresses—which would be considered an analytic success.

The therapeutic frame can be a tool or a disaster when compared to each couple's style of relating in the world. Inevitably, the therapist's approach encounters the couple's bastion (boundaries), and the outcome of the struggle for influence leads to a gradual meeting of minds, a shutdown, a three-ring circus, a calamity, or a catastrophe. The therapist's frame can facilitate or impair therapeutic movement depending on how they adjust to the couple's defenses, impaired object relations, and affect dysregulation. For instance, with couples in a –K situation (knowledge as hard fact, not as symbolized experience), the therapist might explain, "The person you are married to is not the person you know."

The therapist makes the distinction between the shaping effects of unconscious assumptions from *Phantasy*, an earlier mental process that is not de-coded, and *Fantasy*, which are mental processes that are accessible to conscious awareness and therefore subject to revision. Regressed couples have core *Phantasies*. These are usually primitive, such as a hunger for the ideal (which is always absent and sought after though never realized) or a belief/sensory presence that no one cares (as in a painful absence of the nurturing other). The therapist tracks the projective sequences in couple relating, as they directly or indirectly reveal which phantasies operate through their relentless complaints, disagreements, and disappointments. Stuck couples are polarized. Object relations therapists keep in mind they are together and have a history to be experienced along with the polarized positions.

Transference

A factor that often comes into play with problem resolution in therapy is transference. Freud introduced the notion of transference into the psychotherapy nomenclature. **Transference** refers to the client's unconscious projection of emotions, desires, attitudes, and unresolved conflicts from earlier relationships, particularly with significant figures (such as parents or authority figures), onto the therapist. These emotions and expectations are transferred onto the therapist and influence the client's perceptions and reactions within the therapeutic relationship. In object relations therapy, transference can be viewed as the client's projective identification in the therapy room (Scharff & Scharff, 1995). These authors explained this process:

> The therapist is identified with a part of the object or a part of the self that has been projected into him, and the internal object relationship is then re-created between the patient and the therapist, where it can be reworked.
>
> (Scharff & Scharff, 1995, p. 113)

Transference, for the object relations therapist, can also be viewed as an attitude of the clients where they allow themselves to be in the therapeutic space. This entails them feeling safe and trusting the therapeutic process. In some ways, the therapeutic space is created when the therapist fosters a context of safety and security. When this happens, clients can say things they haven't previously felt safe to say as well as listening to each other in new ways.

Whereas the Freudian psychoanalyst tries to be a blank slate so that the client can engage in transference, the object relations therapist views themselves as being neutral so that the client can use them as an object. Through connecting to the client by being present, engaged, and open, the therapist provides the client an opportunity to become an object to be used by the client.

Complex projections are ubiquitous and dwell in all intimate relationships. A careful study of hidden anxieties that lie beneath the crisis or fight of the week in a treatment couple will bring to light the underbelly of projective identifications and their protective and communicative aims. The therapist participates in the field of projective identification, and the triangular situation always brings out developmental problems through projective material. Countertransference is the essential tool for learning about projective identification.

Countertransference

Like transference, **countertransference** was introduced into the psychotherapy nomenclature by Freud. Initially, it referred to the therapist's unconscious unresolved issues, primarily with early significant figures (e.g., father or mother), that emerged in the therapist's therapeutic relationship with the client. When unrecognized or unaddressed, countertransference can interfere with the therapist's ability to be objective.

There are two types of countertransference: positive and negative. **Positive countertransference** occurs when the therapist develops positive feelings for the client based on an association with a past significant relation figure. For instance, the client may remind the therapist, in some way, of their mother, and the therapist tries to please the client as a result. **Negative countertransference** occurs when the therapist experiences negative emotions from their engagement with the client. This could happen, for example, if the therapist has unresolved self-esteem issues from an overbearing parent and is intimidated by a strong-willed client. In traditional Freudian psychoanalysis, the result of experiencing countertransference was that the psychoanalyst needed further analysis of their own so these issues wouldn't rear up during therapy with their client (Scharff & Scharff, 2014).

Whereas countertransference was initially viewed as problematic to the therapeutic setting, it has shifted to be seen as integral to effective psychoanalytic therapy (Freedman, 1998). In object relations therapy, a more totalistic approach is used in understanding countertransference, where the reactions of the therapist aren't so much about their unresolved issues but have more to do with what is happening for the clients (Siegel, 2022). For instance, if the therapist feels defensive in their interactions with one of the members of the couple, this may be a signal that there are similar processes taking part in the couple where one member tends to take a superior position and the other an inferior position. In essence, countertransference may hint at potential projective identification happening for one or both members of the couple.

Understanding and utilizing countertransference adds an extra layer of complexity for the couple therapist. Whereas in other models, therapists are trained to balance their focus on process and content, the object relations couple therapist also has to focus inward because their own reactions in the moment may be pertinent information as to what may be occurring for the couple (Siegel, 2022). This can be harnessed as a resource to allow for deeper insight into the couple's dynamics.

As explained, the therapeutic relationship is key in object relations work. Since the therapist needs to create a holding environment for the clients to engage in transference, the therapist should be as non-reactive as possible. "The therapist is a container and holder of the couple's need to express being together in the room with the therapist" (Bagnini, 2011, p. 66). Given this, the therapist is better equipped to do so when they have the maturity to utilize their internal responses well. Thus, many object relations therapists have their own therapy so that they can be more objective in the therapy room. Scharff and Scharff (1995) explained the importance of the therapist's own psychotherapy:

> The experience of themselves gathered in their personal therapy provides the baseline for knowing themselves well enough so that they can have confidence in knowing when something foreign to their internal reality has been experienced because of the encounter with the patient.
> (Scharff & Scharff, 1995, p. 180)

Transference and countertransference are the psychological centerpieces for studying the specific dynamic elements that are worked with in therapy, beginning from the early contact situation and observed during initial and ongoing sessions. **Projective processes** give the object relations therapist access to hidden struggles about self and other disturbances, and therapist–client analysis is undertaken in the unconscious communication process with the couple. The therapist's decision-making on the uses of self and technique involves a timely and consistent reflecting on the unconscious dimensions of personalities that make up the couple and impact in the moment-to-moment interactions in sessions. These interactions also impact the psyche-soma of the therapist. Understanding how to work from this vantage point requires a treatment model capable of processing how the three minds and bodies are interacting and influencing behaviors and affects in the interpersonal space of a treatment situation.

Effective therapy requires an approach that identifies and works with missing or conflicted individual and couple behaviors. It also considers stunted emotional supplies and the resulting symptomatology. The couple may lack the psychological resources that are requisites for relational stability, growth potential, and individual and couple satisfaction. The therapist "helps them manage conflict through achieving a perspective on the dynamics of their relationship and on what each partner brings to it based on who they are, including their past experience" (Morgan, 2016, p. 200).

Focusing on Couple Types

Couple types—drawing from the Kleinian notions of paranoid/schizoid and depressive positions—are helpful because they can center our observations and modify our techniques when working with couples. However, they can still vary and overlap. The object relations therapist needs to remain attentive to how each couple responds to these approaches based on couple types initially and over time. The therapist should also be aware of small to large shifts between paranoid/schizoid and depressive tendencies within sessions and from session to session.

Couples closer to the depressive position are more accessible to interpretative offerings. They are capable of using knowledge as experience, in contrast to the more regressed who view knowledge as hard fact. Those stuck in the paranoid/schizoid position are least likely to take in the therapist's mental representations of individual and couple defenses, conflicts, and anxieties. One caveat with more primitive types is to refrain from specific references to projective processes and not directly interpret transferences in the setting. These stir the darker aspects of shame-based vulnerabilities that can be too delicate to discuss in the therapy room.

We previously discussed various couple types using a glue metaphor. Now we can talk about the proper technique for making contact with these couple types. With the epoxy type, for example, a surface-to-surface approach is necessary when in the presence of the more insulated couple. Introjected material is what gets communicated since these couples have little tolerance for I-thou in-depth recognition; therefore, surface-to-depth interpretations are premature and off-putting. The couple may initially be cooperative, but they rarely take to analytic exploration. **Analytic exploration** refers to exploring the interiority of experience, either by linking partner to partner projections (unconscious usage of the other's mind) or by moving from current circumstances to their precursors.

Instead, the therapist can utilize the **environmental mother** approach since ventilation is more desirable than stimulation. When the therapist interprets, the client withdraws or flees. The primitive defenses of withdrawal and dissociation are due to the pre-oedipal forces that reside in tightly wound partners, whose psychic and interpersonal worlds are sealed off by a protective coating. They are robotic in speech and affect, demonstrating powerful defenses against the intrusion of a dangerous environment. External stimuli, including the therapist's voice and words, represent the recurrence of traumatic exposures to a collapse of maternal holding. Within the psychic retreat, such couples tend toward speech that stirs very little feeling in each other at first, but a flare-up can occur when one partner becomes aroused in conversation by a trigger. This might be by recalling a life-altering experience (e.g., the birth of a child) that is seemingly unrelated to the content of a present conversation. Abandonment feelings surge with a return of persecutory leftovers embedded in one or the other's core.

With much more regressed couples, the technical approach is as follows:
The therapist does not analyze defenses or unconscious anxieties or go deeply into unconscious motives because of couple vulnerability, persecutory, or annihilative anxieties. Interpretative moves are perceived as intrusive and horrific, like being torn apart, and the therapist is viewed as literally squeezing the defenses out of the couple and shaming them into the light. The therapist approaches defenses from the standpoint of their utility, function, or preventive aims—as survival tools needed for going on being. They enter a slow process of mirroring, with the therapist even joining their fears for a time, legitimizing how exposure in the setting may be their most significant concern. It may appear the therapist is colluding with the status quo, but the opposite can occur by preserving a measure of autonomy in the couple's requirements for self-defense. The therapist counters the fear of being taken over by a powerful tyrant, so the couple can become curious as to other motives for being in relationship. As defenses are lowered, contradictions between means and aims as well as ambiguities and ambivalences can surface. The need to be admired, to feel important, or to be in control of painful rejections can be compared to isolation, being left alone, or lost without the other. Ambivalences may involve the push to flee the other's control, while fearing the loss of one's anchor or stable center for decision-making or self-determination. The partners in a paranoid/schizoid coupling require an identity transfusion from a partner, but rigid, uneven, and unstable individuals make cohesion and continuity difficult to accomplish.

Overall, the object relations couple therapist determines which way of contacting the couple, based on the couple's type/functioning, will likely be most effective. For couples who have a well-developed self and other representations, the field is more open to what techniques and ways of being can be used (Middelberg, 2001). Conversely, for those couples with poorly developed representations of self and relationships, a greater focus on the resolution of splitting and projective identification will be needed.

Interpretation

The object relations therapist can also utilize one of Freud's primary therapeutic tools—interpretation. For Freud, it involved analyzing and interpreting unconscious thoughts, feelings, behaviors, dreams, and symptoms to uncover underlying meanings and conflicts. Object relations therapists tend to have a slightly different definition. For them, **interpretation** involves a range of therapist interventions that serve the purpose of joint understanding (Scharff & Scharff, 1995). These authors described the process of interpretation: "The therapist gathers observations—including the patient's own observations—feeds them back to see if the patient agrees with them, and links or clarifies things that have been diffusely presented but not clearly understood by the patient" (p. 113). However, object relations therapists do not hold their interpretations as truth. The client has an opportunity to agree, disagree, or fine-tune it. When the client disavows the interpretation, the trick is to determine whether they are doing so to make it more accurate or whether they are actually using a defense mechanism.

Resistance to Change

Another common topic among many therapy models is what to do when clients seem to be resisting change. From an object relations perspective, the patterns that have developed—based on each partner's object relations—are strong and enduring. Further, the couple has come together based on these intrapsychic processes to develop an interpersonal process that maintains the projective identification. Thus, the object relations couple therapist factors in that change will likely produce anxiety in one or both partners, usually leading them to utilize regressive defenses (Solomon & Lynn, 2002).

Resistance is not viewed as a negative process but rather as a normal process of people's experiences. Scharff and Scharff (1995) explained that "resistance is the term for the patient's effort to repress painful feelings and fantasies and keep them in the unconscious" (p. 93). When the client engages in resistance, the therapist can use defense analysis where they try to explore and understand the person's fantasies of shame and guilt openly and safely. This process helps them bring forth the repressed material to better deal with it in the conscious realm.

Typically, object relations couple therapy can be successfully completed within 16 weeks; however, working with a couple for 12 to 15 months is not uncommon (Siegel, 2022). Some object relations couple therapists work based on a more short-term format (Donovan, 2003). For most sessions, the couple will be seen conjointly, although there may be sessions when they are seen individually. This is especially the case when the couple is dealing with infidelity, abuse, or severe threats of couple dissolution (Siegel, 2022).

Goals in Object Relations Couple Therapy

We have talked about some specific considerations and approaches that an object relations therapist uses when focusing on problem resolution. We now want to review the general goals of an object relations therapist. Object relations couple therapy is predicated on the therapist's goal of helping each member of the couple to challenge their past meanings of events and develop new ways of responding to those past wounds (Siegel, 2022). This entails digging deep into a client's past and uncovering the intense emotions that are playing out in the present. To do this, the therapist helps the client to foster insight into how their past and present are connected.

One mindset of object relations couple therapy is not trying to meet an individual person's needs but rather to help the couple form a better holding function for themselves. In this place, as a dyad, they can grow up and meet each other's needs. When they do so, they can release their past splitting of parts and become more whole.

Throughout therapy, the therapist doesn't focus on a specific concrete goal. The symptom the client brings to therapy is not the end game. Rather, it is viewed as a sign of the underlying personalities of the members of the couple. For Carissa and Steve, it wouldn't be a mediation process where Steve agrees to scoop the litter however many times per day or week and Carissa agrees to make a date night every other week. These specific actions need to come from the people as they grow developmentally. This will happen when they move beyond their stuck patterns from the far past (their object relationships) to the stuck patterns of their recent present (their projective identifications). Rather, the goal is to help them understand why they are having difficulty being able to emotionally hold for the other person.

In general, there are several goals of object relations couple therapy. These include:

- To recognize and rework the couple's mutual projective and introjective identifications.
- To improve the couple's contextual holding capacity so that the partners can provide for each other's needs for attachment and autonomy, and developmental progression.
- To recover the centered holding relationship that allows for unconscious communication between the spouses, shown in their capacity for empathy, intimacy, and sexuality.
- To promote individuation of the spouses and differentiation of needs including the need for individual therapy or psychoanalysis.
- To return the couple with confidence to the tasks of the current developmental stage in the couple's life cycle.

(Scharff & Scharff, 2008, p. 175)

While these are the primary goals and tools, the object relations couple therapist may at times engage in some forms of psychoeducation, explaining the various processes that people experience and how one or both members of the couple are doing likewise. For instance, the therapist might explain the natural process of splitting and how that influences our thoughts and feelings, which most people would then be able to understand (Siegel, 2022).

Case Transcript

The object relations couple therapist's role during this interview is to allow themselves to empathize with what the partners are suffering with/complaining about and to offer language that can connect the concrete behaviors that cause here-and-now tension to be unspoken. Their role is to also bring forth partially hidden, deeper dependency/autonomy needs that have not been sufficiently negotiated in the here-and-now. Questions the therapist might pursue include:

• What did the couple have in common both at the beginning of the courtship and later after they married? These commonalities may include shared values, attitudes, and beliefs regarding ambition, money, family, individual and couple social needs, sexuality and affection, and of course, parenting a child.
• What are they bickering about? The cat litter relates to "parenting" messy four-legged children.
• Whose cats are they? Who wanted two of them? (if that's the number)
• What type of parent would they each wish to become?
• If pregnancy is not possible, what are their thoughts about adoption?
• They have three years of Carissa trying to become pregnant. Is one or both experiencing sadness? Might Carissa have feelings of being biologically inadequate or injured inside?
• What are the historical and/or current sibling or parental disappointments or unmet needs?
• What are the various losses each has experienced and how have they (if they have) mourned them?

The couple is seen virtually in the same room seated together on a two-seater couch. A black and white cat roams around, and it jumps up onto Carissa's lap as the session begins.

Therapist: Hello. Nice to meet both of you. I'd be interested to talk about whatever it is that you'd want to for this session.

The therapist starts the session by trying to create a warm and caring environment that will become a holding space for the couple to begin to feel safe in tackling their emotionally charged experiences.

Carissa: Well, we've been married for a few years and things were fine. Except this last year or so it hasn't really been good.
Therapist: Okay. So this has been a big change for you. A change that you don't seem to want.
Carissa: No. We were supposed to expand our marriage by having a child. We had some difficulties there. But worse than that is that Steve has pretty much been checking out of the marriage. He goes out a lot with his friends and doesn't spend time with me. He's not loving like he used to be. And he doesn't actively take care of the house. I can smell right now that he hasn't scooped the cat litter like he's supposed to.
Steve: Why is it always me that has to scoop it? If you don't like the smell, you can scoop it.
Therapist: Okay. Hold on one second. This is clearly a charged issue. Before we get into that, Steve, can you tell me a bit about what you are hoping to get from these sessions?

Here, the therapist sees that there is a quick flare-up and potential escalation between the couple. If left unchecked, they could easily spend a large portion of the session taking shots at one another. Rather, the therapist acts as a referee, not letting a fight escalate.

Steve: I want us to just be happy with one another. She is always on me, "Have you scooped the litter?" "Where are you going?" "What about getting pregnant?" It can be overwhelming. I feel like I can't please her anymore.

Therapist: That's a difficult position to be in. To feel like you aren't living up to your wife's expectations. Where do you think that comes from?

Steve: I don't know. It wasn't always like that.

Therapist: What has changed?

Steve: The litter problem isn't completely solved.

Therapist: (*Waits attentively*).

Carissa: (*Looking tense and then smiles down at the cat, who is now nuzzled against her chest*) Nothing changes, Steve does what he wants, and doesn't care about the smell.

Steve: There she goes. If I don't follow her exact demands, I'm the bad one.

Therapist: I wonder about the couple litter you each leave for us to address.
            There are very difficult tensions between you about stinky differences and individual priorities, and one of the results is the increased time you each spend apart?

The therapist uses metaphor to bring what seems like an individual mundane issue, scooping the litter, to a relational experience. The couple has not been able to scoop the litter of their relationship, leaving them both with a rotten smell which neither wants to experience anymore.

Carissa: He seems to not want to be home.

Steve: I don't think I am spending any more time away from home than I used to. You are just focusing on it more. Especially with the pregnancy thing: "Hey, I'm ovulating. It's time!"

Therapist: Is the baby issue being unresolved to date the only influence on how you're distancing? I notice neither one of you feels you have a say in what is important to address. Blaming or defending yourselves gets in the way of compromise.

The therapist continues to provide a holding space for them to be able to sit with their experiences. Neither one is to blame. They just feel blamed by the other. Or feel they need to defend themselves. It may be too early in the session to explore where that comes from in their personal histories. However, the therapist knows that at some point this will play a pivotal role in the therapy.

Carissa: We are not getting along! (*Carissa is snuggling up with the cat. The therapist hypothesizes that this might be for comfort and self-soothing.*)

Steve: I can't take any time for myself. She wants me around, but then I shouldn't see my friends or have any fun.

Carissa: I don't see us doing anything fun together. (*Tense and almost angry/tearful*)

Therapist: Both of you are suffering and finding fault with each other. Say more about what is missing now that used to bring you together in a good way.

Carissa: He couldn't wait to see me. Had his hands all over me as soon as I came in. (*Smiles sheepishly, looking over at Steve*)

Steve: (*Embarrassed look*) We were younger and very attracted to each other. This isn't the honeymoon anymore. Life gets more serious.

Therapist: Like?

The therapist is trying to get the couple to elaborate on the early attachment process. Later in the session or the therapy process, this will be used to examine the loss of the exciting object/ sexual bond.

Steve: The baby issue. I feel like sex is only to make a baby. It's like a demand now. No fun, just do it and make it into a pregnancy. I have to make an appointment. (*Slow burn*)

Carissa: (*Gently moves the cat onto the floor*) He doesn't come to bed and falls asleep in the living room.

Therapist: I noticed the cat was cozying up and you liked that. You moved it away after Steve expressed his disappointment and frustration about what's changed your sex lives.

The therapist is interested in the difference between Carissa's need for comfort, perhaps to reduce anger and sadness, and Steve's feelings of being inadequate while not being allowed to have a separate life. The therapist has now adopted a role more like that of a detective, beginning an exploration for insight.

Carissa: We aren't close for some time. No affection from Steve. If I want something I have to ask. It feels desperate.

Therapist: And for you, Steve?

Steve: (*Looking at Carissa with sadness and frustration*) I was not raised to be that affectionate. My parents did not show it. Vanessa, my sister who was five years older, played with me a little and came into my room at bedtime. When mom and dad fought, she stayed with me awhile.

Therapist: And how was that for you when things were tense in the home?

The therapist is exploring what nurturing they each might have received when they were infants and children.

Carissa: Steve never talks about that with me. He just got horny and always wanted to start doing it.

Therapist: You were talking about the difference between sex and affection earlier. In Steve's childhood, could he feel the old neglect and worries about his parents' relationship breaking down, so Vanessa at least was attentive, when he was anxious, maybe soothing, like your cat was a while ago with you?

Steve: The cat was Carissa.

The therapist pays attention to what the couple is saying as well as the interpersonal processes between them and involving the cat. Steve is more expressive and interested in what part the cat plays in sensing their growing distance. The cat represents a substitute and a good object for needed couple comfort, but Steve longs for what Carissa can receive yet seems to accept it for her now.

Therapist: Carissa and Steve, you have more than one cat. Steve, what do you do for comfort?

Steve: I can't get the cat to jump up and sit with me.

Therapist: Is the other cat male or female?

Steve: (*Smiles in embarrassment as though his deeper non-sexual longing may be exposed*) She's a girl.

Therapist: What if we named her Vanessa the Second?

Steve and Carissa break up laughing, but Steve is also quiet, deciding what to share.

Therapist: Steve was seeing the reference I offered, but I suspect I hit an old nerve too, the lack of feeling warmth and affection as a child from mom and dad. Sex can be a substitute, but it can't heal the wounds unless we address this other part, the one each of you is holding onto unless you can take a risk with touch. What do you each think?

The therapist engages in an intervention. However, it may be in the form of too deep and premature an interpretation. The therapist wonders to themselves, "Can they handle the implication of my comparing sex with affectionate touching?" Steve is carrying Carissa's feelings of neglect, and he is also feeling neglected, but expressed as a different need for individuation in the form of social fun with friends.

Carissa: I get it. My need for a baby isn't resolved yet, but I do need more in our marriage. I don't want to just be a sex object, but I never thought Steve was not addressing other deprived stuff from his family. I thought he's horny, is all.
Steve: I am, it's that the missing part was embarrassing 'cause Vanessa was the one person who came and showed someone cared. (*Steve is tearing up. He's showing anger now.*) I just went along with my parents' stuff and was a good kid.
Therapist: Anger gives you a voice to address early life experiences in which you were hurt and young with no way to have a say in changing any of it.

This interchange demonstrates the process of interpretation where the therapist functions in an interpreter role as they push for insight. However, the interpretation is mutual, as Carissa and Steve play a role in whether it is endorsed, denied, or modified.

Carissa: I feel badly, Steve. You were so tight-lipped about how you were brought up.
Therapist: And now?
Carissa: It's important. Steve is opening up.
Steve: This is not comfortable to be saying things like this.
Therapist: Steve, you are answering the questions, but I get the sense that you are pulling back. I am feeling a little shut out from you.

The therapist has been experiencing a relationship with Steve where he is there but not fully present. The therapist is processing the countertransference and bringing that to the surface in the interpersonal engagement.

Steve: This whole thing about weekends is bothering me. I feel differently about the couple time Carissa keeps nagging about.
Therapist: I think having friends and enjoying that is ordinary; however, the issue of the time to be a growing couple appears to signal anxiousness and avoidance of being together besides trying to have a baby. We need to discuss that more in detail. Whether or not you can conceive, which is the goal, the issue is still the future of how you two build the relationship and give and get what you need.

The therapist starts with a very brief psychoeducation. They then process their internal experience of Steve pulling back which allows the therapist to wonder about narcissistic wounds, and, in particular, how Steve may be projecting an internalized view of Carissa as a "sister" figure. He identified with his sister Vanessa as a dangerous and gratifying symbiotic attachment substitute for a demanding, neglectful mother. The therapist thinks to themselves: Has Steve internalized the persecution in his parents' conflicted marriage that he is now projecting onto his wife? Is there a fear of maternal closeness that was expressed incestuously between Vanessa and Steve but not attainable between mother and son?

Therapist: (*Addressing both partners*) I have a hunch that Steve needs the anger and distancing in order to safeguard some childhood-based unmet needs for closeness with his mother, while carrying the anger like his father did about mother's demands to be served that father interpreted as overwhelming. And Carissa, you may be fearful of and threatened by Steve's separateness and doubts about the potential benefits of becoming a parent. I wonder how the infidelity in Carissa's family might play a part in not trusting Steve's motives for a social life outside the home.

Carissa: I never thought that being unfaithful could ever be my concern. I didn't let myself go there, although my mother never talked about dad's other woman, and we never felt we could ask questions.

Therapist: And that meant you didn't ask your father either, not ever?

Steve: I don't think I'm cheating on you going with my friends to play golf! (*At first, he's annoyed, then looking down, with a sheepish look*)

Therapist: Carissa, I notice Steve stays away from how closeness with Vanessa could be a substitute to make up for neglected needs. Can the early sexual attraction between you help us understand how the losses of trust and security in each family, that were between your parents, affected each of you and expectations for a new marriage? What would make up for these missing child-based losses?

Carissa and Steve are looking directly at each other, eyes meeting, sadly. The therapist engages in a core affective exchange, helping the couple to gain insight into their projective and introjective identification processes.

Therapist: We're getting into the deeper aspects of how the two of you allowed the excitement of romance take over like a wonderful drug. Any thoughts now as we explore the early troubles?

Steve: Affection is still very difficult. Carissa presses me for more, and I get frustrated and withdraw.

Carissa: My folks did not demonstrate hugs and stuff, but my mom was affectionate with me and my sister.

Therapist: Steve, you and Vanessa didn't realize that the physical bond you had was also uncomfortable. She was five years older, and she bathed you and looked after your physical needs which could be comforting but maybe overstimulating, too?

Steve: This is freaking me out. You think I'm afraid of touching my wife because my sister was too close to me?

Therapist: Think for a moment what Vanessa might have been missing from dad? Was your dad partial to any of you kids?

Steve: My dad was a man's man. He played sports with me. No hugs, maybe a pat on the back when I did well on the field.

Carissa: The pregnancy issue makes sex a necessity, not so much fun anymore. It is pressure for us, Steve. (*Looking at him with awareness that they share the pressure to make the baby so the enjoyment is pushed out*)

Therapist: We have to stop here, but an important sharing occurred today. Let's see where it might lead us and what your life stories have to do with what the relationship has been ignoring or not considering with regard to your closeness issues.

The therapist has been able to set the therapeutic frame for the couple to begin to think in larger ways than they have previously. Instead of the problem being one or the other (Carissa being overbearing or Steve being distant), it has been contextualized as both an intrapsychic and inter-personal dynamic where each member is bringing their family-of-origin experiences into the couple relationship and each is maintaining the "stuckness." New openings and possibilities have begun to arise. While this is just the first session, the groundwork of connection has been made for future and deeper explorations into each of their selves and how those selves have come together.

Termination

Termination occurs in object relations couple therapy when the initial presenting problem has been resolved or has lessened and the couple is okay with where things currently are (Siegel, 2022). This happens after the themes of their early childhood experiences are brought to the surface and it is shown how they are playing out in the enactments of the current intimate relationship. Each partner will have developed new understandings of themselves and the other. Mourning prior object relations impacts is necessary for the couple in reworking the hurts and disappointments that each partner was seeking through projective identification and collusion to repeat, rather than to heal, old wounds (Hewison, 2014).

As stated previously, object relations couple therapy is not specifically about symptom removal. The belief is that the members' changes in intra- and interpersonal processes will lead to a change in the presenting complaint. While termination is a joint decision, the therapist pays attention to various signs that the clients are ready for termination. These signs include an increased capacity:

- To master developmental stress
- To work cooperatively
- To have loving object relationships
- To integrate hate with love and tolerate ambivalence
- To perceive others accurately
- To have empathy and concern for others
- To differentiate among and meet the needs of the individual

(Scharff & Scharff, 1995, p. 146)

Once the therapist observes a variety of these signs, they can broach the topic of termination with the couple.

Criteria for termination include:

- The therapeutic space has been internalized and a reasonably secure holding capacity has been formed.
- Unconscious projective identifications have been recognized, owned, and taken back.
- The capacity to work together with family members or life partners is restored.
- Intimate and sexual relating is now gratifying and satisfying.
- The individual can provide good holding for the self, and the couple or family can provide a vital holding environment for the individual, couple, or family.
- The capacity to mourn the loss of the therapeutic relationship is sufficient to support a satis-factory termination and to prepare the patient, couple, or family to deal with future develop-mental losses and to envision their future beyond therapy.

(Scharff & Scharff, 1995, p. 147)

The object relations therapist understands that termination may not signify that the couple is exactly where they want to be. People continue to grow. They will further develop insight into their own behavior and that of the relationship. Thus, depending on the situation, they may decide to reenter therapy to continue the process of development.

References

Applegate, J. S. (1990). Theory, culture, and behavior: Object relations in context. *Child and Adolescent Social Work, 7*(2), 85–100.

Bagnini, C. (2011). Object-relations therapy with couples. In D. K. Carson & M. Casado-Kehoe (Eds.), *Case studies in couples therapy: Theory-based approaches* (pp. 65–78). Routledge.

Bagnini, C. (2013). *Keeping couples in treatment: Working from surface to depth*. Rowman and Littlefield.

Bucci, W. (2002). The challenge of diversity in modern psychoanalysis. *Psychoanalytic Psychology, 19*(1), 216–226.

Dicks, H. (1967). *Marital tensions*. Basic Books.

Donovan, J. M. (2003). *Short-term object relations couples therapy: The five-step model*. Brunner-Routledge.

Edmundson, M. (2018). *Self and soul, a defense of ideals*. Harvard University Press.

Freedman, E. (1998). Secrets, status and countertransference in object relations based couple therapy. *Journal of Analytic Social Work, 5*(2), 47–75.

Hewison, D. (2014). Projection, introjection, intrusive, identification, adhesive identification. In D. E. Scharff & J. S. Scharff (Eds.), *Psychoanalytic couple therapy: Foundations of theory and practice* (pp. 158–169). Karnac.

Ludlam, M. (2022). Lost — and found — in translation: Do Ronald Fairbairn's ideas still speak usefully to 21st-century couple therapists? In S. Nathans (Ed.), *More about couples on the couch* (pp. 141–155). Routledge.

Mendelsohn, R. (2014). Five types of "couple object-relations" seen in couple therapy: Implications for theory and practice. *Psychoanalytic Review, 101*(1), 95–128.

Middelberg, C. V. (2001). Projective identification in common couple dances. *Journal of Marital and Family Therapy, 27*(3), 341–352.

Morgan, M. (2016). An object relations approach to the couple relationship: Past, present, and future. *Couple and Family Psychoanalysis, 6*(2), 194–205.

Scharff, D. E., & de Varela, Y. (2005). Object relations couple therapy. In M. Harway (Ed.), *Handbook of couples therapy* (pp. 141–156). John Wiley & Sons.

Scharff, J. S., & Scharff, D. E. (1995). *The primer of object relations therapy*. Jason Aronson.

Scharff, J. S., & Scharff, D. E. (1997). Object relations couple therapy. *American Journal of Psychotherapy, 51*(2), 141–173.

Scharff, J. S., & Scharff, D. E. (2008). Object relations couple therapy. In A. S. Gurman (Ed.), *Clinical handbook of couple therapy* (4th ed., 167–195). Guilford.

Scharff, J. S., & Scharff, D. E. (2014). *The therapist's internal objects*. International Psychotherapy Institute.

Siegel, J. P. (1992). *Repairing intimacy: An object relations approach to couples therapy*. Jason Aronson Inc.Siegel, J. P. (2020). Digging deeper: An object relations couple update. *Family Process, 59*(1), 10–20.

Siegel, J. P. (2022). Object relations couple therapy. In J. L. Lebow & D. K. Snyder (Eds.), *Clinical handbook of couple therapy* (pp. 151–174). Guilford.

Slipp, S. (2014). *Object relations: A dynamic bridge between individual and family treatment*. International Psychotherapy Institute.

Solomon, M. F., & Lynn, R. E. (2002). Object-relations couples therapy. In J. J. Magnavita (Ed.), *Comprehensive handbook of psychotherapy V. 1: Psychodynamic/object relations* (pp. 387–406). John Wiley & Sons.

Sussal, C. M. (1993). Object relations couples therapy with lesbians. *Smith College Studies in Social Work, 63*(3), 301–316.

Zinner, J. (2008). Psychodynamic couples therapy: An object relations approach. In G. Gabbard, (Ed.), *Textbook of psychotherapeutic treatments in psychiatry* (pp. 581–601). American Psychiatric Publishing.

4 Adlerian Couple Therapy

Len Sperry and Jon Sperry

History of the Model

Adlerian Therapy is a form of psychotherapy developed by Alfred Adler (1870–1937). Early in his career, Adler was invited by Freud to join the Viennese Psychoanalytic Society and remained friendly with Freud for some 10 years. In time he came to view Freud's approach as increasingly inflexible and overly focused on death and sex. Accordingly, Adler broke with Freud in 1911 and continued to develop and refine his own approach. Subsequently, Adler influenced many including Gordon Allport, Aaron Beck, Viktor Frankl, Karen Horney, Rollo May, and Abraham Maslow. Maslow, May, and Frankl studied under Adler and credited him with influencing their own views as did Beck.

Adler's view of therapy emphasizes the individual's life style, belonging, meeting the life tasks, and social interest. He considered that all behavior is purposive and that individuals are motivated to seek "belonging" or significance and meaning as they function in their community. Adler also postulated that within their family constellation individuals first learn how to belong and interact. He emphasized how an individual's "private logic" can contrast to common logic or common sense. This logic serves as a reference for attitudes, private views of self, others, and the world, and behavior which he called the "life style" and "life style convictions." He noted that people form their life style as they relate to others, find a sense of belonging, and overcome "inferiority feelings." Furthermore, Adler believed that healthy and productive individuals are characterized by "social interest"—the hallmark of positive mental health—while those with limited adjustment or psychopathology demonstrated less social interest and tend to be self-focused (Ansbacher & Ansbacher, 1956).

Key Concepts

Key concepts and basic terminology in Adlerian Therapy include:

- **Belonging**—refers to an individual's need to feel connected to and loved by those around them.
- **Early recollections**—specific memories associated with childhood but remembered as vividly as though they were happening in the present. They are understood to be projections of the present-day self onto the past.
- **Family constellation**—the early developmental influences on an individual including siblings, parents, peers, neighbors, and other key individuals like teachers.
- **Gender guiding lines**—an individual's understanding of masculinity and femininity and what it means to be a man or woman, based on the influence of their own family.
- **Inferiority feelings**—the emotional reaction to a negative self-appraisal.

DOI: 10.4324/9781003369097-4

- **Life strategy**—the predictable manner in which an individual deals with problems and resolves conflicts. It reflects one's self-view and world view and is essentially the same as one's basic pattern.
- **Life style**—one's beliefs and convictions about belonging and finding a place in the world.
- **Life style convictions**—the assumptions, beliefs, and attitudes that direct an individual's sense of belonging.
- **Life tasks**—the main challenges—love, work, and friendship—that life presents to all individuals.
- **Private logic**—convictions that run counter to social interest and fail to foster a constructive sense of belonging with others.
- **Safeguarding mechanisms**—the behaviors and attitudes that individuals select to evade responsibility and not meet the life tasks. Safeguarding is also referred to as the defense mechanism by other psychological orientations.
- **Social interest**—the behaviors and attitudes that display an individual's sense of belonging, concern for, and contributions to the community.

Conceptualization of Problem Formation

Adlerian Therapy fosters the process of change by stimulating cognitive, affective, and behavior change. Although an individual may not be aware of their own individual dynamics, patterns, and goals, through analysis of their family dynamic, early memories, and coping efforts, the clinician infers their pattern and goal as a working hypothesis. Recognizing these limiting beliefs and patterns, the clinician helps the client to change. Change occurs when the client can view their problems and concerns from another perspective so that they can explore and practice new patterns of functioning and a new philosophy of life (Ansbacher & Ansbacher, 1956).

Besides eliciting traditional intake material (e.g., present concerns, mental status exam, and general social, occupational, and developmental history), the Adlerian psychotherapist collects information on and analyzes the client's family constellation and life style convictions. The family constellation consists of the client's birth order, identifications with parents and peers, family values, and family narrative (Ansbacher & Ansbacher, 1956). Life style convictions can be inferred from both habitual coping patterns and early recollections. Because a client's recollection of their earliest memories reflects past childhood events in the light of current life style convictions, early recollections are a powerful projective technique that quickly and accurately provides a working hypothesis of the way clients view themselves, others, and the world. The clinician elicits two or more memories, and the description of these memories are analyzed according to themes and developmental maturity, and from these the clinician derives the client's life style convictions which reflect the impact of the client's family constellation. Information from the family constellation and life style convictions is useful in specifying a case formulation, including a diagnostic formulation and a clinical formulation; that is, an explanation of why and how the client perceives, feels, and acts in a patterned and predictable fashion.

Individuals develop three life style convictions: (1) a *self-view*—beliefs about one's identify and sense of worth; (2) a *world view*—beliefs about how the world treats them and what it expects of them; and (3) a *life strategy*—the predictable manner in which one deals with problems and resolves conflicts. The life strategy reflects one's self-view and world view and is essentially the same as one's basic pattern (Ansbacher & Ansbacher, 1956).

The goal of treatment is not just symptom reduction, but the adoption of a contributing way of living. Adlerians view pain and suffering in a client's life as the result of choices made. This value-based theory of personality hypothesizes that the values a client holds and lives their life by, are learned, and when they no longer work as evidenced by suffering or lack of happiness, the client can re-learn values and life styles that work more "effectively." Some Adlerians believe that a client's life style is best viewed as personal schemas or narratives. Because such maladaptive schemas or basic mistakes are believed to be true for the individual, the individual acts accordingly. Adler noted that these basic mistakes are overgeneralizations; for example, "people are hostile," "life is dangerous"; or misperceptions of life, such as "life doesn't give me any breaks" which are expressed in the client's physical behavior, language, dreams, values, etc. (Ansbacher & Ansbacher, 1956). The goal of intervention in Adlerian Therapy is re-education and reorientation of the client to schemas that work "better." The actual techniques employed are used to this end. Adlerians tend to be action-orientated. They believe the concept of insight is just a proxy for immobility. Insight is not a deep understanding that one must have before change can occur. For Adlerians, insight is understanding translated into action. It reflects the client's understanding of the purposeful nature of behavior.

Adlerian Couples Therapy

The Adlerian Therapy approach to couples therapy pre-dates the formal development of the field of marital and family therapy. In fact, it was a "forerunner to the field" (Sperry & Peluso, 2019, p. 165). Adler is credited with being among the first, if not the first, to utilize conjoint sessions with couples. Adlerian Couples Therapy has a long tradition of successfully working with couples, and elements of its theory and interventions have been incorporated within the field of couples therapy (Sperry & Peluso, 2019).

Essentially, the practice of Adlerian Therapy with couples is an optimistic approach that focuses on strengths, protective factors, and health rather than on deficits, risk factors, and pathology. The therapeutic relationship is characterized by mutual respect and equality. Couples and clinicians work together as collaborative partners in the therapeutic endeavor. It is expected that couples will assume an active role in the change process.

Evolution of Case Conceptualization in Adlerian Therapy

Unlike Cognitive Behavior Therapy wherein the importance of the clinical value of case conceptualization is widely discussed and utilized, much less has been written about its clinical value in Adlerian Therapy. Exceptions are the work of Sperry (1989, 2005, 2019, 2022), Sperry and Sperry (2012, 2020a, 2020b), Maniacci et al. (2017), Bitter (2021), and Bitter and Corey (2024). The importance and clinical value of case conceptualization in the practice of Adlerian Therapy could not have been made clearer by these authors and researchers.

The importance of establishing a case conceptualization and maintaining a treatment focus consistent with that conceptualization has also been cited as a contribution to positive outcomes (Sperry, 2024). Moreover, one of the main benefits of the case conceptualization is that it informs the explanation given to clients and couples regarding their presenting problems and concerns. In addition to explanation, an effective Adlerian case conceptualization will also guide the therapy process and anticipate challenges and obstacles in the treatment process. Predictably these include engagement issues, transferences, countertransferences, ambivalence about complying with therapeutic tasks (i.e., homework), and problems with termination including leaving treatment prematurely (Sperry, 2024).

While Adlerian case conceptualizations share a number of common elements with other approaches, three signature elements of Adlerian case conceptualization make it unique. These three elements are predisposition, treatment goals, and treatment interventions. Predisposition in

Adlerian Therapy emphasizes family constellation, early recollections, and life style convictions. The unique treatment goals involve increasing social interest and constructive action. Finally, treatment interventions unique to this case conceptualization approach include early recollection analysis, interpretation, encouragement, the push button technique, and acting "as if" (Sperry & Sperry, 2020b).

Pattern-Focused Adlerian Case Conceptualization

This Adlerian case conceptualization approach has evolved to be more integrative and inclusive. It is called the **Pattern-Focused Adlerian Case Conceptualization approach** (Sperry, 2021; Sperry & Binenstzok, 2019). Typically, it comprises seven Ps: Presentation, Precipitants, Predispositions, Patterns, Perpetuants, Predictive Factors, and Plan (goals and interventions for treatment). Bitter and Corey (2024) succinctly describe the first five:

> Initially, clients *present* [presentation] themselves for therapy, because of emotional/behavioral symptoms or conflicts that feel overwhelming to them. These symptoms are usually triggered by some *precipitant* that reflects the client's orientation and pattern of coping and living. Biological, social, and cultural histories reveal *predispositions* to both precipitants and *patterns* just as current *perpetuants* or external reinforcers keep the problem going. Even though second- and third-order change are the ultimate goal, literally the adoption of an adaptive pattern to living, it is not uncommon to start with interventions designed to interrupt the maladaptive pattern.
>
> (Bitter & Corey, 2024, p. 136)

Furthermore, pattern links the client's presenting concern to the precipitating event, and is driven by predisposing factors and reinforced with perpetuants. Pattern will also influence the plan with regard to treatment strategies, interventions, and challenges or obstacles to treatment.

Adlerian Assessment

Adlerian Couples Therapy begins with an assessment of partner and relational dynamics. This section describes the process of conducting this dual-focused assessment. Just as in Adlerian Therapy, a life style assessment is completed for each partner. The assessment also involves couple relational dynamics which, along with each partner's life style dynamics, are incorporated into the couple case conceptualization.

Partners' Life Style Assessment

The assessment and case conceptualization process in Adlerian Couples Therapy begins with the life style assessment of each partner to identify the individual dynamics that drive their thoughts, feelings, and actions. Typically, the assessment takes place in a conjoint session with both partners and the clinician. Each partner is interviewed while the other listens. However, it is possible for separate assessment sessions to be scheduled with each partner and then a conjoint session is scheduled in which the case conceptualization is shared.

This assessment is a process in which the clinician interviews the couple about the influences that they experienced from childhood. Some clinicians supplement this focused interview with psychological instruments or relational inventories. However, the family constellation and early recollections are the essential aspects of this assessment.

Family Constellation

The family constellation includes information about a client's relationships with other family members, psychological birth order, family values, and the way the client found a sense of belonging in their family. Useful questions to elicit information on the family constellation are:

- What was it like growing up in your family?
- What was it like to be the youngest (oldest, middle, or only) child in your family?
- Describe your relationships with each of your parents. Which one were you most like? Among your siblings who was your father's favorite? Mother's favorite?
- Describe your parents' relationship. Were they openly affectionate? Who supported the family financially? Who made the major decisions? How did they solve problems? Conflicts? Who disciplined? Who did you go to when you got hurt or were frightened?
- What were your family values? What were your parents' expectations of you as you grew up?
- What was your relationships like with your siblings? Who got the best grades? Was the most athletic? Had the most friends? Got in the most trouble? What are they doing now?

The family constellation is assessed with questions focused on the sibling constellation that reflects each partner's personality and basic pattern originating in childhood. Adler's basic premise of the family constellation is that each partner learns to "find a place" in their family-of-origin by taking on one or more areas of significance (Ansbacher & Ansbacher, 1956). They then endeavor to enact this out later in their couple's relationship.

This assessment includes siblings, stepsiblings, and other children with whom each partner grew up. It is not the actual chronological order that matters, but each partner's perception of what it means to occupy that position in this family. Assessed are such characteristics as the number of friends, the extent of mischievousness, the degree of responsibility exhibited, etc. These characteristics reflect the chosen role that each partner created.

Parents, grandparents, and others who influenced each partner—either positively or negatively—are described in detail. The nature of the relationships between these adults takes on great significance in couples' work: how they showed affection, how they resolved conflict, and how they shared family responsibilities. The impact of these early relationships' influences on the couple's functioning is a key component of the resulting Adlerian couple case conceptualization.

Early Recollections

Early recollections are a projective technique used to determine a client's self-view, view of others, world view, and their overall strategy in dealing with others and life's challenges. Early recollections also reflect the client's level of social interest and their life style convictions.

Early recollections also suggest the individual's basic movement in relation to others. There are four such types of movement (Bitter & Corey, 2024). They are movement toward, movement against, movement away from, and ambivalent movement which can be toward-against or toward-away from. These basic types of movement are suggestive of basic personality styles or personality disorders. For example, movement toward suggests the Histrionic Personality or Dependent Personality, while movement toward and against is suggestive of the Obsessive-Compulsive Personality or the Passive Aggressive Personality (Sperry & Sperry, 2022).

Here is a useful strategy for eliciting early recollections:

- "Think back to your early life—before the age of eight or nine—and tell me your first memory. It should be a single experience that you specifically recall, rather than an event that you were told happened to you. It should be a single one rather than a repeated experience."

- If they have difficulty identifying a memory, prompt them by asking for a birthday or holiday that was memorable, the first day of school, or a specific vacation.
- Ask their age for each recollection. Ask them to describe it as if it were captured on a video: how it began, who was involved, what each individual said or did, and how it ended. Then ask about the most vivid moment in the sequence. Ask what they felt during the most vivid moment and what they were thinking.
- A minimum of two early recollections is usually necessary to identify the pattern.

First Encounters of the Close Kind (FECK)

FECK stories are a variation of the early recollection process, but these stories are specifically about the recollector's relationship to one other significant person (Belove, 1997). The strategy is specifically used in Adlerian couples' work. Rudolph Dreikurs (1946) described a moment of "love at first sight," as a time when each partner communicated to the other, "untold impressions, opinions and promises ... (and came) ... to understand without either becoming aware of his participating in the game" (p. 66). His description highlighted the moment that each partner intuitively recognized the other's attitudes toward life and how those attitudes would complement their own. FECK stories are obtained from both partners and often reveal unspoken agreements or expectations of their partner. Part of Adlerian couples counseling will endeavor to find the mistakes in each partner's FECK stories as well as the basic mistakes in each partner's early recollections.

Life Style Convictions

Life style convictions are conclusions about the individual's inner world derived from the family constellation and early recollections. They represent the individual's basic pattern and manner in which they solve problems, and approach and perceive the world around them. Clinicians find the following formula a clinically useful way to summarize these convictions into a pattern:

- I am ... (self-view)
- Life is ... People are ... (world view)
- Therefore ... (life strategy)

Individual Dynamics and Systems Dynamics

Complementing the life style assessment of each partner is the assessment of the couple's relational pattern. The reason for this is that effective couples therapy is based on both partner and relational dynamics. When working with couples, effective therapy focuses on both individual and systems dynamics. A basic premise is that each partner's behavior reflects their own life strategy or pattern (Sperry, 2010). A second premise is that, irrespective of whether a partner reports an individual symptom or a relational issue, the symptom or issue is embedded in the couple's dynamic and serves to maintain the homeostasis or sense of normalcy of their relational pattern (Gehart, 2018).

Couple's Relational Pattern

Partners commonly display one or two habitual and cyclical patterns of relating that each has learned over time—often from their parents—to cope. These patterns are referred to as **couple interaction patterns** or **relational patterns**. When indicated, couples therapy can change or replace these patterns with more adaptive ones. Here is a brief description of six common relational patterns (Christensen & Shenk, 1991).

DEMAND/SUBMIT

This pattern develops as one partner blames the other or demands that they change. Predictably, the other partner complies or surrenders. Also referred to as the pursuer-distancer pattern, it is the most common relational pattern. It is a predictor of aggressiveness, dissatisfaction, and divorce.

DEMAND/WITHDRAW

This pattern develops as one partner accuses, criticizes, or demands change from the other partner. Predictably, the other partner is silent, avoids, or refuses to discuss the concern. It is also a relatively common interaction pattern.

WITHDRAW/WITHDRAW

This pattern develops after efforts to maintain the demand/withdraw pattern are exhausted. Because both partners are hesitant to face conflict, both withdraw further. Continued withdrawal may lead to separation.

ATTACK/ATTACK

This high-conflict pattern involves a sequence in which one attack is responded to with another, resulting in an escalation of relational discord. Often this is a variant of the demand/withdraw pattern in which the withdrawing partner becomes sufficiently provoked and erupts in anger.

REACTIVE DEMAND/WITHDRAW

This pattern develops as a couple reverses a previous long-standing pattern. This can occur when the demanding partner gradually gives up and stops or limits investment in the relationship and increasingly withdraws. The other partner reactively responds by frantically pursuing the other to prevent a separation.

CONSTRUCTIVE ENGAGEMENT

This pattern develops as one partner is willing and able to express bothersome issues in a non-attacking manner and the other partner listens even when they disagree. This pattern facilitates effective communication and problem-solving.

Developing the Couples Case Conceptualization

From an Adlerian Therapy perspective, the couples case conceptualization incorporates each individual, their common relational pattern, and their unique couple dynamics. The clinician first identifies and summarizes the individual dynamics of each partner. The focus is on each partner's basic approach to life; that is, their "convictions" about the self, other people, the world, and the resulting "life strategy" or pattern for dealing with life as well as "finding a place" in the world. The life style convictions and life strategy are unique to each partner and can facilitate or hinder the development of healthy functioning in the couple's relationship.

It is not uncommon for two individuals to be attracted to each other based on the complementarity of their individual patterns. It is also not uncommon for the patterns of each partner to be reflected in one of the six relational patterns. Accordingly, one way to develop a clinically useful couple case conceptualization is to match partner patterns against the various relational patterns. In short, the clinician first identifies each partner's pattern and then identifies how these two patterns match a particular relational pattern.

For example, it is not uncommon for a partner whose individual and family constellation dynamics fostered a pattern of avoidance when faced with demands and fears of being out of control to be attracted to and marry a partner whose individual and family dynamics fostered a pattern of control and protection. It is also not surprising that this couple engages in a demand/withdraw relational style. For example, in Steve's family, conflict was often avoided and his father often would make unilateral decisions based on his own needs that did not consider his wife's input. This family dynamic influenced Steve's manner in solving problems in his own relationship.

A Strategy for Conducting the First Couple Session

The assessment and case conceptualization process in Adlerian Couples Therapy begins with the life style assessment of each partner to identify the individual dynamics that drive their thoughts, feelings, and actions. Typically, the assessment takes place in a conjoint session with both partners and the clinician and is scheduled for a 90-minute session. After introductions, the clinician describes the assessment and treatment process, boundaries, and the consent process. Preferably each partner is interviewed while the other listens. While less desirable, separate assessment sessions can be scheduled with each partner and a conjoint session is scheduled afterwards in which the case conceptualization is shared.

This assessment is a process in which the clinician interviews the couple about the influences that they experienced from childhood. This process is facilitated with each partner filling out a Family Constellation Form and an Early Recollections Form before the first session. Some clinicians supplement this focused interview with psychological instruments or relational inventories. The family constellation and early recollections are two key aspects of this assessment (for the former, see "Family Constellation" section above).

Early recollections are single-occurring events recalled before the age of eight. Each partner fills out an Early Recollection Form on which they describe the event along with supporting details. In the conjoint session, the clinician reads from the form and asks questions to clarify who was present, what happened, what was the most vivid moment of the incident, and what the partner was thinking and feeling at that moment. A minimum of two early recollections are elicited. Identifying the couple's relational pattern comes from history—identification of parental pattern, direct observation of the couple interaction, and is derived from each partner's life strategy or pattern.

The final step in this assessment and conceptualization process involves the clinician sharing the case conceptualization—based on this assessment process—with the couple. This case conceptualization is often shared in the form of **collaborative interpretation** in which the therapist offers their hypotheses, and the couple can modify or confirm the interpretations offered. As the therapist shares the conceptualization, each partner is asked to comment on or clarify any points. In the process, couples learn more about how family influences contributed to a partner's personality development and relational functioning. This leads to a greater awareness of the couple's recurring issues and conflicts.

Following this discussion, the case conceptualization may be modified as needed so that the couple not only understands it, but accepts and "owns" it. Then the clinician suggests a course of treatment based on this conceptualization, and following the couple's input, a mutually agreed-upon treatment plan can be implemented.

Clinical Example: Couple Case Conceptualization of Steve and Carissa

This section illustrates the Adlerian case conceptualization process in the case of Steve and Carissa. Each partner's life strategy and pattern are described as well as their relational pattern.

STEVE: FAMILY CONSTELLATION, EARLY RECOLLECTIONS, AND LIFE STYLE CONVICTIONS

From Family Constellation Form:
Steve is:

—Caucasian male.
—Middle child.
—High parental expectations for achievement.
—He felt his parents' disappointment—he didn't measure up to his sister.
—He is more like his father who didn't live up to parental expectations.
—Parents viewed themselves as a typical couple.

From Interview:

—At age 10, Steve's father left the home, divorces, and remarries.
—Steve's mother wanted more kids, but after two miscarriages and two more children, parents argued about having more kids → father got vasectomy → more arguing → divorce.

Family Constellation Statement:
Steve is a middle child and Caucasian. He is more like his father than his mother in that Steve did not live up to his father's parental expectations. Steve felt he had disappointed his parent by not achieving what his older sister had. He did reasonably well in school, and with his siblings and friends. Even though Steve indicated that his parents viewed themselves as a typical couple, when Steve was 10, his father left the family, divorced, and remarried. It is noteworthy that Steve's mother had wanted more than three children, but his father did not. He then got a vasectomy which led to more conflict and the subsequent divorce.

From Early Recollection Form:

Age 7: When I got my first semester report card, I had four Bs and two Cs. My sister had all As. I could tell my parents were disappointed. I thought they should be happy I didn't get any Fs.
  I told them I would do better, but secretly I told myself I wasn't going to work as hard as my sister and not have any time to be with my friends or play video games.
Age 8: I was at recess and saw an older kid take a dollar bill away from a kid in my class. Two of my friends saw it and smiled and didn't do anything. I thought about telling the teacher but decided not to because I was afraid the older kid would find out and come after me.

Life Style Convictions:

Self-view: I'm pretty good but not that good.
World view: Life is demanding and unfair and others can be unappreciative.
Life strategy: Therefore, have fun and resist others' expectations and demands.

Steve's Pattern:
Steve's movement is both toward and against others, suggestive of a passive aggressive pattern. Accordingly, he is likely to indirectly resist others' expectations and demands which he does not find enjoyable.

CARISSA'S FAMILY CONSTELLATION, EARLY RECOLLECTIONS, AND LIFE STYLE CONVICTIONS

From Family Constellation Form:

Carissa is:

—A highly acculturated African-American female.
—Younger of two girls.
—Best friends with sister.
—Very close to mother and grandmother.
—At age 10, her parents separated for two weeks—then reconciled—stayed married.
—A very good student, many friends, involved in college clubs/organizations.

From Interview:

—High parental expectations for her achievement.
—Parents are reasonably close with limited emotional expressiveness.
—Because Carissa's parents reconciled and remained married, she expects the same outcome with Steve.

Family Constellation Statement:

Carissa is the younger of two sisters and is a highly acculturated African American. She was very close to her grandmother and more like her mother than her father. She and her sister were best friends although they occasionally clashed. Growing up, Carissa was an excellent student, had many friends, and met her parents' expectations for achievement. Her parents remain married although they separated for two weeks when she was 10 years old. She describes their relationship as reasonably close although not very emotionally expressive.

From Early Recollection Form:

Age 5: I remember going to my grandma's house on my birthday. She had a big cake and two presents for me. The presents were perfect. They were just what I wanted. But my sister scooped some of the icing off my cake and ate it. I was so mad that she ruined my party.
Age 7: One day I saw my parents arguing and my father told my mother that the man of the house is supposed to get his way. My mother said nothing and just looked away. I was silent too, but I didn't think what he said was right.

Life Style Convictions:

Self-view: I'm competent, proper, and righteous.
World view: Life is unpredictable, and others can be unreliable.
Life strategy: Therefore, be in control, right, and proper.

Carissa's Pattern:

Her movement is both toward and against others and herself, suggestive of an obsessive-compulsive pattern. Accordingly, she is highly conscientious and initially agreeable up to a point at which she may express righteous indignation.

Steve and Carissa's Relational Pattern

Demand/Withdraw: As Carissa raises expectations, is righteous, and makes demands, Steve is likely to pull back and passively resist.

Couple Case Conceptualization Statement:

Steve and Carissa present for Adlerian Couples Therapy seeking to understand their unresolved conflict about bearing children. Reportedly, they have yet to have an open conversation about their growing tension even though Carissa is contemplating divorce. What is clear from the assessment is that this couple demonstrates a Demand/Withdraw relational pattern. Accordingly, as Carissa raises expectations and makes demands, Steve is likely to respond by pulling back and passively resisting. Their relational pattern is triggered and reinforced by Carissa's pattern to be right and to demand, and Steve's predictable pattern of passive non-responsiveness demonstrated by leaving, sulking, procrastination, or when he feels pushed to the limits, argumentativeness. While this is a mixed-race couple, there are no obvious ethnic or cultural factors at this time that will impact the treatment of this couple. The therapist will monitor culturally bound factors that influence the therapeutic process and further assess the influence of racism and other cultural factors in both families.

Conceptualizing Diversity

Adlerian Therapy can be quite sensitive to multicultural concerns. It has been noted that:

> [m]any of the core aspects of Adlerian psychotherapy mirror recommendations for effective multicultural psychotherapy. These include the importance of an egalitarian, respectful, and cooperative counselor-client relationship (therapeutic alliance); the focus on social equality and social justice; taking a holistic approach that considers, mind, body, and spirit; the need to view people contextually, in their family, social and cultural contexts; and the emphasis on strengths, optimism, encouragement, empowerment, advocacy, and support.
>
> (Carlson & Englar-Carlson, 2017, pp. 106–107)

Furthermore, "the characteristics and assumptions of Adlerian psychology are congruent with the cultural values of many racial-ethnic, minority groups and … the Adlerian therapeutic process is respectful of cultural diversity" (Carlson et al., 2006, p. 32). It has also been observed that the

> individual's unique subjective interpretation and perception are part of Adlerian theory, and the client's culture, values and views are honored and accepted. Adlerian [therapy] goals are not aimed at deciding for clients what they should change about themselves. Rather, the practitioner works in collaboration with clients and their family networks.
>
> (Arcineiga & Newlon, 2003, p. 436)

Diversity issues will likely influence the couples counseling process when working with Carissa and Steve given that they are an interracial couple. Given Steve's father's approach to Carissa and Steve getting married, some overt racism is a consideration. Adlerian Couples Therapy is a useful model for couples that experience racism, oppression, and cultural stressors since the process examines systems, private logic, and family dynamics that influence relational patterns. The Hogarth's therapist will assess their gender guiding lines and will seek to determine their family influence on gender role expectations. Further, the couple's therapist will seek to understand both Carissa and Steve's phenomenological view of what it means to be a male, female, White, Black, heterosexual, a couple, a parent, and other identities and intersectionalities that are part of their lives.

The Role of the Therapist

It is the therapist's role to act as detective, encourager, and (where appropriate) humorist as the couple is guided through the therapeutic process toward a more equal and just solution to their problem (Carlson & Sperry, 2000). The therapist will seek to facilitate a collaborative process that will help the couple enhance their cooperative skills in an egalitarian and democratic environment. Therapeutic processes utilized by the therapist will include interpretation, encouragement, insight, and psychoeducation. Bitter and Corey (2024) identify that the client–therapist relationship is based on cooperation, trust, respect, collaboration, and alignment of goals.

Therapists should seek to model social interest and effective communication with the couple. Working with couples can often lead to emotional and difficult conversations. The therapist should seek to facilitate those difficult moments through effective communication, self-care, empathy, support, and efforts to increase cooperation among the couple. Developing a strong therapeutic relationship with each partner is essential to the outcome of Adlerian Couples Therapy. When working with Steve and Carissa, the therapist should aim to help both partners better understand some of their unhelpful strategies and beliefs as well as offering support as they seek to better understand their partner. The use of therapeutic support, encouragement, insight interpretation, and reorientation/re-education will also place the couple's therapist in the role of collaborator and educator. The Hogarths' therapist will be active and facilitate the couple in learning about themselves and each other while also encouraging them to increase their cooperation. Careful consideration should be monitored when working with the Hogarths to avoid aligning more closely with one of the partners about a specific issue or conflict.

Conceptualization of Problem Resolution

As mentioned above, the relational dyad forms a system that is influenced by each partner (and vice versa). The individual choices of each partner have a unique bearing on the functioning of the system. Thoughts, feelings, and attitudes all influence the behavior of either partner as well as the direction of the couple system. Therefore, according to Adlerian theorists, the choices that a couple makes are not accidental and are directed toward the goal of communication and respect as equals (Carlson & Englar-Carlson, 2017). However, this does not always occur, as individual private logic, goals, and life style dynamics can uniquely guide the system into function or dysfunction.

Treatment Goals

Adlerian theory is neither deterministic nor fatalistic. Instead, at any time, either partner can effect change by making different choices and thus impacting the system. The ability to make changes within a system, however, requires insight, courage, and a sense of humor about oneself and life. Couples' harmony is a function of such factors as individual self-esteem, social interest (ability to give and take), and a sense of humor about life. Treatment goals need to be cooperatively developed with the couple, since a lack of goal alignment from the couple could lead to confusion and early therapeutic termination. Given the egalitarian nature of this approach, both Steve and Carissa will be asked about what they hope to get out of therapy, and they will both be encouraged to examine strengths in their relationship, as well as what attracted them initially to each other.

Treatment Stages

Adlerian Therapy uses some variation of the four-stage model outlined by Dreikurs (1967) of relationship building, assessment, interpretation, and reorientation. In the first stage of relationship building, it is incumbent upon the therapist to create a solid therapeutic alliance with the couple, demonstrate fairness in dealing with both partners, and provide a secure base from which to work. In the next phase, assessment, life style analyses of each partner are conducted and this includes an examination of family-of-origin dynamics (psychological birth order, family atmosphere) and early recollections. From this analysis, the couple's private logic and goals can be determined. Interpretation allows the therapist to juxtapose the life styles of both partners and reflect on how the dynamics and behavioral choices of each partner are contributing to the disruption in the marital system. The insight into the couple's relationship allows the therapist to begin interventions and help the couple make some different choices in relating to one another. The reorientation phase is the aspect of therapy where the couple, under the guidance and encouragement of the therapist, creates an action plan based on the result of the life style assessment and in light of the presenting problems (Robey & Carlson, 2011). The couple makes specific changes in their interactions with each other and evaluates the effect on the relationship. Termination is usually based upon mutual agreement between client(s) and therapist once the main goals of therapy have been accomplished (Carlson & Sperry, 2000). Sessions can range from 1 to 25 since the needs of each couple vary depending on the presenting issues.

This four-stage model (Dreikurs, 1967) will be incorporated in each session with the Hogarths. The first session will include efforts to connect with both Steve and Carissa and to assess their life styles, their patterned responses to conflict, and their style of dealing with problems and others. As the therapist gathers information about each partner's life style pattern, interpretations will be utilized and offered to each partner. Reorientation and re-education will be utilized as Steve and Carissa seek to learn about themselves and each other while practicing new behaviors and managing conflict, as well as meeting their own needs on a daily basis.

Ongoing Assessment

In addition to family constellation and early recollections data at the outset of therapy, Adlerian therapists use structured marital inventories that identify specific relationship domains as treatment targets (Sperry, 2019). Assessment occurs not only in the initial stage of working with couples, but is an ongoing process as well (Carlson & Sperry, 2000). In this era of accountability, clinicians are increasingly expected to assess progress as well as treatment outcomes. **Routine outcome monitoring** (ROM) is becoming commonplace in individual as well as couples therapy. Adlerian therapists can use various ROMS to assess progress and outcomes (Sperry & Binenstzok, 2019). The Social Interest Index, Short Form (SII-SF) is an 11-item measure of social interest and is a key Adlerian indicator of overall well-being (Leak, 2006). Some therapists use the SII-SF at the beginning and at the end of therapy while others use the form at every session. In addition, Adlerian therapists can elicit a second set of early recollections at the end of therapy. Comparing the life style convictions derived from the first set with those derived from the second set provides a useful and reliable measure of treatment progress.

Given that Steve and Carissa will examine their family patterns and their own relational tendencies, ongoing life style assessment will naturally be a primary therapeutic strategy that will inform the Adlerian couples counseling process. The therapist will assist Steve and Carissa to understand their basic mistakes in thinking and responding to each other, while helping them to increase their cooperation and social interest toward each other. Formal assessment strategies will serve to monitor therapeutic outcomes as well as assess various life style concepts such as social interest and life style convictions.

Case Transcript

Therapist: It's really nice to meet you both. I appreciate that you both completed the intake forms before our meeting today. I had a chance to briefly look at each of your responses and would like to now follow up on some of them. I'd also like to learn more about what brings you both here and hopefully to work toward some mutual goal. Before we get started, do you have any questions for me?

The therapist begins the session by orienting the couple to the process and then asks if they have any questions before starting. Allowing the couple to ask questions communicates a collaborative process in which Steve and Carissa can make decisions about the therapeutic process.

Carissa: I don't have any questions so far.

Steve: Same here.

Therapist: Okay, great. Tell me about what brings you in for couples therapy and also what you are hoping to get out of this experience. Who would like to start?

Since Adlerian Couples Therapy is an optimistic and strengths-based approach, the therapist seeks out both the problems and goals from the couple. Focusing on strengths, resources, the positive intentions of unhelpful solutions, and hopes are essential in the first meeting.

Carissa: To be honest, we really need help. We've been fighting more than ever. I have been spending less time at home during the weekends because I feel like we are totally stuck and sometimes I just need to get away from Steve.

Steve: Yeah, we keep fighting about everything. It seems like we both don't know where to go from here. It's like our relationship is running out of gas.

Therapist: I can hear you both are both feeling stuck and a bit discouraged. Steve, is the gas tank totally empty, or are there still a few miles left?

The therapist joined in Steve's metaphorical description of his view of the relationship running out of gas. Adlerian couple therapists often utilize metaphors to discuss client issues in a non-linear and creative manner. Metaphors are used in Adlerian Therapy because they highlight the client's perception of their story.

Steve: It's getting close, but there is some gas left.

Therapist: What do you think, Carissa?

The therapist probes Carissa's response to include her in the unpacking of the presenting narrative.

Carissa: Yeah, we've been dealing with infertility issues over the past three years, and we are putting everything into it, even the majority of our finances. Our feelings for each other seem to have dimmed during this time. To be honest, it does feel like we are running out of gas, we haven't even spoken about any of this at all. The only time we bring up this topic, it's just yelling at each other about household chores.

Therapist: Yeah, I can hear how hard this is. Infertility issues often put a lot of stress on couples and major stressors often have the tendency to pull couples apart or somehow push them together. I am guessing that you are both experiencing the former.

This response normalizes stressful experiences that impact couples differently.

Steve: You are correct, it has pulled us apart. I feel like Carissa has become out of control over the past few months. I really get bent out of shape when she needs to dictate every move we make as a couple.

Carissa: Wow, tell us how you really feel. (*becomes tearful and moves a few inches away from Steve*)

Therapist: I can hear that you both feel many emotions about how the past few years have gone, financially and emotionally. I am curious if you both might be able to tell me how a typical conflict goes. Can you think of the last time you both had a conflict over the past week?

The therapist is asking this question to probe for further evidence of their life style and interpersonal dynamics, as well as to determine if the conflict that just unfolded in the session matches the same pattern.

Steve: Easy. Yesterday, Carissa confronted me about my approach to cleaning the cat litter box. I told her that I took it out the night before and she yelled at me for not taking it out twice a day. I told her that she could take it out if she wanted it to be taken out more than that. She then said, "You want our house to smell like cat shit? What's wrong with you?"

Therapist: Is that how you recall the conversation going, Carissa?

Carissa: Basically, I just think it's easy to do and I don't understand why he can't just clean it more than once per day.

Steve: Not all people obsess about the cat litter box on a daily basis. Carissa can pitch in if she would like it to be monitored more than that.

Therapist: I see that the cat litter box gets both of you activated quite a bit, how about we shift to how you both first met? (*pause*) Can you both tell me about that?

The therapist shifted focus to continue to the intake process but makes note of their conflict pattern. Eliciting how they first met was done to assess their initial attraction to each other and to learn more about both of their life styles.

Carissa: I'll go, we were both attending the University of Florida and met at a club. Steve walked up to me and asked if he could buy me a drink and we instantly clicked.

Steve: Yeah, we immediately connected and started a relationship.

Therapist: Sounds like there was an intuitive connection and you both felt comfortable quickly while getting to know each other. Most couples have a story that they share about their first encounter. Do either of you have a way of telling that story to family or friends?

The therapist assesses the FECK story to learn about any unspoken expectations, rules, or conditions.

Carissa: Yes, for sure. I remember Steve totally making me laugh the entire night. He made me feel like I was the only person in the room. He made me feel special and it seemed like he knew exactly how to attend to my needs and make me feel comfortable.

Therapist: Sounds like it felt wonderful to feel so connected to Steve back then. Steve, do you have a story that sticks out to you about your first interaction in meeting Carissa?

Assessing the FECK story with both partners can further clarify their relational themes.

Steve: Yes, I remember her being very confident and seeming comfortable in her own skin. I remember thinking, "She is the most beautiful Black woman that I have ever seen, my dad is not going to like this!"

Therapist: So, your father's view of her being Black popped into your mind right in the beginning of the relationship?

Following up about the FECK story to make meaning of Steve's experience and to probe for additional information.

Steve: Yeah, my father has always lived in a sheltered view of reality and grew up in a time where racist slurs were flying out of his family members' mouths. I've felt like he didn't understand me very well, and as a result, I tended to do the opposite of what he expected of me (*with a smile and laugh*).

Therapist: Sounds like you're attracted to Carissa's strength and a part of you even felt attracted to her even further because you anticipated your father not being okay with you dating a Black woman. Does that fit or make sense to you?

The therapist offered an interpretation about his tendency to resist expectations from his father, but checked to see if Steve concurred with this idea.

Steve: I guess so. I have always been a little bit rebellious. At this point in my life, my father's opinion doesn't really matter to me. Carissa's demeanor was easy-going but also very confident and it was exactly what I was looking for. I had previously dated some women who were very needy and had low self-confidence.

Carissa: Yeah, Steve has a way of disagreeing with people in subtle, yet powerful ways. With me, he is often subtle but, in many cases, he is very direct about getting his way. That is where we get hung up.

Steve: This is true.

Therapist: I wonder if either of you see a connection with your early encounter memory and today.

The therapist made an effort to bridge the FECK story to current relationship dynamics.

Carissa: I guess the thing that sticks out to me is that Steve made me the center of his universe and put his entire being into the early part of our relationship. I had never had someone show such a high level of interest in me that I was attracted to, so his enthusiasm and presence highly appealed to me. Unfortunately, these days, I don't feel his enthusiasm and presence very often since he often spends most weekends doing things with his friends. I want him to want me around and to make efforts to make plans for us to be together on the weekends. So, I guess the memory is highlighting what I feel is missing in our relationship right now, quality time together.

Steve: She is right. I have always been a very social person, so I like being active on the weekends. Carissa just wants to sit home all day on the weekends and binge-watch movies and her favorite TV shows.

Therapist: So, Carissa, your recollection of the early encounter was an indicator of what feels missing in the relationship today. I hear you stating what you would like to see more of in the relationship.

Summarizing and clarifying Carissa's desire for her and Steve to spend more time together on the weekends.

Carissa: Yes, exactly. I want his presence and he doesn't seem to want to give it to me.

Steve: I mean, we do our weekly date nights and I like those nights with her.

Carissa: Steve, are you serious? We've basically done date nights once a month for the past year.

Steve: Okay, maybe we need to get back to that. I'm sorry that I haven't prioritized that.

Therapist: I am glad to hear that you both have tried date nights, that is so important in relationships. I also appreciate your efforts (*to Steve*) to try to repair that part of your relationship. Going back to the early encounter story, Steve, is there a connection from your memory of Carissa's confidence and the idea that your father would be unhappy with you dating a Black woman?

The therapist utilizes encouragement and therapeutic support to emphasize useful strategies that are already occurring and attempts to bridge Steve's FECK story to their current relationship dynamics.

Steve: I am not sure I see the connection.

Therapist: I have an idea. Would you like to hear it?

The therapist asks for permission to share an interpretation.

Steve: I'm all ears.

Therapist: It looks like you sensed a specialness in Carissa. She was exactly what you were looking for at that time in your life, and part of that included finding a person that your father would highly disapprove of because of the color of her skin.

The therapist offers an interpretation of Steve's FECK story.

Steve: You aren't wrong. (*laughs anxiously*)

Therapist: I wonder if your tendency to be a bit rebellious shows up in your relationship with Carissa.

The therapist checked in with Steve about one of his hypotheses about Steve's life style.

Carissa: I'm glad that somebody else sees this!

Steve: Yeah, I do tend to do my own thing when I feel that other people are pushing me too much or trying to control me.

Therapist: Okay, awareness of our patterns is often the first step toward changing them. I have another addition to my guessing here. I think Carissa feels like the opposite of her first encounter story. She doesn't feel that presence and attention that she once had from you, Steve. So, it's sort of like a contract was broken in the relationship, and now the relationship is running out of gas. (*pause*) What do you both think?

The therapist offers a second interpretation and uses the metaphor that Steve initially used to describe the relationship. The therapist checks in to see Carissa's and Steve's reaction.

Carissa: I agree, I want to feel like Steve wants to be around me and I want us to have a family together.

Steve: I didn't know Carissa was feeling this way. I thought she just wanted to spend more time with her family on the weekends because she was feeling sad about our lack of success with the pregnancy situation. I want to fix this, I guess we just need to figure out how to find a balance in our social lives.

Therapist: Carissa, are you up for working on this with Steve?

The therapist seeks to elicit Carissa's commitment to working on some mutually agreed-upon goals in couple therapy.

Carissa: Yes, I want us to have what we originally had together. I want us to have a family and be a couple that wants to be around each other again.

Therapist: I can see your love for each other is still there, but even more than that, I can see that you are both choosing each other by coming here to meet with me. (*pause*) Let's shift to another question about a memory. I often ask couples about their earliest memories so that I can learn more about the way they show up in life. Carissa, can you think of a memory that sticks out to you sometime before the age of seven or eight that happened one time?

The therapist asks about an early memory to elicit life style themes.

Carissa: Hmm, I remember going to my grandma's house on my birthday. She had a big cake and two presents for me. The presents were perfect. They were just what I wanted. But my sister scooped some of the icing off my cake and ate it. I was so mad that she ruined my party. I think I was five then.

Therapist: What was the most vivid part of that memory and how were you feeling in that moment?

Seeks the most vivid part of the emotion and the feeling as it informs the life style assessment.

Carissa: Yeah, it was my sister eating the icing on my cake. I was mad and angry.

Therapist: Okay, great, can you think of any other memories?

The therapist endeavors to elicit a second memory to further assess Carissa's life style.

Carissa: I remember when I was seven. One day I saw my parents arguing and my father told my mother that the man of the house is supposed to get his way. My mother said nothing and just looked away. I was silent too, but I didn't think what he said was right.

Therapist: What was the most vivid part of that memory and the feeling or feelings with it?

Carissa: Seeing the look on my mother's face and feeling sad and angry that my father thinks that women are less than men.

Therapist: Thanks, Carissa, for sharing these. I wonder if you see any link between these memories and your relational pattern? Specifically, when you raise expectations, are righteous, and make demands that Steve pulls back from and resists.

The therapist attempts to bridge the memories to her relational pattern with Steve.

Carissa: Well, for one, I still think that men and women are equal, so I can see how my memory shows that I care about seeing myself as an equal with my partner. It sort of reflects how I get annoyed with Steve for being so social on weekends and not considering how I feel about this. I can also see that in the cake memory that I really like for things to go my way. (*pause*) Sometimes I get angry if Steve does things that don't meet my expectations and then I increase my demands on him. (*pause*) I don't like the thought that I can be so bossy.

Therapist: That makes sense. (*pause*) So, might the pattern in these memories be something we can address in our sessions?

The therapist seeks to elicit possible therapy goals with Carissa.

Carissa: I imagine that my tendency for things to go my way should be considered.
Therapist: Okay. (*pause*) So, what might be the purpose of that tendency which we could call
             your life strategy? As I see it, our personality becomes a pattern of solutions that are
             designed to minimize pain and discomfort and to maximize feeling good. So, your
             effort for things to go your way is a very human tendency that occasionally could back-
             fire, like when life doesn't go as planned but you insist that it does. The great part of
             this strategy is that you are effective in solving problems and are very persistent.

*The therapist is offering an interpretation of Carissa's life style and her role in the relational
pattern with Steve.*

Carissa: Yeah, I've always known that I tend to get impatient with things not going as planned.
             I could try to work on being less of a control freak, maybe by practicing what I truly
             need, to let things be.
Therapist: That is a great awareness to have, perhaps we can see how that can inform our work in
             these sessions. (*pause*) Steve, can you think of a memory that sticks out to you some-
             time before the age of seven or eight that happened one time?
Steve: I was thinking about mine when you were asking Carissa. I think I was about seven
             when I got my first semester report card. I received four Bs and two Cs. My sister
             had all As. I could tell my parents were disappointed. I thought they should be happy
             I didn't get any Fs. I told them I would do better, but secretly I told myself I wasn't
             going to work as hard as my sister and not have any time to be with my friends or play
             video games.
Therapist: How about the most vivid image and the feeling?
Steve: I remember the disappointment on my parents' faces, feeling sad, and I also remember
             my plan to proceed as I already had been, even though I told my parents that I would
             work harder.
Therapist: Steve, do you see any connections between that memory and the issues occurring in
             your relationship more recently?
Steve: Absolutely. It's sort of embarrassing to admit, but I see that my memory shows my ten-
             dency to ignore expectations that other people put on me. So I guess it relates in how
             I feel today about Carissa asking me to take out the cat litter or even pushing me to
             stay home on weekends and also to keep pumping money into the in-vitro fertilization
             procedures.
Therapist: There seems to be a connection there. Can you think of another memory?

The therapist seeks to obtain a second memory to gather more life style information.

Steve: I was probably eight and I was at recess and saw an older kid take a dollar bill away
             from a kid in my class. Two of my friends saw it and smiled and didn't do anything.
             I thought about telling the teacher, but decided not to because I was afraid the older kid
             would find out and come after me.
Therapist: And the most vivid memory and emotion?
Steve: Probably was seeing the older kid taking the dollar bill away and feeling bad for the
             kid in my class. It felt like no one cared and that bothered me.
Therapist: Does that memory connect to today?
Steve: I don't really know. (*pause*) Do you have any ideas?

Therapist: Maybe it just reflects how you feel about the world, that it is sometimes unfair, and that people are often unappreciative or even self-centered. It also seems to reflect your relational pattern with Carissa. (*pause*) As she increases expectations and makes demands on you, you are likely to pull back and passively resist. (*pause*) Does any of that fit you?

The therapist suggests Steve's role in their relational pattern.

Steve: Yeah, I do think that the world is unfair.

Therapist: Okay; and do you ever pull back when she makes demands of you?

Steve: To be honest, yes, I feel that since we've been focusing on the IVF process, she doesn't seem to want me around, it just feels that way at least. Her main way of communicating with me is through complaining or just asking me to do things for her. It doesn't motivate me to want to be around her, so I sort of pull back from her and try to focus on things that make me happy, like spending time with friends or focusing on the parts of my job that I like.

Carissa: Steve, I didn't know you felt that way. I just thought you wanted some space. I feel bad that I didn't know this. I can see that we just simply didn't talk about all of these feelings over the past few years and resentments have been building.

Steve: You're right, we haven't wanted to put all of this into words until now.

Therapist: It sounds like this process has opened some communication about some important issues and topics. How are you both feeling about these conversations being initiated?

The therapist uses immediacy to check in with the couple to examine the process of the meeting so far.

Carissa: I think this is much needed. I had no idea how much we had just avoided and put off all these issues.

Steve: I feel a bit relieved and am hoping this can help us fight a lot less.

Therapist: Great, I'm glad to hear that this is a helpful process for you both. Well, after reviewing your intake forms, I have a few hypotheses of why you both would not want to deal with these challenges directly. Would you like to hear my guesses?

Steve: Please, do share.

Carissa: Yes, please! You've been pretty accurate so far.

Therapist: So, I'm basically playing the role of investigator and am trying to uncover what led to the gas running low in the relationship and to understand the dance in your conflict styles and also to understand how your personalities fit together. So far, I can see that you both still have a lot of love for each other, or these conflicts wouldn't be happening, you would both just walk away from each other if the gas was completely out. Steve, I learned that you are a middle child and you had quite a bit of expectation from your parents to perform at a high level, but you secretly decided to ignore those expectations, like in your early memory. I imagine that today when Carissa puts expectations on you to comply or do something that you don't want to do, like the cat litter, you also ignore those expectations. Does that sound remotely close to what is actually happening?

Steve: (*laughing out loud*) You're spot on!

Carissa: I am guessing that you are going to say that I am just perfect and have zero flaws. (*laughs loudly*) Just kidding, I know that I was always a strong student and often had my parents' approval, so I have high expectations of myself and of other people.

Sometimes this looks like me being a perfectionist and expecting things to always go my way.

Therapist: Okay, that seems like some great awareness. I noticed that you mentioned in the intake forms that your parents were not very emotionally expressive; does that influence show up in your relationship with Steve?

Carissa: I saw that dynamic in my family as not very effective so I might have over-corrected when learning how to deal with conflict. I sort of jump right in and voice my feelings and my preferences rather strongly.

Steve: Sometimes to a fault. I'd say she is incredibly direct, but it sometimes is like going to a drinking fountain and planning to take a sip and the fountain sprays with the force of a fire hydrant.

Carissa: (*laughs*) He isn't wrong.

Therapist: (*laughs*) Well this sounds like an opportunity for growth. How can we take this awareness and help you both have more productive/cooperative disagreements?

The therapist attempts to elicit treatment goals and workable strategies.

Carissa: I could try taking a five-minute break before going into conversations in which I'm super upset or emotional.

Steve: That sounds like it could be useful.

Therapist: Steve, is there anything that we discussed today that could help in working toward a more cooperative and productive way of communicating?

Steve: Yeah, I need to work on being less rebellious.

Therapist: How might you do that in the coming days?

Steve: I'll think about that and try to come up with something.

Therapist: Okay, that is fine. How about putting some more gas in your relational gas tank? I wonder how you might both work on this between now and our next session.

The therapist seeks to elicit engagement and cooperation from both partners, and also uses the gas metaphor that was used throughout the session.

Steve: Gas is expensive these days, so I'm not sure.

Therapist: Letting the gas run out on a car could seriously damage the engine.

The therapist redirects back to the discussion at hand by confronting Steve's joke about gas prices.

Carissa: I would be willing to make Steve's favorite meal this week.

Steve: Really? You haven't made it in over a year!

Carissa: I want us to work, so I will try to show you that I want you around.

Therapist: So, to summarize, I hear a goal of reducing conflict in the relationship as well as Carissa planning to try to work on "letting things be," and Steve is going to come up with some ways to be less rebellious. Would you mind if we tried one more thing before we finish up?

Summarizes the currently discussed goals and initiates a closing activity.

Carissa: Sure.

Steve: Okay.

Therapist: Can you turn toward each other and look each other in the eye and complete the following sentence: "I just want you know that… ." You can fill in the sentence.

The therapist uses this therapeutic strategy to initiate some supportive and cooperative movement for the couple.

Carissa: Steve, I just want you to know that you are so incredibly important to me, and I really appreciate everything you do to help around the house.

Steve: Aw, you are so sweet. I just want you to know that I love you beyond words and I want us to work on us! I love you.

Carissa: Aw, I love you too, Steve. I am going to cry. (*smiles with tears in her eyes*)

Therapist: That was so kind and loving of you both. Thank you for making an effort to do this important work. Let's schedule a follow-up for next week.

Concluding Note

Adlerian couples counseling is an integrated, systemic, optimistic, and humanistic approach. This approach can help couples learn about their rules of interaction through an investigation of their family constellation, early recollections, and relationship history. Through encouragement, insight, and reorientation, each couple can learn about themselves and their partner through examining their approach to solving problems in life, especially the love life task. Termination in Adlerian couples counseling is determined based on the level of cooperation built during the therapeutic process and status of the mutual goals being achieved. The future of Adlerian couples counseling will likely be more integrated with apps, telehealth, and evolving technology to meet the needs of couples in our ever-changing society.

References

Ansbacher, H. L., & Ansbacher, R. R. (Eds.). (1956). *The individual psychology of Alfred Adler.* Basic Books.

Arciniega, G. M., & Newlon, B. J. (2003). Counseling and psychotherapy: Multicultural considerations. In D. Capuzzi & D. F. Gross (Eds.), *Counseling and psychotherapy: Theories and interventions* (3rd ed., pp. 417–441). Merrill/Prentice Hall.

Belove, P. L. (1997). First encounters of a close kind (FECK): The use of the story of the first interaction as an early recollection of a marriage. In J. Carlson & S. Slavik (Eds.), *Techniques in Adlerian psychology* (pp. 362–379). Taylor & Francis.

Bitter, J. R. (2021). *Theory and practice of couples and family counseling* (3rd ed.). American Counseling Association.

Bitter, J. R., & Corey, G. (2024). Adlerian therapy. In G. Corey (Ed.), *Theory and practice of counseling and psychotherapy* (11th ed., pp. 109–157). Cengage.

Carlson, J., & Englar-Carlson, M. (2017). *Adlerian psychotherapy*. American Psychological Association.

Carlson, J., & Sperry, L. (2000). Adlerian therapy. In F. M. Dattilio & L. J. Bevilacqua (Eds.), *Comparative treatments for relationship dysfunction* (pp. 102–115). Springer.

Carlson, J., Watts, R. E., & Maniacci, M. (2006). *Adlerian therapy: Theory and practice.* American Psychological Association.

Christensen, A., & Shenk, J. L. (1991). Communication, conflict, and psychological distance in nondistressed, clinic, and divorcing couples. *Journal of Consulting and Clinical Psychology, 59*(3), 458–463.

Dreikurs, R. (1946). *The challenge of marriage.* Duell, Sloan & Pierce.

Dreikurs, R. (1967). *Psychodynamics, psychotherapy, and counseling: Collected papers.* Alfred Adler Institute.

Gehart, D. R. (2018). *Mastering competencies in family therapy: A practical approach to theories and clinical case documentation* (3rd ed.). Cengage.

Leak, G. K. (2006). Development and validation of a revised scale to measure Adlerian social interest. *Social Behaviour and Personality, 34*(4), 443–450.

Maniacci, M. P., Carlson, J., & Sackett-Maniacci, L. (2017). Neo-Adlerian approaches to psychotherapy. *Journal of Individual Psychology, 73*(2), 95–109.

Robey, P. A., & Carlson, J. (2011). Adlerian therapy with couples. In D. K. Carson & M. Casado-Kehoe (Eds.), *Case studies in couples therapy: Theory-based approaches* (pp. 41–52). Routledge.

Sperry, L. (1989). Integrative case formulations: What they are and how to write them. *Individual Psychology, 45*(4), 500–508.

Sperry, L. (2005). Case conceptualization: A strategy for incorporating individual, couple, and family dynamics in the treatment process. *American Journal of Family Therapy, 33,* 353–364.

Sperry, L. (2010). *Core competencies in counseling and psychotherapy: Becoming a highly competent and effective therapist.* Routledge.

Sperry, L. (2019). Assessment and case conceptualization with couples and families. In L. Sperry (Ed.), *Couple and family assessment: Contemporary and cutting-edge strategies* (3rd ed., pp. 20–32). Routledge.

Sperry, L. (2021). *Pattern focused therapy: Highly effective CBT practice in mental health and integrated care settings.* Routledge.

Sperry, L. (2022). Adlerian case conceptualization and therapy: The pattern focused approach. *Journal of Individual Psychology, 78*(4), 465–478.

Sperry, L. (2024). Adlerian case conceptualization. In L. Sperry, J. Sperry & M. Bluvshtein (Eds.), *Psychopathology and psychotherapy: DSM-5-TR diagnosis, case conceptualization and treatment* (3rd ed.). Routledge

Sperry, L., & Binensztok, V. (2019). *Learning and practicing Adlerian therapy.* Cognella.

Sperry, L., & Peluso, P. R. (2019). *Couple therapy: Theory and effective practice* (3rd ed.). Routledge.

Sperry, L., & Sperry, J. (2012). *Case conceptualization: Mastering this competency with ease and confidence.* Routledge.

Sperry, J. & Sperry, L (2020a). Case conceptualization: Key to highly effective counseling. *Counseling Today, 63*(6), 50–56.

Sperry, L., & Sperry, J. (2020b). *Case conceptualization: Mastering this competency with ease and confidence* (2nd ed.). Routledge.

Sperry, L., & Sperry, J. (2022). *The 15-minute case conceptualization: Mastering the pattern-focused approach.* Oxford University Press.

5 Bowen Family Systems Couple Therapy

Christopher Burnett

History of the Model

Bowen Family Systems Theory was developed by the psychiatrist Murray Bowen. His work on the theory began during the 1950s and early 1960s and continued to develop throughout the 1960s and 1970s. Born in Tennessee in 1913, Dr. Bowen trained as a psychoanalytic psychiatrist after a brief foray in surgery. The late 1940s and 1950s were a pioneering period of "systems thinking," and emergence of what was to become the field of family therapy. Many systems theorists of the time employed models derived from general systems and/or cybernetics ideas. These thinkers applied concepts like feedback loops, homeostasis, complexity, isomorphism, and circular causality to understand family relationships and behavior.

Bowen and his approach remain unique in their conceptualization of the human family as a naturally occurring emotional unit (Bowen, 1976) that governs the behavior of the individuals within it. His assumptions were based on his intense and extensive work with schizophrenic patients and their families. Not satisfied with conventional psychoanalytic conceptualizations of both the onset and resolution of the syndrome (which he believed were fraught with excessive subjectivity), he began immersing himself in readings about biology, evolution, and the natural sciences in order to understand how those sciences, grounded in empirical data, had tackled novel and difficult problems. His conclusion was that any *science* of human behavior would have to be consistent with the *facts* of evolutionary theory. During this period Bowen used the term "theory" as a shorthand reference to natural systems theory in general, and Darwinian evolutionary theory in particular (Titelman, 1998).

After a few years at the Menninger Clinic in Kansas where his psychiatric career began, he started looking for another institution to support his developing hypotheses about the interpersonal nature of the syndrome. He eventually moved to the newly created National Institute of Mental Health (NIMH) in 1954 where his study of the family would become the basis of his family system theory (Bowen, 1978). His research at the NIMH initially focused on mother–child relationships in families with schizophrenic children (Titelman, 2008). It expanded to encompass ways to work more effectively with these families, and to describe and understand other patterns of behavior in family relationships over generations. From this, Bowen articulated a series of concepts that represented the entire family as an emotional system, and schizophrenia as a family process, not simply an individual disease. Furthermore, Bowen came to postulate that the concepts he used to describe emotional processes in his research families applied to all families, not simply clinical populations.

DOI: 10.4324/9781003369097-5

Conceptualization of Problem Formation

Theoretical Framework

Bowen Family Systems Theory (BFST) is grounded within the larger framework of natural systems thinking (Bowen, 1976; Kerr & Bowen, 1988). **Natural systems theory** holds that there are forces which exist in the world and are there to be discovered. Such forces are said to be a part of the *natural world* and exert themselves throughout it. Evolution is understood as a natural force impacting all living things. Examination of the fossil record shows that these forces impacted life on earth long before the emergence of *homo sapiens* (Wilson, 1975). Darwin's theory of evolution is the leading exemplar of a natural systems theory, in that it holds that all living things continue to be subject to the *forces* of evolution (Darwin, 1979). Seen inthis light, *survival* and *reproduction* are forces understood as underlying a good deal of both individual and group behaviors.

In the same way that the laws of physics and the laws of nature are inferred by observing interactions, Bowen sought to articulate similar law-like forces that operate on and shape human relationship systems. Bowen and his followers have done this through the observation of interaction patterns in both human and non-human relationship systems (Noone & Papero, 2015). The resulting synthesis of these observations and theory has been a set of principles that lay out the fundamentals of human relationship regulation and management.

The Emotional System

The **emotional system** functions to organize and process information from inside and outside of an organism. Such a concept makes it possible to help *explain* and not simply *describe* the fundamentals of human relationship processes. Imagine the concept as being roughly akin to a hybrid between the concept of the unconscious mind and the concept of instincts. It exists outside of the realm of conscious awareness, but it is different from the unconscious mind in that it is a cumulative phenomenon, shared across multiple participants over generations. Each participant shapes the course that this system has on every other member. In this way, it is antithetical to simple, singular individual diagnosis. The concept of the emotional system assures that all individuals must be understood within the context of the biological, psychological, and social relationship systems they are, and have been, an ongoing part of. Kerr and Bowen (1988) further described this seminal concept:

> The emotionally determined functioning of the family members generates a family emotional "atmosphere" or "field" that, in turn, influences the emotional functioning of each person. It is analogous to the gravitational field of the solar system, where each planet and the sun, by virtue of their mass, contribute gravity to the field, and are, in turn, regulated by the field they help create. One cannot "see" gravity, nor can one "see" the emotional field. The presence of gravity and the emotional field can be inferred, however, by the predictable ways planets and people behave in reaction to one another.
>
> (Kerr & Bowen, 1988, p. 55)

Working on the marriage relationship of Steve and Carissa, a Bowen Family Systems informed clinician needs to understand the context of each of their respective family emotional systems. BFST holds that any marriage or significant emotionally committed relationship is an amalgamation of two different family emotional systems, much like the confluence of two tributaries into one river. In any such co-mingling, some elements persevere and others dissipate in the tumult of the crosscurrents. The challenge most young marriages face is the question of what elements of whose family culture, customs, and practices will survive and live on in the newly forming emotional system and any of its progeny. For Carissa, pregnancy and childbearing are very important, likely not just for herself, but probably also for other significant members of her own extended family. For Steve, the question of children and childbirth in his family has a very different emotional valence. His mother wanted a large family, but after his younger brother was born, Steve's father had a vasectomy, unilaterally ending the reproductive phase of the marriage. While not causal, it seems that this played some role in his parents' later divorce. It is not too much to say that this likely has had some impact on Steve regarding his attitude toward the pregnancy difficulties he and Carissa have experienced.

More about the Concept of the Emotional System

Bowen's theory uses natural systems thinking to both describe as well as explain the interactions of the emotional unit. His work at NIMH had a tremendous impact on the mental health field's thinking about families and pathology. It was no longer sufficient to simply think of schizophrenia as due to problems in the early years of the mother and child. His focus included the mother, father, child, and siblings. Moreover, it was not just the early years that were seen as fundamental. Current and historical family relationships that ebbed and flowed in intensity over time were also seen as crucial for contextual understanding. Levels of emotional intensity over time were seen to be constitutive of general family functioning (Kerr & Bowen, 1988). If the family is an emotional unit, then the people who make it up often function in ways that reflect the circumstances around them.

Kerr and Bowen (1988) emphasized that to observe the larger family systems process, one must shift focus from the parts (individuals) to the relationship between the parts (interactions). Admittedly this can be a difficult task. A therapist has gained this perspective when they can focus simultaneously on (a) the influence of each family member's thinking, feelings, and behavior on the family atmosphere, as well as (b) the reciprocal influence of the atmosphere on any one member of the family's thinking, feeling, and behavior. If one emphasizes only one side of this equation, a family systems perspective is lost.

Seeing the family as an emotional unit implies a deep, multigenerational connection between family members that significantly influences everyone's relational behaviors (Kerr & Bowen, 1988). Such influence is, however, largely outside of one's awareness. Seeing the family as an organism means that dysfunction, in whatever form it takes (physical, behavioral, social), is a symptom of disruption to the overall system's functioning. Individuals may be more vulnerable to developing difficulties if they are part of an emotional system that is unable to adequately manage the level of relationship anxiety experienced by its members.

For Carissa and Steve this means neither one of them can be said to be *the problem*. Together they are at a moment in time where the anxiety of being in relationship with one another is sufficiently high that it generates automatic responses from each of them. The threat that the relationship could be in danger brings each of them to call on things they learned in their families of origin, where the fundamentals of relationship survival were first learned, experienced, and practiced.

The Concept of "Anxiety" in a Bowen Family Systems Framework

In physics, the largest known natural force impacting the order of the world is gravity. Nothing seems to be unaffected by the power of this force in nature. It is so ubiquitous that this force of nature is accounted for and taken as a given by most people. In fact, it wasn't until Newton and his famous apple that the force was even named. In BFST, the organizing force of the emotional universe can be said to be **anxiety**. Unfortunately, the use of this term has led to enormous amounts of consternation and confusion for those who employ it. It is a term that gets easily confused with the medical and DSM-5-TR (APA, 2022) definitions of a pathological condition that needs to be ameliorated. A case can be made that eliminating this kind of anxiety is the goal of most psychotherapy.

In *Family Evaluation* (1988) Kerr and Bowen attempted to draw the distinction between "acute" and "chronic" anxiety. **Acute anxiety**, they claimed, was mostly of a short-term, incident-specific nature. Within a given period it resolved itself as the perceived threat receded. **Chronic anxiety** is such that a specific point of initiation is often not possible to discern. Chronic anxiety can, and often does, emanate from completely imagined or simply feared circumstances. It is:

> assumed to have manifestations on levels ranging from intracellular systems to societal process, is influenced by many things, but it is not <u>caused</u> [original emphasis] by any one thing. It is most accurately conceptualized as a system of process or actions and reactions that, once triggered, quickly provides its own momentum, and becomes largely independent of the initial triggering stimuli. While specific events or issues are usually the principal generators of acute anxiety, the principal generator[s] of chronic anxiety are <u>people's reactions</u> [emphasis added] to a disturbance in the balance of a relationship system.
>
> (Kerr & Bowen, 1988, p. 113)

The theory holds that such anxiety can be transmitted over long periods of time, sometimes generations, to multiple descendants of any given family line. A *re-conceptualization* of chronic anxiety as the residual force generated in and by a world absent of guaranteed safety allows us as clinicians to see it as a part of all human relationship systems. Doing this moves it out of the established framework of a pathology to be healed and into the more mundane realm of an existential condition to be understood and managed.

This transformation of the sweep, scope, and understanding of the concept makes it possible to see chronic or relational anxiety as a primary organizing principle of family emotional life. This is especially so when viewed over generations. Its sources, transmission, and management are as central to the family relationship process as gravity is to the order of the cosmos. It is this concept that sets Bowen Family Systems thinking apart from all other approaches in mental health. Transforming the concept of anxiety into a *natural* part of family relationship functioning makes it possible to approach families from an entirely different clinical horizon. Kerr and Bowen (1988) explained,

> The ability to act on the basis of more awareness of relationship process (not blaming self or others, but seeing the part each plays) can, if done repeatedly in important relationships, lead to some reduction in emotional reactivity and chronic anxiety.
>
> (Kerr & Bowen, 1988, p. 132)

Carissa and Steve can each express their so-called "reasons" for the current problems in their marriage. Carissa is *anxious* about the prospect of getting pregnant with Steve, and Steve is *anxious* about their continued efforts to try. If a therapist makes the resolution of their respective anxieties the focus of therapy, the result will resemble simultaneous individual therapy. This might bring temporary relief, but soon another "reason" for discontent would likely appear between them. When one assumes that all relationships are shaped by responses to the *relational anxiety* generated by being in them, a larger perspective can be achieved regarding the complaints of any couple or family member.

Individuality and Togetherness in Bowen Family Systems Theory

Another foundational concept for Bowen is that of individuality and togetherness. **Individuality** and **Togetherness** are said to be two countervailing forces of nature that exert themselves on human as well as non-human relationship systems. Kerr and Bowen (1988) write:

Individuality is a biologically rooted life force (more basic than being just a function of the brain) that propels an organism to follow its own directives, to be an independent and distinct entity. … Togetherness is a biologically rooted life force (more basic than being just a function of the brain) that propels an organism to follow the directives of others, to be a dependent, connected, indistinct entity.

(Kerr & Bowen, 1988, pp. 64–65)

This concept creates a continuum upon which human relationship systems can be assessed. It is a concept that allows one to assume that all people, and most animals, have automatic, non-brain driven responses to the ebbs and flows that are part of any relationship system. For most people trying to understand human relationships, these responses are often comprehended in terms of "feelings." The term *feelings* is often used interchangeably with the term *emotions*. Both are often the central focus of psychotherapeutic interventions aiming to "fix" relationships. Kerr and Bowen (1988) hypothesize that an evolutionary function served by the feelings we often refer to as emotions is to control the balance between contact and separateness in a relationship. Love, hate, anger, sadness, jealousy, remorse, etc., these feelings are often what clients are hoping will be changed by the process of psychotherapy.

Bowen assumes that in every human dyadic relationship, both parties seek some measure of emotional closeness and emotional distance (Kerr & Bowen, 1988). Furthermore, this is a dynamic subject to constant fluctuations. It is impacted by internal as well as external factors. The concept of closeness and distance does not refer to feelings. Many couples express a wide range of negative *feelings* about one another, and yet stay in the relationship for years on end. Emotional closeness and distance refer to the sense of safety and security provided by being in relationship. Closeness equates to safety and security for some, while for others it is distance and space which provide that same sense. Moreover, these dynamics are never set once and for all. They are contingent upon the level and intensity of relational anxiety that exists in and around a given relationship system at any point in time.

Individuality and togetherness are contextual *forces* which impact individual behaviors. These two pulls exist side by side in any relationship system and exert themselves on it throughout. When the terms *distancer* and *pursuer* are used to describe two people in a relationship, this treats each of them as individual actors imbued with specific traits. Understanding individuality and togetherness as forces in nature, occurring across multiple and various forms of life, we can understand human relationship conflict using a much larger contextual lens.

The concept of individuality and togetherness allows a clinician to understand there are deeper functions being served by a couple's movements toward or away from each other. Time and its passing naturally create ebbs and flows in any relationship. It is the duration and intensity of relational anxiety, as well as the individuality and togetherness forces, that together predict how or if a relationship system can continue as sustainable. With enough distance and the proper perspective (which is the position a BFST therapist aspires ideally to occupy) one can see that the individuals involved, and the roles they play, can and do transform over time. This is exactly what can be seen using a family diagram, and why it is so useful as a clinical tool. (More about this below.)

In this situation, it would be easy to label Carissa as a pursuer, and Steve as a distancer. Stepping back, however, we can see the ebb and flow of these pulls in their relationship's history. When he had the chance to take a position in North Carolina, Steve instead chose to work for a company in Orlando, putting him closer to Carissa's school in Gainesville. During this time, Steve also spent a lot of his weekend time with Carissa at her family's home in Bushnell, establishing good relations with her parents and deepening their relationship. When they eventually moved in together, Steve then liked to spend more of his weekend time with his friends while Carissa did homework. This arrangement only became problematic when she finished her degree, and his friends became less available because of their own growing families. This was when Carissa started saying that she too wanted to become pregnant, to which Steve agreed, but with somewhat less enthusiasm. Where once Steve could be described as Carissa's pursuer, some years later he looks to be the one seeking distance, and she the one pursuing more closeness from him.

The concepts of the emotional system, anxiety, and individuality and togetherness are understood to be expressions of the *natural* forces which in Bowen Family Systems Theory appear to operate in all levels of family life. Taken together, they have exerted themselves throughout evolutionary history, and have led to human relationship life as we now know and live it.

There are multiple contexts to be considered in any assessment of both individual and family levels of functioning. It is this foundation upon which Bowen Family Systems Theory and its eight major concepts rests.

Bowen's Eight Concepts

After decades of studying, research, and clinical experience, Bowen articulated the eight principles he "discovered" as necessary for understanding human family relationships. Each concept interlocks with every other one, and all of them are grounded in natural systems thinking. None of these concepts can be adequately understood independent of any of the others. Bowen's eight concepts are: (1) Differentiation of self, (2) Emotional triangles, (3) Nuclear family emotional process, (4) Family projection process, (5) Multigenerational transmission process, (6) Emotional cutoff, (7) Sibling position, (8) Societal emotional process (Kerr, 2019).

In the scope of this chapter, there is not time enough to properly review each of them. What follows are a few introductory notes to guide the reader regarding a few of the key ideas for couples counseling.

Differentiation of Self

This is the most well-recognized, and almost certainly the most difficult of all of Bowen's concepts. Most practitioners agree that an adequate understanding of the concept and its power takes years. Titelman (2014) explained that togetherness and individuality underlie the concept of differentiation of self. **Differentiation of self** is a concept that encompasses individual, family, and even societal dimensions. It is said to relate to the abilities of individuals or groups of people to distinguish between intellectual and emotional processes as the drivers of behavior. There is no adequate single definition of such an encompassing concept. It remains a fluid construct, even for those who use it often. Here are some of Bowen's (1976) own early comments on the construct and its relationship to therapy:

> The differentiated person is always aware of others in the relationship system around him. … [O]ne has to get a broad panoramic view of the total human phenomenon in order to be able to see differentiation. … The therapy based on differentiation is no longer therapy in the usual sense. The goal is to help the motivated family member to take a microscopic step toward[s] a better level of differentiation, in spite of the togetherness forces that oppose… . The togetherness forces are so strong in maintaining the status quo that any small step towards differentiation is met with vigorous disapproval of the group. This is the point at which a therapist or guide can be most helpful.
>
> (Bowen, 1976, p. 370)

When applied to couples therapy, it may be most useful to think of differentiation of self as the quality most important for *the therapist* to possess. Each member of the couple in distress is eager for the therapist to see things from their side of the argument. Many therapists in their zeal to be helpful have a hard time resisting this siren's call. Usually, this failure to resist means looking at the *root* of the *problem*, often in the behavior(s) of one or the other partner. Once the root issue has been identified, the therapist suggests exercises or interventions designed to alleviate it. The therapist's suggested interventions often have the goal of improving communication, expressing greater intimacy, or achieving a better distribution of family responsibilities.

From Bowen's point of view, such an approach demonstrates a lack of differentiation on the part of the therapist. The therapist's motivation to be helpful gets in the way of their being a thoughtful, non-reactive presence for the couple. Bowen (1974) writes:

> I believe and teach that the family therapist usually has the very same problems in his own family that are present in families he sees professionally, and that he has a responsibility to define himself in his own family if he is to function adequately in his professional work.
>
> (Bowen, 1974, p. 468)

Bowen came to believe that there is no real distinction between client families and any other families. For him, the struggle to define oneself in the face of social and emotional pressures is universal. Hall (1991) explained that the concept of differentiation of self doesn't involve reference points of "normal" or "abnormal." We have all had experiences both of trying to get closer with someone and trying to maintain a healthy distance from someone. These are relationship positions that all people inevitably occupy. Being able to look thoughtfully at their place in their own family helps a therapist to understand something about the plasticity of relational position and function. Bowen thought a therapist was of best service when they could successfully begin to apply this knowledge to the family systems of others.

If a therapist failed to maintain a vantage point that kept an emotional distance and perspective greater than that of the client, Bowen believed it was only a matter of time before the client's emotional system would incorporate the therapist into their original ongoing processes. Doing so rendered the therapist incapable of being useful, as they then could no longer offer perspective on that process. Giving and maintaining perspective is accomplished largely by the therapist's ability to recognize, and then successfully navigate, the emotional triangles that exist in a client's emotional system. "To be objective and to promote differentiation in others is directly related to the being of the therapist, not to his/her technical skills" (Friedman, 1991, p. 138).

In the case of Carissa and Steve, this means being able to hear, acknowledge, and understand the complaints that each has made about the other and their relationship. It means granting each of them the dignity and respect of trusting that they have the capacity themselves to be able to make decisions about the course of their relationship. The skill that the therapist brings to this process is the skill of being able to offer perspective, be it intellectual, emotional, or relational. This perspective is most usefully given with knowledge about and respect for the emotional systems that each of them comes from. Doing this requires a good working knowledge of the emotional processes and triangles that exist for them, as well as those that exist within the therapist's own emotional system.

Emotional Triangles

The concept of the **emotional triangle** is another fundamental element in a BFST understanding of human relationship systems. It is a concept that helps us to see that the anxiety produced in all human relationships is automatically regulated. It is regulated by the ways that the people in those relationships move closer to and away from one another in regular understandable and predictable ways over time. Kerr and Bowen (1988) explained the concept of triangles when they said:

> The thinking on which the concept of a triangle is based illustrates the thinking on which the entire family systems theory is based. The theory is an attempt to define *facts of functioning* in human relationships—facts which can be observed to repeat over and over so consistently that

they become knowable and predictable. *What* and *how* and *when* and *where* are facts about a relationship that can be observed. Conjecture about why something happens is not fact and so the inclusion of such conjecture in the theoretical concepts was avoided as much as possible. While it is a fact that human beings speculate about *why* people do what they do, the content of those speculations is not fact. The triangle describes the what, how, when, and where of relationships, not the why. [All original emphases retained.]

(Kerr & Bowen, 1988, p. 134)

The concept of emotional triangles is another way of saying that all human relationship systems are understandable in the structure and function of their component parts. Doing this removes any unnecessary and subjective speculation about motives. Bowen believed that any effort to discern individual motives only distracted from the efforts to account for relational facts.

On the concept of emotional triangles, Bowen (1974) writes:

The theory states that the triangle, a three-person emotional configuration, is the molecule or the basic building block of any emotional system, whether it is in the family or any other group. … A two-person system may be stable as long as it is calm, but when anxiety increases, it immediately involves the most vulnerable other person to become a triangle. When tension in the triangle is too great for the threesome, it involves others to become a series of interlocking triangles.

(Bowen, 1974, p. 373)

It is through this concept that we see the predictable pathways anxiety takes in human relationships. Once these pathways have been illuminated, variations in the level of anxiety throughout a family system can be traced over time. Accurately tracking these variations illuminates the malleability of functioning throughout a given relationship system. "A triangle has different characteristics during moderately anxious periods than calm periods" (Kerr & Bowen, 1988, p. 136).

Seen from a natural systems point of view, emotional triangles act as a regulatory mechanism. They help keep the natural anxiety generated in human relationships manageable. When relational anxiety rises, it spreads and activates other people in a contagious way. Bowen (1974) called this phenomenon "**interlocking triangles**." Those being secondarily affected in turn involve more and more others. Understanding this dynamic goes a long way toward comprehending the ebb and flow of symptoms in a given relationship system.

Bowen (1976) and Kerr and Bowen (1988) suggest that the process of emotional triangula-tion has been observed in several species of primates and other animals. By assuming emotional triangles exist outside of human relationship systems, the concept illuminates how structure, function, and nature are amalgamated in this theory. The primary emotional triangle happening for the Hogarths is that when the anxiety between Steve and Carissa increases, Steve draws in a friend or Carissa a family member.

Nuclear Family Emotional Process

The concept of **nuclear family emotional process** speaks to the idea that there are predict-able patterns of relating between spouses, parents, and children (Kerr & Bowen, 1988). In all family systems, excessive anxiety in the emotional system results in predictable, specific patterns of behavior in the nuclear family unit. Bowen originally identified these as (a) Marital conflict, (b) Dysfunction in one spouse, (c) Transmission to one or more children, and (d) Emotional dis-tance (Kerr & Bowen, 1988). In his more recent work, Kerr has revised his description of these patterns in this way: (a) Emotional conflict, (b) Dominant-adaptive (deferential), (c) Triangles, and (d) Emotional distance (Kerr, 2019). Kerr explained these patterns thus:

If emotional conflict is the dominant pattern between the spouses, marital conflict is the presenting clinical problem. If the dominant-adaptive (deferential) pattern is the principal pattern at work, dysfunction in a spouse will be the presenting problem. Emotional distance consistently operates with both of those patterns. Marital conflict (emotional conflict) and dysfunction in a spouse (dominant-adaptive) are different ways of managing the chronic anxiety generated … in a marital relationship.

(Kerr, 2019, pp. 26–27)

What we see with Steve and Carissa can very easily be described as emotional distance as a way of managing the anxiety in the marriage. Steve's desire to spend weekends with his friends, and Carissa's spending increasing amounts of time with her family at their home are ways whereby both of them are seeking to avoid conflict in the marriage. Her increasing desire to become pregnant may also be seen as an attempt to overcome this emotional distance in the marital relationship, as motherhood is certainly one way to always feel emotionally connected to someone in the nuclear family.

Family Projection Process

Bowen (1976) described the **family projection process** as "the patterns through which parents project their problems to their children" (p. 308). This concept recognizes that the anxiety parents experience in their own lives, and their strategies for managing said anxiety, cannot help but be transmitted to and through the children they produce. The common experience most of us have of this phenomenon is when in early full adulthood we find ourselves doing or saying the things our parents did and said to us that our younger selves vowed never to replicate. For some, this is simply an accepted part of "growing up." For others, such recognitions spark a renewed need for rebellion and renunciation of such legacies. For Steve, it is interesting to know that his father has very strong prejudicial attitudes toward race. Nonetheless, he married across racial lines. However, in the same vein, he can also be seen as being like his father in the way he is managing the issue of pregnancy and potential fatherhood by emotionally distancing himself in the marriage. Carissa is the child of a mother who went to great lengths to remain married despite her husband having an affair. It is not unreasonable to assume that Carissa feels that she too has gone to great lengths to keep her young marriage viable during this time of difficulty.

Multigenerational Projection Process

The **multigenerational projection process** describes how chronic relational anxiety has been managed, manifested, triangulated, and transmitted over the course of multiple generations of a given family system. Kerr and Bowen (1988) explained that "the intensity and characteristics of the emotional patterns in one generation are significantly influenced by the intensity and characteristics of the emotional patterns in the previous generation" (p. 225). This dimension of a relationship system is one of the aspects of a family that is revealed and assessed through the use of a genogram. When three generations can be mapped out, the therapist can begin to get a sense of the general levels of adaptability and flexibility that have been demonstrated historically. This can give them a rough working sense of how much or how little of these characteristics are likely to be in play in the client's here-and-now situation.

Without knowing a great deal of the specifics, we can nonetheless make some working assumptions about the relative levels of chronic anxiety Steve and Carissa each bring to this marriage. In Steve's family, there is a good deal more distancing, emotional cutoff (see below), and intense triangulation than we see in Carissa's. From this, it is possible to hypothesize that in this marriage, Steve is likely to be the one who is most likely to respond to relationship problems with distancing, triangulation, and cutoff as the level of anxiety in the relationship increases. This is not to pathologize him. It is simply to recognize what is likely to actually happen, based on what has actually happened in the past. The assumption is that we all first learned from the families we grew up in how to, or how to fail to, recognize and deal with relationship-related problems.

Emotional Cutoff

Emotional cutoff happens when anxiety in any relationship system becomes too much to manage, and meaningful contact among some of the elements of the system ceases. This cutoff can last briefly, or it can span generations. The consequence of emotional cutoff on a given emotional system is, however, something that does have predictable consequences. Kerr and Bowen (1988) explained cutoff in this way:

> Many people "escape" their families of origin determined to be different from them. … They marry, invest strongly in their "new" family, and "know" (or hope) things will be "better" than in their original family. … Cutoff may relieve immediate pressure and lower anxiety, but the person's basic vulnerabilities to intense relationships remain unchanged.
>
> (Kerr & Bowen, 1988, p. 272)

We see this process clearly in Steve's family and the way that his father left the marriage with Steve's mother. While this cutoff is not complete, in that Steve and his father, Ethan, still have some contact with one another, there is clearly a desire on Steve's part to be different in his marriage to Carissa than his father was in his marriage to Melanie.

Sibling Position

Sibling position is another way of recognizing that families operate as units composed of component parts. Individuals often perform functions within the unit simply as a result of (a) when in time they were brought into it (i.e., periods of relatively high or low anxiety) and (b) the functional positions available when they were born into it (i.e., if one is born as a younger sibling, it is not possible to have the same relationship to one's parents as that of an oldest child). Bowen based this concept on the work of Walter Toman (1961), who did research to establish that certain personality traits could be directly attributed to birth order. Bowen built on this work by saying that an additional dimension, that of differentiation of self, needed also to be considered when assessing the functions that are assigned to various siblings in any given family system.

Steve is a middle child, but he is also the oldest male child in his nuclear family-of-origin. Carissa is two years younger than her sister. Neither of the Hogarths describes themself as being a decision-maker growing up, as Steve described growing up with a very decisive older sister, and Carissa described how her older sister "protected her" from knowing about their father's affair for several years. This kind of larger perspective is helpful when the therapist is trying to assess the people in front of them, and it can be used to generate all manner of hypotheses to be tested through careful and considered questioning of each partner.

Societal Regression

Societal regression is the last of Bowen's concepts and needs to be seen as yet another "context" from which family systems emotional processes can be viewed and understood. Bowen asserted that the overall functioning of family systems is not unrelated to the overall functioning of the societies in which those families exist. Indeed, the emotional processes that underlie family functioning are, for Bowen, the same processes that underlie the constellation of families we call a society.

> The emotional process in society influences the emotional process in families, but it is a background influence affecting all families. ... [T]he concept of societal emotional process describes how a prolonged increase in societal anxiety can result in a gradual lowering of the functional level of differentiation of a society. The lower the functional level of a society, the greater the incidence of "social symptoms..."
>
> (Kerr & Bowen, 1988, p. 334)

This concept leads directly to our discussion in the next section.

Conceptualizing Diversity

Any relationship of significant emotional investment between two people can be understood as an encounter between two "cultures." Understanding culture in the broadest sense, from a natural systems point of view, allows us to see that any group connected by shared and common survival interests can be said to be bound together in a *culture* of survival. A marriage or similar intimate pairing is likely the smallest expression of this kind of culture of survival. A sense of "us" is developed in rejoinder to a sense of "them," whoever "they" may be. The next level of culture in this way of thinking expresses itself through one's family of origin. "We Smiths are different from you Joneses because... ." The increasing sizes of one's identified member grouping (from student or graduate, West side or East side, laborer or management, red state or blue state, European or Asian) also imply this notion of belonging through culture. Any relationship system of mutual interdependence can be seen in this light. From small community social organizations to business enterprises all the way through to patriotic national identities and racial identification, *culture* and its many manifestations can be understood as a product of the emotional system whereby the survival of the group is an unseen but organizing dynamic that impacts all the members of the association.

Defining culture and exactly what it means across its many contexts continues to consume enormous amounts of societal intellectual and emotional energy. Seen from a natural systems point of view, culture can be understood as one more among the many ways in which survival and reproduction are the inviolate goals of all living things. A natural systems informed view allows one to transcend the constraints that relativism places upon seeking the "right" understanding of the concept. If culture is understood as one more among the many ways in which relationship systems respond to the anxiety of simply being and staying alive, then we can see it as a characteristic of all human relationship systems. Focusing on either the "White" culture that Steve came from, or the "African American" culture that Carissa came from, is not wrong, as they are both "cultures" which helped to shape their views of the world and how to survive in it.

The fact that Steve's father, Ethan, warned him not to marry someone outside his own race could be made to be a racial issue and addressed as such. However, from a Bowen Family Systems Theory point of view, the fact that a parent cast doubt on the suitability of their child's potential partner is not news. The "reasons" parents give for such doubts span the spectrum from the reasonable to the absurd. The goal of the therapist is to stay focused on the process of the relationship dynamic, and not get caught up in issues of content. Culture, in all its forms, can be seen as one of the many ways in which emotional systems and their various multiple vectors have *evolved* to manage the anxiety of survival. Culture is yet another way whereby groups exert pressure on their individual members to work for the preservation of the group against threats, whether those threats be real or imagined.

The Role of the Therapist

For clinical practice, the therapist must first and foremost recognize that any couple seeking therapy is, by definition, seeking to involve the therapist in an emotional triangle. This is not a disparaging comment on either the couple or the therapist. Rather, it should be understood as simply a fact. The relationship anxiety that exists between Carissa and Steve is simply a fact. It has always existed. The therapist's work consists primarily of recognizing this fact, and then staying "**detriangulated**." Kerr and Bowen (1988) explained this concept:

> A basic tenet of systems therapy is that the tensions in a two-person relationship will resolve *automatically* [original emphasis] when contained within a three-person system, one of whom is emotionally detached. In other words, despite togetherness urges to the contrary, a problem between two people can be resolved without the "well intentioned" efforts of a third person to "fix" it. It only requires that the third person be in adequate emotional contact with the other two and able to remain emotionally separate from them. The process of being in contact and emotionally separate is referred to as "detriangling."
>
> (Kerr & Bowen, 1988, p. 145)

Getting and then staying detriangled, the therapist can see, recognize, and then discuss the emotional structures behind the content of the couple's complaints. Being an effective therapist means working actively to not take sides, for doing so creates yet another interlocking triangle in the couple's relationship. When this happens, it severely limits the therapist's ability to have, and give, perspective.

Gaining access to and accurately identifying the structures and functions of any family relationship system takes time and requires patience. The shifting alliances of family emotional triangles, the levels, pathways, and history of anxiety in a relationship system, the development and dissipation of symptoms over time; these are not things that openly announce themselves in a session or two. It takes time, discipline, and patience on the part of the therapist to allow these phenomena to emerge from the everyday descriptions that clients give them.

It also requires the therapist to keep their "fingerprints" off those structures as much as possible. The training and discipline of a Bowen Family Systems therapist requires them to identify and recognize the part they play in any triangulation efforts. An effective therapist knows how to respectfully deflect and decline these efforts. The human impulse to offer advice and intervene is tempered through the active implementation of theory for understanding both one's own, and other people's, family systems.

For Carissa and Steve, their descriptions of family relationship process come in the form of *complaints* about and *explanations* of one another. Carissa initially complains that Steve is lousy at cleaning the cat box, and that he needs to do it more often. She complains that he is more interested in spending time playing golf with his friends than he is with being with her. She explains that if he is going to do that, she is going to spend more time at her parents' home. She has not yet expressed her complaints that Steve is not as enthusiastic as her about her getting pregnant. Steve explains that they have already put so much money and energy into trying to get Carissa pregnant that he doesn't want to do so anymore. He explains that he thinks he is being a good husband, and that Carissa is the one creating problems in the marriage. There is little point in trying to discern who is right in any of their claims. It is the job of the therapist to be able to see beyond the explanatory "whys" of their relationship situation and keep track of the relationship processes underlying them.

Identifying relationship structures and functions takes thoughtful, reflective discussion. Such discussions can be punctuated by "what ifs" offered by the therapist or the clients. Ideas, connections, patterns, potential outcomes of changed behaviors are offered and dismissed by the client(s) and the therapist in an atmosphere of mutual exploration. One of the keys to allowing this to happen is resisting the need for intervention on the part of the therapist. Once the function and structure of certain family dynamics and interactions are recognized or acknowledged, the process then becomes one of mutual hypothesis testing and exploration regarding alternate, more adaptive responses. The important stance for the therapist is to maintain emotional neutrality even in the face of the family's attempts to draw them into the family drama (Bowen, 1976). In the session transcript at the end of the chapter, the reader will see the efforts that the therapist undertook to keep themself in a position outside of Steve and Carissa's ongoing emotional process. There were many invitations to get involved that were recognized and passed up.

Conceptualization of Problem Resolution

The Family Diagram in Bowen Family Systems Work

The family diagram is a tool that Bowen used in his family research, clinical practice, and in training other professionals. The term **family diagram** has gradually been used interchangeably with the term **"genogram"** over the past few decades, and both terms are employed interchangeably here. A family diagram is a graphic depiction of both the facts and functioning of a family emotional system over several generations. It is a tool for graphically seeing the family as an emotional "unit." It is used in recognizing patterns of behavior and emotional reactivity that impact individual family members. It is also used to take the overall emotional temperature of the family system.

Family diagrams usually start with indisputable facts, such as dates of birth, death, marriage, divorce, illness, employment, education, and geographic location. Once the major factual matters of the family system are known, they are represented graphically in a kind of family tree format. After this, the therapist may then start to inquire about such things as the nature, quality, and history of some of the relationships between people. These inquiries often start with the here and now, but may quickly move to historical instances where similar issues or patterns may have also occurred. This assemblage of facts, factors, and observations is used to illuminate, illustrate, and hypothesize about some of the processes operating within the emotional system at hand. It allows both the therapist and the clients to understand how issues such as differentiation of self, emotional triangles, emotional cutoffs, chronic anxiety, birth order, and multigenerational processes impact the emergence and expression of behavioral, social, and emotional symptoms. Figure 5.1 shows the genogram for Steve's family; Figure 5.2 shows the genogram for Carissa's family.

The family diagram is also an important way to help a client see themself as part of a larger family system. The mutual creation of a genogram provides a framework for people to see problems from a broader and more factual perspective. Kerr and Bowen (1988) held that "to act on the basis of more awareness of relationship process (not blaming self or others, but seeing the part each plays) can, if done repeatedly in important relationships, lead to some reduction in emotional reactivity and chronic anxiety" (p. 132). Figure 5.3 shows the genogram for Steve and Carissa's families.

Viewing Steve and Carissa's relationship situation through a family diagram makes it easier to move away from simple cause-and-effect thinking. This can be true for both the client and the therapist. When a systems shift is achieved, it makes it possible for people to move away from blaming self or others. In the transcript below, Carissa moves from a blaming stance to one of more mutual understanding. When people can assume greater responsibility for their actions, and stop blaming others for their problems, this allows greater curiosity to emerge. In an atmosphere of greater

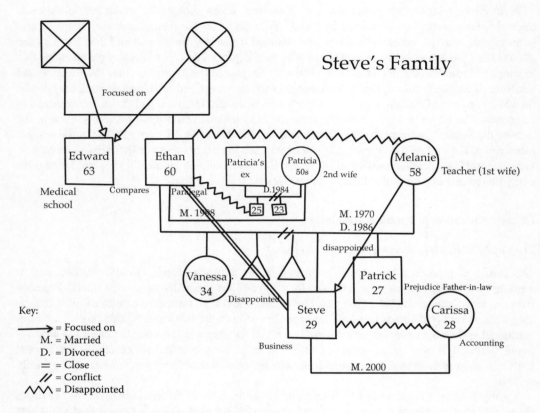

Figure 5.1 Genogram of Steve's family-of-origin.

curiosity, both Carissa and Steve can become more interested in the relational nature of their family life and come to more thoughtful decisions and resolutions about it.

When applied to couples therapy, Bowen Family Systems Theory is not a technique-focused model, incorporating specific descriptions of how to structure therapy sessions. Rather, it is the application of a way of thinking designed to help each member of a relationship system operate at a higher level of "emotional functioning." This is to say they operate more from a "thinking" frame of reference, and less from an automatic or reactive one. Friedman (1991) stated that "in Bowen theory, the differentiation of the therapist is the technique" (p. 138). The emotional level of reactivity of the therapist, when sufficiently low, serves to help the client(s) also become less reactive. At its best, doing this allows each member of the couple to better manage their automatic, emotionally driven processes. Slowing down the automatic reactions and processes already in place in the relationship makes space for one or both of their intellectual system(s) to function more effectively. However, this is not a cause-and-effect dynamic. Reducing automatic responses and behaviors is no guarantee that thoughtful ones will replace them.

Case Transcript

The detailed description of Steve and Carissa's relationship and family histories contained in the general case description is exactly the kind of information gathered by doing a family diagram. Experienced clinicians can collect historical family information while conducting therapeutic

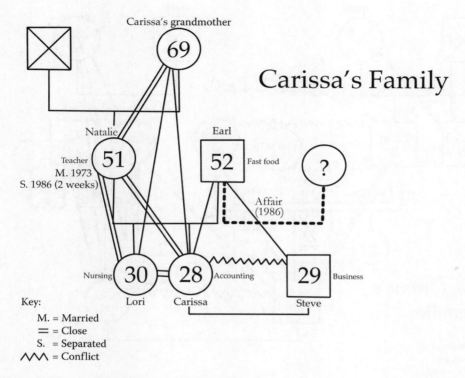

Figure 5.2 Genogram of Carissa's family-of-origin.

conversations. There is no one correct way to gather this information, but it is important for a therapist to have access to it in order to be able to understand the family as an "emotional unit."

Therapist: So, Steve and Carissa, let me review with you what I have in my notes. You two have been married for five years. Steve, you're 29 years old, Carissa, you're 28 years old. You met at college, eventually moved in together, then Steve, you proposed to Carissa after she finished her Master's degree. The first couple of years of marriage were quite happy. Then there was some talk of having a baby. There's been some difficulties in Carissa getting pregnant, and it seems there has been some friction in the marriage due to that. Carissa, you've kind of been going back to your family a bit more often these days, spending more time with your family again. It seems as if you're a little bit upset because you're not sure what the problem has been with the relationship. And it's kind of come to a head where last week the two of you snapped over something as simple as doing the cat litter. Is that an accurate description of things?

This recap of prior knowledge is done with as much factual recapping and as little emotional reactiveness as possible, to help set the tone for the session that facts are to be prioritized over feelings.

Steve: Yeah, not the cat litter, but that we're not on the same page.

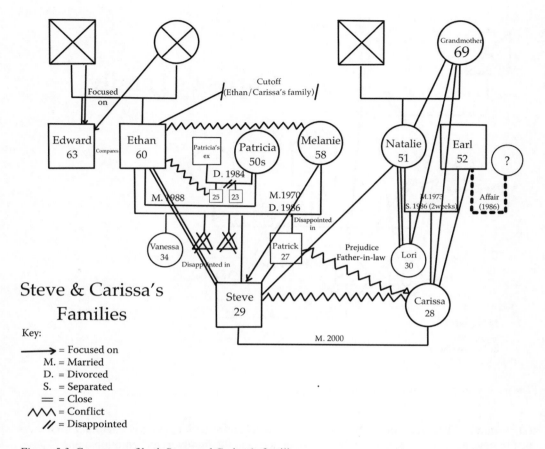

Steve & Carissa's
Families

Key:

⟶ = Focused on
M. = Married
D. = Divorced
S. = Separated
═ = Close
∧∨∧ = Conflict
// = Disappointed

Figure 5.3 Genogram of both Steve and Carissa's families.

Carissa: I think that's fairly accurate, but I don't want to say that I don't know what the problem is, because I feel like I have a fairly good idea of what the problem is, and it's that I'm the one that's doing the heavy lifting in this marriage and this partnership.

Therapist: Okay. And Carissa, the conclusion that you've reached is based on what?

Again, the effort is to have the conversation dwell as much on factual information as possible, in order to promote thoughtfulness and reduce the level of automatic reactivity that is already present in the relationship.

Carissa: So, the cat litter. I don't know why you said, Steve, that the cat litter is not relevant. It's just one small reflection of everything else that you're not doing in this marriage that I'm having to do instead. And the other thing that's really causing a problem in our marriage is the lack of having a pregnancy.

Therapist: Carissa, is this general disconnection something that you've noticed has changed? Or has this been kind of the way the marriage has been from the beginning?

This is an assessment of the level of change in the relationship over time. If this is the way the relationship has always been, that is a very different matter than if this is seen as a new development.

If this is perceived as being a change, then it can be assumed that it is reflecting some kind of an increase in the level of anxiety in the relationship.

Carissa: In the beginning, I was kind of in that honeymoon stage, so I didn't have as much of a problem taking care of him as I do now. I think I figured that he would eventually grow up and start taking care of himself, and that just hasn't happened.

Therapist: Okay. It's not like something is completely different about it in terms of what he does and what he doesn't do. It's just that you've become a lot less tolerant of the things that he's not doing. Is that accurate?

This is confirmation that Steve's behavior is not so much different, but the emotional energy and context around it is. This is understood to be an indicator of an increased level of anxiety in the relationship, and as a relatively recent development.

Carissa: Yes.

Therapist: Steve. Is that accurate? From your point of view?

The therapist here is being careful to make sure that Steve's point of view is also being given space to be recognized, and that the therapist isn't going to get caught up in any single point of view on the relationship.

Steve: No, I take a lot of offense to what she said. It sounds like she's treating me like a child, that I need her to take care of me, which I don't. I'm an independent person. I don't have to be there because I don't need her. I'd be there because I'd wanna be with her.

Therapist: I'm just trying to get a sense of whether that independence is getting read by one or both of you differently now than maybe it was in the first couple of years of your marriage?

The therapist is trying to make the point that while both of them may have been fine with Steve's "independence" earlier in the relationship, the issue currently has a very different emotional impact in the marriage. "Independence" is not made to be the issue, it is understood as an indicator of the relative level of the "togetherness" force in the marriage.

Steve: Like me going out hanging out with my friends? From early on, she'd say, "Go have fun with your friends." Now it's, "Hey, I thought you were gonna spend time with me. And why are you leaving me home alone?"

Carissa: I've been saying that since the beginning. I didn't say it as often because our relationship was pretty new, and I didn't want to strain it by being needy. But I've absolutely said from the beginning that I need more time with my partner. And you just haven't given it to me.

Therapist: Carissa, if I'm hearing you right, when he wasn't giving it to you in the beginning of the marriage you were willing to overlook that. But nowadays you're somewhat less able, less willing to do just that?

Carissa: Yes, and I'll never want to say that I was ever willing to, but I almost feel like the risk of saying no outweighed the reward.

Therapist: And now, would you say what? That that calculation in your head is shifting or is different?

Carissa: I don't care about the risk anymore. These things need to be said, because they haven't been said for years.

Therapist: If the risk profile is changed now and you're saying, "These things need to be said," what is it you're hoping will be accomplished when you say them?

This is a very important inflection point in the session, as at this point the therapist is being invited to join in the heightened emotional process occurring between the couple. The invitation is deflected and redirected by asking Carissa exactly what she is hoping to accomplish by raising the stakes in this way. This keeps the conversation on a more "thoughtful" and "goal directed" plane, and keeps the therapist from being emotionally triangled into the couple's reactivity to one another.

Carissa: I need you to step up as a partner! I can't have two children at the same time.
Steve: I still don't understand what you're talking about. I can make my own food; I can clean my own clothes.
Carissa: You can. But do you?
Steve: Do you give me an opportunity to?
Carissa: In the past when I have, it hasn't gotten done. So, the only way that it will get done is if I do it.
Steve: Yeah, I guess maybe it hasn't gotten done in the timeline that you want. Now, now, now.
Carissa: I think that a week and a half is enough time to do the dishes.
Steve: Exaggeration there. But that's okay.
Therapist: Steve, looking at your history in your family, you're the middle of three children. You have an older sister and a younger brother.

The therapist declines the invitation to get caught up in the "content" of the couple's argument, and instead tries to direct the conversation to some larger process. The therapist has access to this larger process via the family diagram. Steve is a middle child who grew up with an older sister. This relationship dynamic, living with an older sister, can be explored as it may or may not relate to the present situation. Regardless of whether it does or doesn't, it moves the conversation between them away from blaming and finger pointing, thus reducing automatic reactivity.

Steve: Yes.
Therapist: I'm just really curious as to what being a middle child, or what being the younger brother of an older sister has taught you about how to deal with women in your life?

The assumption being made here is that sibling position has a fundamental impact on the ways people learn to function in their relationship system with others. Being a younger brother to an older sister has likely had some impact on the way that Steve responds to Carissa, even if the specifics of this are still unknown.

Steve: I don't view it as like my relationship with her is like my relationship with my wife.
Therapist: I don't either. But my premise is that in our families-of-origin is where we learn how to deal with other people. It's kind of the foundation of how we begin relating with other people. I know myself, being an oldest brother of a younger brother, has kind of set certain ways I manage people and the way I do things. So, one of my assumptions is the kind of family that we're born into, and especially our position in that family, also kind of sets a certain kind of parameter for how we deal with other people. I'm just wondering if that might have any application in this situation or not?
Steve: I don't know. I had a closer relationship with my brother because we tended to play sports together and things like that.

Therapist: Okay. Now I am only assuming this, because I don't know anything for sure, but an older sister who liked to "boss you around." I know that's not true of all older sisters, but…

Steve: She likes to be controlling and stuff like that.

Therapist: How do you manage her when she's trying to tell you what to do and how to do it?

Steve: I try not to. I've kind of decreased my contact with her. Now it's kind of texting and stuff. I don't see them face-to-face that often. And I talk much more with my brother, either on the phone or texting, than my sister.

Steve's response here is taken as a confirmation that his preferred way of dealing with conflict is through cutoff. This, of course, may not always be the case, but it does allow for certain hypotheses to be further explored in the conversation.

Therapist: Would it be fair to say, then, that one of the ways your family has taught you to deal with family difficulties is that distance is a way to keep things kind of calm and regulated?

Steve: There were lots of fights and stuff like that. My brother and I, we play basketball with one another and had that sort of sibling rivalry thing. But there were issues with my parents and divorce and stuff like that.

Therapist: That makes some sense. Carissa, you were talking about your experience of being the younger sister of a bossy older sister. What was that like for you?

Carissa: She was bossy, but I love her very much. We were always very close growing up, and I've always had somebody to look out for me and protect me. I think that I developed the expectation that I would also have that in my marriage. And, so far, that hasn't seemed to pan out.

Therapist: Okay. With your older sister that has been your experience. Did you always feel like she was kind of there to protect you, in your corner when you needed her? That kind of thing?

Now, both Carissa and Steve have moved out of a blaming/defensive conversational mindset. The conversation has moved to how each of them learned to manage other people from their experiences in their respective families-of-origin. The entire dynamic of the conversation that all three people are engaged in is now one of reflection and exploration as opposed to who does what right and who does what wrong.

Carissa: Yes, everyone in my family. My whole family was very close. But … you know my dad cheated on my mom when I was about 10 years old, so we also had our fair share of problems here and there.

Therapist: Do you mind talking a little bit about that experience for you when your parents separated? Did they separate, or was there just an affair?

This question is aimed at getting Carissa to describe in detail some of the larger family systems dynamics that helped shape the emotional system of her nuclear family. This helps the conversation stay on an exploratory track, as Carissa is now being invited to speak about herself, and not simply to complain about Steve and his behaviors. This conversation will also give the therapist some idea about the differences in their two family systems with regard to the pull of togetherness in each.

Carissa: There was just an affair. I didn't know what happened until the time I was in college. All I remember is that when I was 10, my dad just moved out of the house for two weeks. Mom just said that he was on a vacation. She wouldn't answer questions about where he was. He was just gone, and then he came back two weeks later, and things were a bit tense in the house, but I didn't think that anything was terribly wrong. So, it really came as a great shock to me when I found out all that time later that it was really an affair that had been behind that two-week vacation.

Therapist: I think that is a remarkable story because that's not the way those kinds of things always play out.

This is an invitation for Carissa to discuss further how the force of togetherness has impacted relationship dynamics in her family-of-origin, and perhaps also colored her expectations within her own marriage.

Carissa: It's not. And so, when you asked Steve what role distance plays in his family and he said he doesn't really know. I think that it plays quite a big role in his family because his parents divorced when they didn't go through anything like what my parents did.

Steve: But are you thinking that I'm cheating or something?

Carissa: No, I don't think that you're cheating.

Therapist: I don't hear that in any of the conversation here at all. What I hear, I guess, Carissa, is that you grew up in a household where your mother was pretty good at covering up your father's affair and protecting her children from it. Would that be an accurate statement?

Steve was hearing what Carissa was saying through his own heightened emotional lens and was misunderstanding the point of what Carissa was saying. When she mentioned his parents' divorce, he leapt to a conclusion about his own fidelity. It was important for the therapist to clarify this misunderstanding for the conversation between them to be able to continue thoughtfully. Otherwise, things might easily go off the rails again, with accusations and counter accusations that had no bearing in facts. This is one of the ways that the therapist is there to "absorb" anxiety in the emotional triangle that exists between the three of them in the room. By not reacting and staying thoughtful themself, the therapist is able to help the couple do the same. Additionally, the therapist is also trying to expand the perspective that they both have on each of their families-of-origin.

Carissa: I suppose so, when you put it that way.

Therapist: This is what I'm thinking. I've seen a number of families, where, if a spouse has an affair, the other spouse can't wait to drag them through the mud and make them feel bad and embarrass them and make them live with that scarlet A for the rest of their lives. And that does not sound like what your mother did.

The therapist is trying to get Carissa to further describe how her mother went to great lengths not to make a bad situation worse by triangulating her children into the adult's relationship problems. It is seen as an indication of a level of differentiation that the therapist may be able to draw upon later in the process.

Carissa: Those families don't know what love is.

Therapist: There's lots of ways that families express love, but I'm more interested in the way that yours does. For me, it's very interesting that your mother was able to kind of swallow a lot of things for the sake of what she thought was the family's overall good. Did she ever talk to your sister about it or did both of you find out at the same time?

Again, the therapist is trying to keep the conversation away from generalities and to focus on issues of specific family dynamics. If Carissa's mother was able to put aside her own personal hurts for the sake of keeping the family intact, what lessons, implicit or explicit, might Carissa have learned about doing the same? The timing to ask this specific question of Carissa is too soon and too abrupt, so the therapist puts it on the back burner. However, another dynamic that can be explored is the dynamic between sisters. This too gives some indication of how Carissa came to expect to be treated by intimate others.

Carissa:	My sister knew for a little while before I did, and I didn't know about that until my mother told me about the affair. It was hard to find out that the whole family, except me, knew this secret, but I did eventually find out.
Therapist:	So, whether I might be right or not I don't know, but can we say even in this situation, your older sister again was serving a certain kind of protective function for you, and she knew it. But she wasn't going to be the one to tell you?
Carissa:	Again, when you put it that way, I suppose so.
Steve:	But she's making it like I'm not protecting her. When have I never protected you? I would protect you for whatever.
Carissa:	You would protect me when your friends weren't around, when there wasn't something that was more enjoyable or fun for you to be doing.
Steve:	When have you been in a place that I didn't protect you? And from what I don't know. You know I'm your husband.
Carissa:	You're not protecting me from the pain of not knowing what it feels like to be a mother.
Therapist:	That's kind of a big one to be protected from, don't you think? I don't think finger pointing is really going to do anything to help understand this situation. You've been trying to have a baby for three years is it, the two of you?

The temptation for people under emotional distress to point fingers and blame others is pervasive and completely understandable. Carissa is trying to bait Steve into assuming a defensive position in the conversation. The therapist is actively trying to create an atmosphere between them that promotes thoughtful, and not automatic, responses between them. The conversation is redirected to a topic that can be discussed factually, where Steve doesn't have to defend himself or his actions.

Carissa:	Yes, and he wants to stop trying.
Therapist:	And I'm assuming that that's not acceptable to you?
Carissa:	Absolutely not. I was born to be a mother, a biological mother, and my life will not be complete without having that experience.
Therapist:	Steve, what's the thinking behind your wanting to stop trying?

The therapist is trying to get Steve to talk, thoughtfully, about his reluctance to pursue pregnancy at this time. The way the question is phrased, "What is your thinking," is very deliberate and designed to help avoid tit-for-tat kind of responding which is likely what happens when the two of them are talking alone with one another.

Steve:	For three years we haven't been successful; meaning something's wrong. There's also the cost of in-vitro, which is a lot of money. We're still young. I know some stories of people who try so hard and couldn't, and then when they stopped trying, then they got pregnant.
Carissa:	I don't even know if I want to get pregnant with you anymore.
Therapist:	Hmmmm! That's a different matter entirely, then.

Arguing about the mechanics of getting pregnant is a very different thing than arguing about the desire to get pregnant, and this is the turn the conversation has just taken. Instead of the therapist making this the point of the therapy conversation, it is left open to the couple whether or not to pursue this dimension of the question.

Carissa: And I wish it hadn't taken this long for you to finally begin to listen to that. Because this is not a new thing that I'm saying to you, Steve.

Steve: This is kind of out of the blue.

Carissa: This is the first time you're hearing me for what I'm saying.

Steve: No, no, I've heard you, you know. "I want you around the house more." And I have made some accommodations to that, which I don't think have been acknowledged by you.

Therapist: If you don't mind my asking, Carissa, is this idea of not wanting to get pregnant, or thinking about not wanting to continue in the marriage, something you've talked about with your family?

This revelation is apparently something brand new to Steve, and he has yet to be able to fully process it. He still thinks Carissa is upset about his being out of the house. Asking Steve to respond more fully and directly to what Carissa has just said is likely to only increase the level of anxiety he is already feeling about the situation, a situation that he clearly is not fully comprehending just yet. By asking Carissa who else she has shared her concerns with, the therapist is tracking both the paths and the intensity of the anxiety she is feeling about this decision as it has been expressed back into her own family-of-origin. The therapist is assuming that this is likely to be the place where her unspoken frustrations with Steve are most likely to find verbal expression.

Carissa: My mother, a little bit, because I'm spending so much time over there now. She's started asking questions, and I've told her a little bit here and there about how his time with his friends is more important than his time with his wife, and how I'm not just gonna sit around and wait for him to come home anymore. She thinks I should work it out.

Therapist: Well, given the history of what she's been through and what she's done with her husband, that advice doesn't surprise me.

In this comment, the therapist is acknowledging the power of the togetherness force in her family-of-origin.

Carissa: It's a lot to live up to, having your mother be the someone that made a marriage work through an affair.

Therapist: Yeah, it is. Is that the kind of pressure that you're trying to live up to? Or live away from, I guess, would be one of the questions I have.

This comment gets the question of whether to stay or leave the marriage away from the issue of what Steve is going to do and how he is going to do it, and puts it more squarely on what she is going to do. This helps both of them to get out of the blame game and helps Carissa see her own role in the marriage's current challenge.

Carissa: I don't know. I want to have a happy family like the one that I grew up in, but I don't know at what price I'm willing to pay for that happiness.

Therapist: That's really very reasonable. That's not an answer I think you need to come up with on the spot. It's a powerful thing when you look back on your life in terms of what I did or didn't do, the choices I did or didn't make. Steve, Carissa described how her family weathered a difficult time in their marriage. Your parents sound like they had a different kind of experience. Can you talk a little bit about what you know about their divorce?

This comment is designed to get Steve to reflect on the impact of his family-of-origin on his marriage in the same way that Carissa has just done. The therapist, armed with information gleaned from the family diagram, suspects that the pull for togetherness that Carissa has described in her family may not play as strong a role for Steve in his. This question also gets the focus off Carissa for the moment and helps to illuminate the idea that both of them are bringing the influences of their respective family experiences into their current marital situation.

Steve: I don't remember much. I was pretty young at the time.
Carissa: I'm surprised that you don't. What happened was your mom had two miscarriages. She really wanted a big family like I do, and like you, her husband was dragging his feet. He didn't want that large a family, and so what he did was after they had three kids, he had a vasectomy without telling her, and then came home and said, "Surprise, no more children," and there was no discussion.
Therapist: I think there's plenty of material to chew on there.

What to do with this information has to be left to the couple themselves. The therapist is trying to stay as neutral as possible, so there can be the maximum flexibility with each of them going forward.

Steve: For my parents, not only was it an issue of having more children, but, my father's a … I don't wanna say an a'hole, but there's a bit of an a' hole in him.
Carissa: He's an a'hole.
Steve: My mom, she's pretty nice. They had some issues with one another, and they're better apart. Between Carissa and me, I've never yelled at her. Never hit her. She makes it seem like I'm never home. But I'm home most of the time. I just work a lot. I work hard. I spend time with her, and then I wanna have fun. I'm still a young guy. I've asked her if she wants to go. She doesn't wanna be around all the guys. I don't know what she wants, just me and her to be alone in the house, with our cats. And then I know she wants kids. But God's not shining down on us right now for that.
Therapist: Have you talked to anyone in your family about that fact?
Steve: No.
Therapist: No, okay. If you were going to, who might you think you might wanna talk to first?

This is a probe to see who in his family-of-origin Steve might feel closest with.

Steve: Either my brother or my mother. My mother likes Carissa. Part of the reason you get married is to have a family, and probably Carissa wants a family more than me. I'd be okay with just us as a couple going through life, but also having our own interests and our own friends while being a couple.
Carissa: And I would love that too. But I need the baby, too.
Therapist: Steve, what does your mother think about Carissa in general?
Steve: She thinks she's nice and sweet, and that we actually make a good couple. I'm trying to think, like has my mom ever said anything bad about Carissa? I don't think so.
Carissa: Do you wanna tell him how your father feels about me?
Steve: He didn't ask that.

Therapist: Well, it's on the table. Might as well put it on the table now.

Clearly this is a point of friction for Carissa, and she wants it to be acknowledged. Doing so recognizes another emotional triangle in the system. If the therapist fails to acknowledge this, the issue will go "underground" for a time, but likely will resurface again. The effort to promote transparency in communication makes it important to offer the space to have this element of the ongoing family dynamic "put on the table" for everyone to be able to view and discuss it thoughtfully.

Steve: My father comes from the South, and he's still trying to get into the 21st century. So, seeing a Black/White couple is not something that he was used to. He came to the wedding. He's still getting used to the idea.

Carissa: He came to our wedding, and he didn't speak to a single member of my family, myself included, on my wedding day.

Steve: Okay, that's my father. That's not me.

Therapist: Did your father ever say anything to you about this idea of an interracial marriage?

Steve: He said, "Look where we live. You know there will probably be issues from society." And I didn't listen to what he said because he's not that advanced. We've been together for a long time, and I can't really remember ever having an issue. We live in the South. But we live in a big city, and where we met was a university town that was fairly progressive.

Carissa: When I think about having babies, and the grandfather of my children being repulsed by their skin color. That makes me sick. That makes me not wanna have a baby. That makes me not wanna stay in this marriage.

Steve: Well, one, he won't have that much interaction. Just like we don't now. And two, it's gonna be his grandkids. So I'm sure he's gonna love his grandkids.

Carissa: He doesn't love his daughter-in-law.

Steve: That's not his grandkid.

Therapist: I can clearly tell, Carissa, this is something you're feeling very strongly about.

Carissa: Yes.

Therapist: And is this part of what's weighing on your thinking that maybe this marriage isn't for you anymore?

Carissa: I feel like there's so many things that are just layered on top of each other, that it brought me to that conclusion. No matter which way that I look at it, all roads point to "This is not going to work out in the long run."

Therapist: Okay.

This is a possibility that must be considered by the therapist as well. If the therapist gets themself in a "rooting position" for one outcome or another, they have lost their ability to stay emotionally differentiated and have likely become a part of the ongoing emotional system of the couple, making them no more able to keep a larger perspective on things than all the other members of the couple's emotional circles.

Carissa: And I only have so much time to become a mother and to have babies. And I don't wanna waste that time waiting for him to get his act together.

Therapist: I hear that. I'm guessing, Steve, this is some of the first times you're hearing it?

Steve: I think so, and I'm not too happy about it.

Therapist: There's nothing to be happy about for either one of you. But it sounds like this is the situation that you find yourselves in.

This is another affirmation of the therapist's commitment to objectivity and perspective. It is not the job of the therapist to make either of them feel better with promises that things will improve.

Steve:	She makes it seem like I haven't done anything nice in the relationship. We've had lots of good times. It's like the more she focuses on this the worse it gets between us.
Therapist:	I'm not hearing that you haven't had good times. You have. What I'm hearing is that the relationship is simply at a point now where the idea of bearing children together, raising them together, has put a pretty good strain on the relationship. I can see where some of the differences that both of you have as individuals, maybe some of the differences that come from both of your families, are making it difficult to see the road forward.

This is the therapist allowing the conversation to take a much broader perspective on the marriage than the blaming stance where the session started. The problem isn't Steve's or Carissa's alone; it is theirs together now. The relationship is at a point where decisions must be made, and the consequences of those decisions have to be lived with. Not everyone is able to make such consequential decisions at the same rate or with the same levels of confidence, and both are coming at it from different family-of-origin experiences. This kind of "perspective giving" has the effect of reducing the anxiety both are experiencing about this phase of their relationship. Hopefully, it allows them to be more thoughtful and less reactive in their respective understandings of it.

Carissa:	I think that's fair.
Therapist:	I don't think it's unusual for any marriage to come to certain points where you must make some decisions about what it's gonna look like from this point forward. Jobs, money, education, babies, relatives. All those kinds of things come into every family, through every marriage, at some point, and decisions wind up getting made. And the relationship simply changes as a result. This is how I understand what's going on here. That doesn't make it easy. But I don't think you're going through anything that most people in a long-term committed marital relationship don't go through in some shape or form.
Carissa:	I guess that's true of both of our parents.
Therapist:	It sure is. That's what I understand of them. Your parents certainly went through a hard time with your father's affair, and maybe there's even other things that they went through that you still don't know about. And then, Steve, it sounds like in your family, they came to a certain decision point, and they came to a different conclusion than Carissa's family. They decided staying together just wasn't an option.
Steve:	Well, it seems like roles are reversed now, because she wants to be out of my family and I want to keep it together.
Carissa:	I don't want to end things; I want things to be different than they look now. I still love you.
Therapist:	For me, this is a miniature kind of re-creation, Steve, of what your family went through with your father and mother, when she said she wanted more babies. Your father at that point simply took it upon himself to say, "Nope, that's not happening," right?
Steve:	I don't think I'm saying that. I'm just saying it's not happening for us *now*. We've put in the money and time. It's tough on me, too, to go through that, and then tough to see her go through that, and the disappointment that she has.
Carissa:	I think sometimes I get so caught up in my own disappointment that I forget to consider yours as well.

Steve: I know it's different. You have the urge to be a mother. Not so much for me. Being a father would be nice, but I could see a life without it. So I understand we differ in that.

Therapist: Becoming a parent would be a big change for both of you. It's something you cannot go back from. It is a big leap into the unknown, and it is a great source of anxiety. You may not have the freedom that you now have. Look at how many of your friends' lives have changed that way. And I don't begrudge anybody having doubts about it. The question becomes how can this marriage manage the idea that the two of you are not seeing eye to eye on this very important issue?

This summary and disquisition by the therapist are designed to show a larger perspective to both Steve and Carissa about their "in the moment" disagreements. Putting their fighting about household chores into the larger emotional context of the difficulties, and irreversibility, of the decisions all couples make together can have the effect of draining immediate concerns of their urgency.

Steve: I guess that's now the unknown. My friend group, a bunch of them are also married, and they're, like, "Oh, you two seem to have the best marriage." And I thought so too.

Therapist: Until this hour it sounds like you were pretty much of that same opinion.

Steve: I knew there was tension and stuff in the last some months, but not to this degree.

Therapist: Understood. Again, I don't know how this is going to resolve itself, either. I will say it's not that unusual for people like yourselves to be in this situation. I've seen these kinds of situations break all kinds of ways. I've seen where the couple actually gets closer together because of it, or the marriage is not able to survive, or they kind of continue pretending like nothing is happening for the next couple of years until something does happen. So, I don't know what the resolution for the two of you is going to be. Based on your family histories, it sounds to me, Carissa, like your family has kind of been of the mind, and maybe has taught you, that you kind of stick out the hard times, and you get yourself through it one way or another. And in your family, Steve, it sounds like when the going gets tough, sometimes the tough just get going. That doesn't mean that that's a guarantee for either one of you. I don't think it is. But those are the kinds of relationship things you've seen in your own lives that have prepared you for this moment.

Many therapists at this point would emphasize the positives, and minimize the negatives, to build on the goodwill that has now entered the conversation. By talking about all the different ways that their relationship might go, the therapist here is trying to reinforce the notion that the outcome is in the hands of the couple, not the therapist, and the process is far from over.

Steve: I haven't been preparing to go. This is why I'm here. Carissa is my wife, and we're going to figure it out.

Therapist: Hmm. Carissa, for that to happen, what would you need to see from Steve?

This question helps make things less abstract and more concrete for both Carissa and Steve to think about a path going forward.

Carissa: Well, you did show up today, and I haven't acknowledged that. So, I want to say thank you for caring enough to put your friends on hold for a bit and come take this time here for therapy. I would like more presence because you're physically there, but you're not emotionally with me. I can't feel like I'm living with a roommate. I love what we have together, but I really don't think that I can compromise about being a mother. And it's very scary for me because if I leave this relationship there's no guarantee that the next relationship will have any better luck.

Therapist: That's very true.

Carissa: The problem could be me.

Therapist: Well, I don't see you as the problem. There seems simply to be an issue in this marriage at this point in time. I don't think anyone has a problem here. I think this is just one of those things in relationships that must be figured out for the relationship to continue. In every relationship, there are moments where the question of what are we going to do about X occurs. How are we going to manage X? And in doing so, how do we manage to keep the relationship viable? I'm guessing just by what you said here earlier tonight, Carissa, that you hadn't broached the whole idea that you didn't want to be married to Steve until this meeting. That these are not the kinds of conversation that the two of you are going to have an easy time having by yourselves.

It was important for the therapist to maintain the notion that neither Carissa nor Steve is the problem to prevent blaming and scapegoating. The therapist is trying to convey a larger and more removed understanding that the problem exists more in the nature of the relationship at this point in time than it does in either individual. This makes it more difficult to either occupy or accept a blaming posture if it reappears in the future.

Carissa: I haven't said it because I haven't really wanted to pursue it. It's just been a thought. If this doesn't work out, then what else is there?

Therapist: That makes sense. It seems you both came in to fix the problem of snapping at one another. Do either of you think that maybe having these conversations on an ongoing basis with somebody like myself present would make it easier for the two of you to regulate some of that stuff? The anger, the snappiness, the shortness, the smartass-ness that comes out during those difficult-to-have conversations. Might that make it easier for the two of you to kind of figure out what you are going to do and how you're going to do it?

This is the therapist laying out as clearly as he can just what he believes he can offer the couple in terms of ongoing couples therapy. An emotionally reduced atmosphere for them to be able to talk reasonably about how they are going to be able to navigate this time in their marriage. No promises or false hopes, no sense of healing old wounds, just a place for the two of them, as adults, to be able to make decisions about their future. Based on the way that the level of anxiety between them has reduced over the past 50 minutes, it is likely that each of them feels better now than they did coming in, and for that reason alone, they are likely to accede to trying it again, at least for a while. If questioned, neither of them likely could tell exactly why this was. There was no "a-ha moment," but most people do respond to the physical relief they experience when their level of anxiety is reduced. The therapist has been successful in joining them in an emotional triangle if: (a) each of them feels like they can occupy an insider position with the therapist; and (b) the therapist can maintain a position of emotional neutrality such that each member of the couple believes that their point of view is being accurately understood.

Termination

Therapeutic success in this case would likely mean that the couple returned for a few more sessions to be able to continue discussing the issue of pregnancy for their marriage. The hoped-for outcome of these sessions would be that both Steve and Carissa could talk calmly and thoughtfully about the course they wanted their relationship to take from this point forward. Whether that meant actively pursuing pregnancy, putting it off for a time, or deciding that it was no longer desirable for one or both would be a decision for them to make together, not for the therapist to weigh in on. Being able to explore all of these possibilities accurately, clearly, and honestly is the ultimate goal of this approach to couples work. The assumption behind this is that adult couples can decide for themselves what does and doesn't work, if only they can manage to have a chance to think clearly about their options. The job of the therapist is to try to create and reinforce an atmosphere that makes this possible, but to stay out of the business of thinking that they, the therapist, knows what is best in anyone else's relational life.

References

American Psychiatric Association. (2022). *Diagnostic and statistical manual of mental disorders: Fifth edition text revision.* APA.

Bowen, M. (1974). *Family therapy in clinical practice.* Jason Aronson.

Bowen, M. (1976). Theory in the practice of psychotherapy. In P. J. Guerin, Jr. (Ed.), *Family therapy: Theory and practice* (pp. 42–90). Garner Press.

Bowen, M. (1978). *Family therapy in clinical practice.* Jason Aronson, Inc.

Darwin, C. (1979). *The origin of species.* Grammercy Books.

Friedman, E. H. (1991). Bowen theory and therapy. In A. S. Gurman & D. P. Kniskern (Eds.), *Handbook of family therapy*, Vol. 2 (pp. 134–170). Brunner/Mazel.

Hall, C. M. (1991). *The Bowen family theory and its uses.* Jason Aronson.

Kerr, M. (2019). *Bowen theory's secrets: Revealing the hidden life of families.* Norton.

Kerr, M. & Bowen, M. (1988). *Family evaluation.* Norton.

Noone, R. & Papero, D. (2015). *The family emotional system: An integrative concept for theory, science, and practice.* Lexington Books.

Titelman, P. (1998). *Clinical applications of Bowen family systems theory.* Haworth.

Titelman, P. (2008). *Triangles: Bowen family systems theory perspectives.* Haworth.

Titelman, P. (2014). *Differentiation of self: Bowen family systems theory perspective.* Routledge.

Toman, W. (1961). *Family constellation.* Springer.

Wilson, E. O. (1975). *Sociobiology: The new synthesis.* Harvard Press.

6 Cognitive-Behavioral Couple Therapy

Norman B. Epstein

History of the Model

Cognitive-behavioral couple therapy (CBCT) is a widely used treatment model that has evolved since the 1960s and is well supported by research (Baucom et al., 1996; Baucom et al., 2023; Epstein & Baucom, 2002; Fischer et al., 2016; Lebow & Snyder, 2022). There is substantial evidence of its usefulness for a variety of relationship problems (e.g., infidelity, mild to moderate partner aggression), as well as facilitating therapeutic gains with individual partners' mental and physical health challenges such as depression, anxiety, eating disorders, and coping with cancer (Fischer et al., 2016). It addresses major components of people's experiences in their intimate relationships: internal cognitions, emotions, and physiological responses, as well as behavioral responses. It also focuses on past and present experiences and characteristics of the two partners, as well as the present dyadic qualities of their relationship and contextual factors (e.g., outside stressors) that impinge on the relationship. Thus, it is a model that has great potential for integration and clinical applications with other couple therapy theoretical approaches. Northey (2002) noted that CBCT interventions are widely used by marriage and family therapists with other primary theoretical orientations. The following are the historical roots of CBCT, some of which now seem fairly simplistic compared to the more layered current approach, but all of which made important contributions to understanding and treating distressed relationships.

Social Learning and Social Exchange Theoretical Roots of CBCT

The earliest form of CBCT was behavioral marital therapy which focused on types of behavioral interactions between partners that influenced their satisfaction with each other. Developers of behavioral marital therapy (Jacobson & Margolin, 1979; Stuart, 1980; Weiss et al., 1973) applied learning theory principles to understand how members of a couple bring learned patterns from their relationship histories to their current relationship and continuously influence each other's positive and negative actions. Learning theory concepts focus on processes through which an individual learns both constructive and problematic behaviors through interactions with their environment, especially with other people, beginning in their family of origin. B. F. Skinner's (1953, 1971) model of **operant conditioning** focuses on processes in which an individual's actions increase or decrease depending on the consequences that result from them. When an individual's action leads to results they experience as pleasant (**positive reinforcement**), they exhibit that action more. An alternative consequence that increases an action is the removal of aversive stimulation (**negative reinforcement**), as when a member of a couple stops nagging their partner when the partner complies with a request, and the partner subsequently complies more quickly when the individual begins to nag. In contrast to reinforcement that increases actions, **punishment** decreases a person's action by providing an aversive consequence. Another type of consequence is **extinction**, in which another person ignores an individual's action, and the individual eventually stops the behavior.

DOI: 10.4324/9781003369097-6

Behavioral marital therapists described how members of a couple shape each other's behavior by providing those types of consequence, sometimes consciously, but not always. Because members of a couple produce consequences for each other's actions, they develop a circular interaction process that can be positive or negative. This circular causal process is an aspect of a CBCT model that makes it compatible with a systems theory framework.

Another concept of operant conditioning relevant to relationships is **discriminative stimuli**, in which cues occur that an individual is likely to receive reinforcement or punishment by behaving in a particular way. For example, Steve may have learned over time that particular cues from Carissa (e.g., her frowning when looking at handouts from their infertility specialist) indicate that she is unlikely to be receptive to affectionate behavior from him. Sometimes individuals intentionally exhibit such cues, but they also may occur spontaneously, and in either case a person's ability to "de-code" cues from their partner affects their success in contributing to a mutually satisfying relationship.

In order to understand how partners' actions toward each other influence their relationship satisfaction, behavioral marital therapists applied **social exchange theory** (Thibaut & Kelley, 1959), which proposes that people are more satisfied when their relationship provides a favorable ratio of benefits (positive behavior from their partner) to costs (negative partner behavior). An individual's satisfaction also depends on whether the benefit-to-cost ratio they receive compares favorably to the ratio they believe they would receive in an alternative relationship. Research in which members of couples reported frequencies of positive and negative actions by each other on a daily basis demonstrated that their satisfaction was greater when they received a more favorable benefit-to-cost ratio (Jacobson & Margolin, 1979).

Even though learned patterns commonly become ingrained, learning theory proposes that they can be modified through new experiences. Consequently, early approaches to behavioral marital therapy emphasized identifying a couple's exchanges of negative behavior and engaging partners in substituting positive actions. However, even when unhappy partners are aware that they could change a negative pattern by behaving differently, they may lack motivation to acknowledge their own contribution and may blame the other person. Barriers such as this raised challenges for a strictly behavioral treatment of distressing couple patterns.

Early behavioral marital therapy concepts and methods were not restricted to operant conditioning, because the learning involved in shaping an individual's behavior via consequences is quite inefficient for developing the complex social skills that occur in human relationships. Consequently, couple theorists and clinicians also drew on **social learning theory** (Bandura, 1977) that describes how an individual can observe a complex behavior demonstrated by another person and imitate it. Thus, individuals commonly learn ways of interacting with other people by observing other people's behavior, in their family-of-origin relationships, other relationships observed in daily life (e.g., neighbors, friends), and media portrayals such as movies and online social media (Epstein & Baucom, 2002). For example, both Carissa and Steve observed their parents coping with relationship problems by avoiding open communication about them.

Based on learning and social exchange concepts, initial behavioral marital therapy focused on increasing partners' positive actions and decreasing negative ones, using contracts in which each person agreed to enact particular behaviors the other person desired (Jacobson & Margolin, 1979). Observational learning principles (modeling desirable behaviors and coaching partners in enacting them) were used to teach partners skills for positive communication and solving problems together (Jacobson & Margolin, 1979; Stuart, 1980). The expressive and empathic listening skills were based on a tradition of teaching them in relationship education programs (e.g., Guerney, 1977), as well as on research (e.g., Gottman, 1979; Revenstorf et al., 1984; Weiss et al., 1973) and identified specific positive actions (e.g., asking for more information, paraphrasing, validating) and negative actions (e.g., interrupting, invalidating a partner's idea, criticizing), as well as problematic dyadic patterns (e.g., escalating reciprocal exchanges of negative behavior, a demand-withdraw pattern). Because the interventions were developed on the basis of research primarily with samples from Western societies, therapists need to be mindful of adapting skills training for couples whose cultural backgrounds may emphasize different standards for acceptable communication.

The early emphasis in behavioral marital therapy on ways in which partners continuously influence each other's behavior demonstrated the influence of family systems theory. Although simple operant conditioning principles involving effects of reinforcement, punishment, and extinction are linear, when those and social learning concepts were applied to dyadic interactions, assessment and interventions with circular causal processes became obvious foci. Interventions targeting one member's behavior might produce change in the other member, but ingrained responses on the latter person's part could undermine change. Theorists and clinicians recognized the need for conjoint therapy, consistent with Gurman and Kniskern's (1978) finding that individual therapy for relationship problems had limited effects.

In spite of the focus on partners' behaviors toward each other, early practitioners of behavioral marital therapy began to address the fact that the impact of an individual's behavior on their partner depends on cognitive processes, such as selectively noticing some actions while overlooking others, and the meaning that the recipient attaches to the actions. Jacobson and Margolin (1979) noted that distressed partners tend to "track" each other's displeasing acts and overlook pleasing acts, a process that can increase one's overall negative view of the other person. They also described how blaming one's partner for relationship problems and attributing the partner's displeasing behavior to negative motives is associated with greater relationship dissatisfaction. Gottman et al. (1976) focused on gaps between the intent a speaker was trying to express and the intent the listener perceived. Thus, an individual may have made an effort to behave in ways that their partner requested, but the partner was still dissatisfied with those efforts through attributing them to the person having a negative motive such as trying to look good in front of their therapist. Furthermore, Bandura's (1977) social learning model included attention to individuals' expectancies, predictions an individual makes that particular actions on their part are likely to lead to particular outcomes. For example, an individual who has an expectancy that attempting to discuss relationship issues will result in their partner behaving defensively (based on negative experiences with a former partner or with the current partner) may avoid disclosing areas of unhappiness. Although behaviorally oriented therapists were sensitive to such cognitive factors, at this stage of the development of CBCT, relatively little attention was paid to specific ways to assess and intervene with partners' problematic cognitions. Further development of CBCT required integration of the behavioral model with concepts and methods from other theoretical models that address partners' internal experiences.

Contributions of Cognitive Therapy Models

The development of behavioral models of couple therapy co-existed with the emergence in psychology of cognitive models of individual psychopathology and therapy (Beck, 1976; Ellis, 1962; Meichenbaum, 1977), as an alternative to traditional psychodynamic models. Ellis's (1962) rational-emotive therapy focused on identifying and altering individuals' irrational beliefs that they developed from growing up in a societal context (e.g., that one must attain perfection and be liked by everyone to be a worthwhile person). Ellis's model proposed that failure to attain one's unrealistic standards leads to emotional distress and dysfunctional behavior, both as an individual and within one's relationships with other people (Ellis, 1962; Ellis et al., 1989). Beck's cognitive model of psychological distress also included unrealistic stable beliefs (schemas) regarding characteristics of the self and the world, but differentiated the relatively stable cognitive structures from the transitory stream-of-consciousness automatic thoughts that enter one's mind regarding immediate experiences. In the Beck model, a life event (e.g., taking an exam in school) activates an individual's underlying relevant schema (e.g., perfectionism as a personal standard), leading to stream-of-consciousness automatic thoughts (e.g., "I'm not smart enough to do well on this test. I'm a loser!") (Dobson et al., 2018). The model also includes cognitive distortions or information processing errors (e.g., all-or-nothing thinking) that contribute to distressing automatic thoughts.

Meichenbaum's (1985) cognitive model focused on thoughts that occur during individuals' responses to stressful life experiences. Similar to the Beck model, Meichenbaum noted that those thoughts commonly are automatic and can be beyond one's awareness, and that individuals can be coached in noticing distressing cognitions that can be tested for appropriateness and modified. In particular, Meichenbaum emphasized assisting individuals in developing skills for **"stress inoculation"**—intentional rehearsal of positive "self-statements" about managing stressful experiences. The individual develops coping self-statements for preparing for an anticipated stressor (e.g., "Remember specific things I can do about it."), confronting and handling it when it actually occurs (e.g., "One step at a time. First…"), coping with feeling overwhelmed (e.g., "Relax your body and slow down."), and evaluating one's coping efforts (e.g., "I am happy with the progress I'm making in handling this problem."). Because members of a couple can be stressors for each other, Meichenbaum's stress inoculation model has relevance for couple therapy.

These cognitive models initially were developed to understand problems with individuals' psychological functioning such as depression and anxiety, but they also were used increasingly to treat problems in people's couple and family relationships that often are major stressors in their lives (Beck, 1988; Dattilio & Padesky, 1990; Ellis et al., 1989; Epstein, 1982; Epstein et al., 1988). In a couple relationship, partners continuously perceive and appraise each other's actions, influencing their emotional and behavioral responses to each other. Those appraisals are automatic thoughts that are shaped by each person's underlying schemas such as standards regarding characteristics that a caring partner "should" exhibit (Baucom & Epstein, 1990; Epstein & Baucom, 2002). Some initial publications that applied cognitive models to close relationships mostly extended the Ellis and Beck models, focusing on each individual's distorted or unrealistic cognitions and intervening with each person to modify them. However, a more integrative model emerged that attends to a couple's dyadic behavioral interactions and each member's cognitions and emotional responses to them. For example, a therapist treating a couple for escalating verbal arguments would inquire about each person's thoughts about the other's behavior (e.g., "He acts like he has no respect for me."), the associated emotional responses (e.g., anger), and subsequent behavior toward the partner (e.g., verbal aggression). Although the more comprehensive CBCT model pays major attention to all three realms of cognition, emotion, and behavior, its title that omits emotion has persisted, perhaps contributing to it having an unwarranted reputation for overlooking emotion.

The Experience and Expression of Emotions

Foundational publications by Beck, Ellis, Meichenbaum, and others tended to emphasize associations between particular cognitive themes and emotions. For example, Beck (1976) described thoughts of loss associated with depression, danger with anxiety, and violation of one's rights with anger. This led some readers to conclude that the models only proposed a linear causal direction between individuals' distorted thinking and their negative emotions and behavior. However, more recent writers have described pathways through which emotional states can influence cognitions and behavior. Regarding effects on thinking, emotional states can interfere with cognitive problem-solving and can lead a person to pay attention selectively to particular actions of another person, as when an individual's anger toward a partner focuses their attention on the partner's negative actions. In terms of behavior, emotions motivate people to avoid situations, engage in aggressive actions, behave altruistically toward others, etc. (Leahy, 2015; Nezu et al., 2019; Rizvi & King,

2019). Furthermore, as emphasized by proponents of Emotion-Focused Therapy (EFT) (e.g., Greenberg & Goldman, 2008; Johnson et al., 2023), members of couples commonly "co-regulate" each other's emotions, as when one member's anger elicits emotions such as anxiety and anger in the other member. The CBCT model shares with EFT foci on both deficits and excesses in individuals' emotional awareness and expression, and in couple therapy, key goals involve increasing partners' awareness of their emotions and developing their skills for communicating about them constructively with each other (Baucom et al., 2023; Epstein & Baucom, 2002; Epstein et al., 2016; Epstein & Falconier, 2024; Rathus & Sanderson, 1999).

Family Systems Theory

Core aspects of traditional behavioral marital therapy and later development of CBCT incorporate family systems concepts. Exchanges in which members of a couple elicit and provide consequences for each other's actions (Epstein & Baucom, 2002; Jacobson & Margolin, 1979; Stuart, 1980) capture systemic aspects of the dyadic relationship, including the concept of feedback. When partners reciprocate each other's verbal aggression and escalate their negative interaction, they are providing each other with "positive feedback" in a systems theory sense, amplifying the negative dyadic pattern. Similarly, in a demand-withdraw pattern, the more one partner pursues interaction, the more the other withdraws from it, and vice versa. In dyadic patterns, a CBCT model holds each member of the couple responsible for their own behavior (especially verbally and physically abusive actions), and therapists look for opportunities for each person to make contributions to changing negative dyadic patterns (Baucom et al., 2023; Epstein & Baucom, 2002; Epstein & Falconier, 2024).

A CBCT model also incorporates family systems concepts of boundaries and hierarchy. Boundaries within and around a couple relationship involve partners' overt behavior (who interacts with whom, and in what roles) and their cognitions about what interaction patterns are appropriate (Epstein & Baucom, 2002; Epstein & Falconier, 2024). Thus, Carissa holds a belief that members of an intimate relationship should be the primary people in each other's social life, so she becomes angry when Steve's frequent get-togethers with his friends violate that personal standard about an appropriate boundary between the couple and outsiders. Regarding hierarchy, Steve tends to become angry when Carissa pushes for maintaining their intense and expensive infertility treatment, as he perceives her insistence as violating his standard (and the couple's explicit agreement when they formed a committed couple relationship) that they would engage in democratic sharing of power in decision-making.

Finally, the enhanced CBCT model developed by Epstein and Baucom (2002) applies Bronfenbrenner's (1979) ecological model of multiple levels of contextual factors (nuclear family, extended family, community, jobs, national economic conditions, forms of discrimination within society, etc.) that present both challenges and resources for a couple. CBCT intervenes with ways in which stressors from such factors influence couple interactions (e.g., job demands interfere with couple emotional intimacy), addressing partners' cognitions, emotional responses, and behavioral coping responses in their attempts to deal with them.

Conceptualization of Problem Formation

In a CBCT model, the success of a relationship is influenced by the partners' capacities to collaborate in meeting their basic needs (e.g., emotional connection, security, personal growth) while navigating a variety of challenges they face in life. Those demands originate in the characteristics of the individuals (e.g., personality traits, past traumatic experiences, forms of psychopathology such as depression, physical health problems), the couple as a dyad (e.g., conflicting life goals, cultural traditions, preferences), and the couple's social and physical environment (e.g., conflicts with extended family members, job demands, a child with a developmental disability, discrimination in the community) (Epstein & Baucom, 2002).

Some stressors or demands are relatively normative, experienced by many couples and predictable (e.g., financial issues, job demands), whereas others are non-normative and take a couple by surprise (e.g., a partner's sudden diagnosis with a serious medical condition, an unexpected job loss) (Price et al., 2010). In addition, some stressors are more likely to occur at a particular developmental point in a relationship, such as the shift to parenthood. A couple may be relatively stress-free until circumstances change, and they then may be faced with initiating problem-solving they never needed before. Their ability to manage demands and meet each other's needs depends on their resources as individuals and as a couple, as well as the availability of supportive resources in their environment. **Personal resources** can include characteristics such as intelligence, emotion regulation ability, problem-solving experience, self-esteem, financial resources, and communication skills. Examples of **couple resources** are joint problem-solving and dyadic coping skills (Bodenmann, 2005; Bodenmann et al., 2016), shared values and life goals, mutual trust, and emotional attachment. **Environmental resources** may include emotional and financial support from extended family and friends, services from community agencies, religious communities, and local health providers. The couple's ability to communicate constructively about problems they are experiencing in their relationship, avoid blaming each other, and adopt a collaborative attitude about finding solutions together is crucial to managing conflict about their relationship.

Carissa and Steve experienced relatively little stress and conflict during the early years of their relationship as they engaged in their jobs, moved in together, and spent positive time in the evenings preparing meals, exercising, and watching television together. They experienced some mild to moderate incidents of discrimination from being an interracial couple (people staring at them on the street; Steve's father distancing himself from Carissa's family and telling Steve their marriage would not last). However, they did not share their feelings about it, focusing on happiness with their relationship. Carissa expressed a desire for Steve to spend less time with his friends and more time with her, but he did not adjust his schedule, and the issue was left unresolved.

Initially, Steve agreed to have children, a priority for Carissa. Conflict arose when they were unsuccessful for three years in their attempt for a pregnancy, including infertility treatments, and developed polarized positions about what to do next. This conflict became a higher-level stressor on their relationship than prior ones such as the amount of weekend time Steve spent with friends, and their difficulty resolving it led to broader tension and conflict that was expressed through what they labeled "inconsequential" issues. CBCT clinicians guide couples in exploring ways in which seemingly minor issues often have more significant underlying meanings that elicit negative emotion and behavior. Thus, when the couple argued about Steve's approach to cleaning out cat litter, with Carissa stating that he was failing in his responsibility, this may reflect a sensitive issue for her—of his not taking her priorities and feelings seriously about time with his friends, and more so regarding her strong desire to become a biological mother. It also may have triggered a broader issue for Steve, regarding relative status and power in their relationship and longstanding self-esteem issues. Couples who have not developed good skills for sharing their thoughts and feelings about even lower-level issues and demonstrating empathic understanding are at risk of escalating conflict and distress when they face severe challenges. The risk is greater if one or both members have poor emotion regulation abilities, as quickly rising negative emotions can interfere with one's ability to empathize with one's partner and can lead to aggressive behavior. Steve and Carissa have reported verbal aggression that seems fueled by anger, which may call for anger management interventions. At this point, both partners seem to feel helpless about reducing their arguments.

Information about partners' family backgrounds is relevant to understanding the difficulty they have had with communication. Carissa's family environment was very positive overall, with especially close relationships with her sister, mother, and grandmother. Although this was healthy, it provided her with little experience in resolving conflicts with others. When her father moved out for two weeks, it was only years later that she learned that it was due to his infidelity, and there was no hint of *how* her parents managed that major relationship stressor and reconciliation. On his part, Steve observed much more overt conflict between his parents and had no model of clear and constructive couple communication and problem-solving.

Another aspect of their backgrounds that may have influenced their relationship without their explicit awareness or communication involves their relative levels of self-esteem. In addition to Carissa's generally supportive relationships with her parents and sister, she had a strong academic record and a promising career. In contrast, Steve was aware of performing at a lower level in school than either he or his parents expected, and he believed his career was not what they would prefer. Because self-esteem is a personal resource that can facilitate partners being comfortable negotiating when in conflict, it is possible that Steve felt at a disadvantage when Carissa took a strong stand regarding something she wanted, which could even play out regarding minor issues such as maintaining the cat litter. In CBCT, a therapist formulates hypotheses about factors that might affect a presenting problem and interviews the partners individually and together to gather information that may support or refute the hypotheses.

An additional factor that may have influenced the couple's negative interactions when in conflict involves the messages they may have internalized regarding the potential for stability of marital relationships. As already noted, Carissa witnessed significant trouble in her parents' relationship, and even though they stayed together, the process remained a mystery. Not only did Steve's parents model a high-conflict and aggressive relationship; his father also predicted that his interracial marriage to Carissa was doomed. The couple did not seem to have other clear models of successful interracial marriages (including challenges they typically face and strategies that help them thrive in a society that often discriminates against them). They mentioned no awareness of community resources that could assist them with such important information, validation, and social support.

When the couple's resources for managing stressors together were insufficient for their intense conflict over continuing to try and conceive a child, it is important to note that they had endured chronic stress from trying for over three years, including the expensive and typically intrusive infertility treatments that commonly detract from a couple's intimacy. The case description does not indicate whether their infertility specialists collaborated with couple therapists who could be a resource for a stressed couple, but it seems important for Steve and Carissa to receive therapy from a clinician who has expertise in working with couples experiencing infertility.

This section has focused on identifying characteristics of the individual partners, their dyadic patterns, and stressors and resources (or lack thereof) in their lives that influenced the development of the conflict and distress that brought them to couple therapy. In a CBCT framework, this evaluation included partners' cognitions and emotional responses as well as behavioral interaction patterns, and life experiences from their pasts as well as in the present.

Conceptualizing Diversity

In a CBCT model, a wide variety of forms of client diversity can influence factors contributing to a presenting problem, as well as aspects of treatment that may require some modification from "standard treatment" in order to meet each couple's needs and expectations. These include diversity in age, race, ethnicity, religion, gender identity, sexual orientation, education, etc. In couple therapy, diversity involves the characteristics of each partner as well as the dyad. Thus, Carissa and Steve are Black and White individuals, respectively, and both are cis-gender. As an interracial couple, they are a minority, and Carissa noted that her only models of interracial couples while growing up in a small Southern town were on television. There is no evidence that Steve had such models either. Carissa's parents were both supportive of their relationship, whereas Steve's father reacted negatively. Addressing diversity is important in developing a strong therapeutic alliance with members of a couple, which has been found to account for a significant amount of therapy effectiveness (Sprenkle et al., 2009). This involves demonstrating understanding and respect for both partners' needs and perspectives, as well as the challenges that an interracial couple has experienced.

Cultural sensitivity involves therapists developing awareness of their beliefs, values, and biases about characteristics of their own and other cultural groups, actively learning about their clients' cultural traditions and values, and intervening in ways that reflect that sensitivity (Sue & Sue, 2003). Therapists must understand and be respectful of couples with cultural expectations and traditions regarding romantic relationships that may be different from their own. This includes being aware of implicit values regarding healthy couple functioning that are present in the therapy models they use. For example, CBCT was developed primarily within a Western cultural tradition that values direct, open communication, so communication training is intended to increase the quality of a relationship by replacing hostile and avoidant interactions with constructive exchanges of information and mutual empathy.

However, open communication may not be valued equally across cultures, particularly in those that emphasize maintenance of harmony and avoidance of loss-of-face in relationships, and in which nonverbal behavior and instances of what is *not* said convey key meanings (Epstein et al., 2012; Epstein et al., 2020; Falconier et al., 2016). Carissa and Steve both reported limited communication about sensitive topics in their families of origin, so their therapist needs to be aware that encouraging them to practice open communication skills may elicit significant discomfort. In addition, because both partners minimized their experiences with racial discrimination, the therapist's inquiring about the effects of being an interracial couple within a community in which they are unusual and have been subjected to at least micro-aggressions might be uncomfortable. Furthermore, exploring underlying meanings associated with their "trivial" arguments (e.g., a power differential based on educational and career success) has the potential to create fear that couple therapy is "opening a can of worms" that could harm their relationship. Their therapist needs to discuss these possible concerns with Steve and Carissa, explaining the positive goals of the interventions, but giving them a voice in when and how these are delivered.

Clinicians also must be aware of self-of-therapist issues such as discomfort in working with clients with particular types of diversity (e.g., a different sexual orientation, race), as this can interfere with the therapeutic alliance. This need not preclude working with diverse couples, but it necessitates work by the therapist to counteract biases; for example, seeking clinical supervision.

Role of the Therapist

This writer has read some stereotyped descriptions of CBCT that portray the therapist as mostly challenging clients' distorted thinking and coaching them in practicing communication and problem-solving skills. CBCT is considerably more nuanced than that. At a broad level, the therapist emphasizes collaboration with the couple in setting goals that are meaningful to them, given the factors that motivated them to seek therapy. Assessment begins with a joint interview to gather information about each partner's concerns about their relationship and desired changes, and a history of the relationship: what attracted them to each other, how they formed a close attachment, significant events that affected the relationship positively or negatively, how they interacted when faced with problems, contextual factors that influenced the relationship (e.g., job stresses, relations with extended family, discrimination), what signs appeared that they were experiencing significant difficulty, and what changes each person would like to work toward in therapy (Epstein & Baucom, 2002; Epstein & Falconier, 2024). The therapist begins developing a therapeutic alliance by exhibiting "common factors" characteristics such as balanced attention to the individuals, empathic listening, and "multi-partiality" (Anderson, 2007), and demonstrating understanding of both people's experiences without taking sides. Following the joint assessment interview, the therapist interviews each partner separately, with an explicit agreement that the therapist will not keep secrets regarding factors that directly affect the couple's relationship and the process of couple therapy (e.g., undisclosed infidelity). The individual interview covers personal history (e.g., family of origin; functioning in school; history with peers, jobs, prior romantic relationships, mental health problems and treatments), as well as the individual's current functioning (Epstein & Baucom, 2002; Epstein & Falconier, 2024).

In the following session, the therapist provides the couple with feedback on what was learned about the strengths and challenges of their relationship, the problems that motivated them to seek therapy, and factors that seem to have contributed to their problems. Because partners may disagree about the types or severity of problems or their causes (at times blaming each other), the therapist must maintain multi-partiality in discussing problems and therapy goals. When partners disagree about the existence of a problem, sometimes consensus can be reached by reframing it in dyadic terms (e.g., "A problem is that you disagree about what good extended family relationships look like."). Although Carissa and Steve agree that difficulty with infertility and the associated treatments have been a financial and emotional strain, and have created awkwardness in their interactions, they have different preferred solutions to it and argue intensely over it. Epstein and Baucom (2002) differentiated between forms of "**primary distress**" and "**secondary distress**" in a relationship, with the former being a source of stress on the couple, and the latter being distress they experience when their negative way of interacting regarding the stress becomes a problem in itself. Carissa and Steve are experiencing primary distress from unresolved infertility and disagreement about future efforts to conceive a child, as well as secondary distress from their increasingly aversive arguments about it, which have spilled into arguments about other issues. In CBCT, the therapist's role includes guiding the couple in understanding those types of distress and devising a treatment plan that includes interventions for each type. Often the initial goals center on reducing the negative interactions that produce secondary distress and interfere with solving the primary distress problems.

Overall, the therapist's role is collaborating with the couple in identifying strengths, problems, therapy goals, and appropriate interventions. A key to this process is engaging the couple in shifting from blaming each other for problems to each person taking responsibility for making some contributions to improving the relationship. Although the therapist takes a firm stand that each person is responsible for their own verbally or physically aggressive behavior, the therapist still explores contributions both members can make to reducing overall tension in their daily life (Epstein et al., 2023).

In CBCT, the therapist uses assessment information to plan interventions to modify factors that contributed to development of a problem or its persistence and worsening. Interventions can be categorized as primarily focused on partners' cognitions, emotional responses, or behavior toward each other. Because those three types of response influence each other, a therapist typically will integrate them into sessions, but for the sake of clarity, they are summarized separately in the next section.

Conceptualization of Problem Resolution

When a problem exists in a relationship, the goal of therapy may be primarily to remove it as much as possible, but at times it may involve decreasing the negative impact on the partners by increasing both individuals' acceptance of it as undesirable but "livable" (i.e., "We can have a satisfying relationship even if this problem persists."). Jacobson and Christensen's Integrative

Behavioral Couple Therapy (IBCT; Christensen et al., 2023; Jacobson & Christensen, 1996) emphasizes balancing efforts to produce changes that each partner desires with greater acceptance of conditions that are very difficult or unlikely to change. The former interventions focus on modifying couple behavioral interactions, whereas the latter (acceptance) interventions are more cognitive/affective, such as increasing empathy with one's partner who has a chronic condition that is difficult to change (e.g., trouble focusing on goals due to attention deficit/hyperactivity disorder [ADHD] symptoms). CBCT guides partners in differentiating between behavioral changes that it is reasonable to ask of each other and changes that are likely to be unrealistic (i.e., unattainable standards) and for which they could be satisfied living with the status quo or a compromise level of change. Thus, it can be reasonable for Carissa to request a better balance between the time that Steve spends with friends and with her. In addition, it can be reasonable for Steve to request that they both enter further discussions about infertility treatment with open minds about options, such as how long to keep trying for a pregnancy, so the timeframe does not seem potentially endless to him, while supporting how much Carissa's strong desire to be a biological mother means to her. It also is reasonable for the couple to ask each other to make explicit efforts to stop their contributions to aversive arguments, using guidance from their therapist regarding communication skills and anger management. On the other hand, Carissa may want Steve to confront his father about his racist behavior toward them as a couple and her family; but the couple may need to discuss what they could realistically expect such an approach to produce, based on knowledge that his father has a history of rigidity, unwillingness to discuss the effect of his behavior on others, etc. The couple could consider some level of acceptance that change on his father's part is unlikely and discuss how they can develop the best possible relationships with both sides of their extended family while limiting interaction with his father. They could agree to focus on family relationships that validate them as an interracial couple and make it clear to his father that if at some point he wants a relationship with them, he will need to do some soul searching and deal with his prejudices.

Interventions to Modify Behavior

By the time couples seek therapy, they often have developed fairly ingrained patterns of negative behavioral interaction, such as mutual verbal attack, a demand-withdraw cycle, or mutual avoidance. As a result, some behavior changes often are needed early on, to provide the couple with evidence that change is possible. Therapists commonly introduce expressive and empathic listening skills quickly, followed by coaching in joint problem-solving skills, with the rationale that both members have described feeling discounted by the other, and they need some evidence that both of them are willing to make a contribution to constructive discussions about issues. This section describes core CBCT interventions used to reduce negative behavioral interactions and replace them with constructive behavior designed to meet both partners' needs better and help them manage stressors in their life together.

However, partners' willingness and ability to change negative behavior also depend on how they think about each other and their willingness to cooperate. Individuals in unhappy relationships commonly develop a "frame" (Beck, 1988) or trait attributions (Baucom & Epstein, 1990; Epstein & Baucom, 2002) that their partner possesses broad, stable negative characteristics and motives (e.g., selfishness, insensitivity, desire to control). Individuals who hold negative views of a partner are likely to be pessimistic about the partner's motivation and ability to make positive changes, and experience negative emotional reactions to the partner. Even when the partner exhibits a constructive action, such as reflecting back the individual's feelings in an empathic manner, the individual may experience it negatively based on attributing the behavior to a negative motive (e.g., "She was just trying to impress the therapist.").

Individuals who are unhappy with their partner and relationship also may hold standards for the other's behavior that are extreme, unrealistic, or significantly different from the partner's standards (Baucom et al., 1996; Eidelson & Epstein, 1982; Epstein & Baucom, 2002) (e.g., that a caring partner can mindread the other person's moods and needs without the person needing to tell them; that partners should spend all of their free time together rather than pursuing individual interests). When a therapist identifies members' cognitions that interfere with positive behavior change (as well as negative emotions that they elicit), it is important to integrate interventions for those cognitions and emotional responses early in therapy. Interventions for cognition are described in the next section. This section covers commonly used interventions to modify behavior: (1) improving communication, problem-solving, and dyadic coping skills, (2) replacing negative patterns (e.g., demand-withdraw, reciprocal verbal aggression) with constructive behavior, and (3) increasing positive actions, because only decreasing negative behavior does not necessarily result in partners becoming more satisfied with their relationship.

Improving communication, problem-solving, and dyadic coping skills: CBCT clinicians use procedures to enhance partners' skills for expressing themselves clearly and constructively, listening to each other's expressions empathically, collaborating to solve problems in their relationship, and using dyadic coping with life stressors affecting them as individuals or as a couple (Baucom et al., 2023; Epstein & Baucom, 2002; Epstein & Falconier, 2024). All three types of skill training include psychoeducation about the goals and methods of using constructive skills with one's partner, the therapist's didactic presentation and modeling of the skills (often facilitated with handouts that the couple can use in sessions and at home), and coaching of the couple as they practice those skills.

Goals of **communication skills training** include decreasing misunderstandings between partners, increasing empathy for each other's needs and desires, and increasing the degree to which they perceive caring and respect from each other. Guidelines for expression include describing one's thoughts and emotions as subjective (e.g., "When I ask to talk about my feelings about pursuing pregnancy and you avoid it, it seems to me that you don't care about how important it is to me, and I feel sad."), conveying empathy for the listener (e.g., "I know you worry a lot about the costs of infertility treatments and are bothered by how it takes any spontaneity out of our sexual relationship."), to the extent possible identifying positive actions one would like from the partner rather than just describing areas of dissatisfaction, and being brief and specific so the listener can understand and remember the key points. In turn, guidelines for empathic listening include using nonverbal cues that one is paying close attention (e.g., good eye contact, nodding), focusing on understanding the speaker's experiences rather than formulating rebuttals, and concisely reflecting back what one heard the speaker expressing, without expressing one's own opinions.

Problem-solving steps include jointly defining characteristics of a problem in behavioral terms (e.g., "We both are frustrated by a long history of trying to have a baby and the negative effects it has on closeness between us, and we need to figure out what to do about it."), generating potential solutions, collaborating in evaluating the advantages and disadvantages of each possible solution, agreeing on a solution worth trying, devising a plan to carry out the solution, and continuing or revising it, depending on whether the results indicate that it is effective or not. Throughout this process, the partners should use positive expressive and listening skills to be sure they understand each other and are conveying respect for each other's thoughts and emotions.

Dyadic coping involves strategies members of couples use together when life stressors affect one or both partners, as stressors that affect one member also influence the other member (Falconier et al., 2016). Partners commonly participate in each other's coping in ways that can either enhance or detract from positive outcomes. Successful dyadic coping occurs when a stressed individual effectively communicates their experience to their partner, and the partner intervenes in a way that increases the individual's coping efforts, or the pair cope jointly with the stressor in a way that reduces negative effects on both of them. Carissa and Steve need to be able to communicate about the effects that infertility and its long treatment have on them individually and as a couple, and find ways to assist each other in coping effectively, rather than working at cross-purposes. Examples of positive dyadic coping that might occur in Carissa and Steve's experiences with infertility stress are **emotion-focused supportive coping** (e.g., each partner expresses caring and behaves in ways that soothe the other's emotional distress at least temporarily), **problem-focused supportive coping** (e.g., a partner suggests actions the individual might try to reduce a pile-up of stressors on top of the stress of trying to get pregnant; the couple seeks therapy to re-establish sexual intimacy that was lost during infertility treatment), and **delegated coping** (e.g., a partner offers to take on some of the other's household chores to give the individual more time for relaxation and leisure activities). In contrast, negative dyadic coping might involve **ambivalent coping** (e.g., the partner exhibits an obviously half-hearted attempt to take over some of the other's stressful chores) (Falconier et al., 2016). The therapist uses psychoeducation to teach the couple about dyadic coping, demonstrates the forms, and coaches the couple in practicing enacting them.

Replacing negative interaction patterns with constructive behavior: The therapist points out a negative pattern such as mutual criticism, discusses evidence of its negative consequences (with examples from the couple's relationship), and encourages them to experiment with ways whereby each partner can contribute to a new pattern. For example, when Steve and Carissa begin to blame each other for a stalemate about future attempts to conceive a child, the therapist can coach them in using problem-solving skills to generate possible solutions and discuss each solution's pros and cons. The therapist then interrupts further instances of the negative pattern during sessions and coaches the couple in substituting the alternative positive behavior (Epstein & Baucom, 2002; Epstein & Falconier, 2024).

Increasing positive, pleasing actions: Because couples often express relief when negative interactions decrease, but still experience limited happiness when mutually pleasing interactions are lacking, the therapist discusses the importance of increasing actions that produce pleasure. One option is to arrange a behavioral contract in which each member identifies actions they desire from their partner, and they commit to enact those behaviors for each other. This process can be refined with **guided behavior change** procedures (Baucom et al., 2023; Epstein & Baucom, 2002; Epstein & Falconier, 2024) that focus on increasing particular types of behavior which address specific needs of a couple, such as actions that increase feelings of intimacy. For example, Carissa and Steve described a deficit in experiences of togetherness and intimacy, exacerbated by infertility treatments that made sex feel pressured and awkward. Their therapist could provide psychoeducation about diverse ways of creating intimacy in a relationship (e.g., sharing their thoughts and emotions about life goals using communication skills, walks together in pleasant outdoor settings, listening to music they both enjoy, non-demand mutual sensual touching), and then guide them in selecting activities to try to discover any that make them feel closer.

Interventions to Modify Cognition

The goals of interventions for cognition focus on increasing each individual's awareness of ways they perceive, interpret, and evaluate events in their relationship, and their ability to consider the degree to which those cognitions are accurate and realistic. The goals also emphasize increasing partners' knowledge about each other's cognitions and associated emotional responses, and demonstrating empathy, whether or not they agree with the other's views. For example, the therapist can interview Carissa and Steve about the standards each person has about behaviors that demonstrate caring for one's partner, as well as their beliefs about what constitutes a good balance between time together and independent activities, beliefs that appear to be related to their conflict over Steve's involvement with his friends.

Furthermore, it is important to intervene with negative attributions that individuals make about the causes of each other's distressing behavior, such as Carissa inferring that Steve's desire to discontinue efforts for pregnancy are due to his not caring about being a parent or to his not understanding how important becoming a biological mother is to her. In turn, Steve may infer that Carissa's insistence on continuing efforts to become pregnant is due to her caring more about herself than their happiness as a couple. Although CBCT clinicians do not assume that all negative attributions are inaccurate, they engage the couple in exploring alternative causes of upsetting partner behavior. The therapist works to foster an atmosphere in which partners do their best to reduce criticism of each other's beliefs as well as defensive responses, and increase a collaborative partnership in identifying ways to resolve their differences (using communication and problem-solving skills). A therapist's positive alliance with members of a couple facilitates their openness to input in examining ways in which their thinking affects their emotions and behavior toward each other.

Two broad categories encompass most interventions for modifying cognitions: Socratic questioning and guided discovery (Baucom et al., 2023; Epstein & Baucom, 2002; Epstein & Falconier, 2024). The following are brief descriptions of those interventions, which may be combined.

Socratic questioning: This involves guiding clients in considering the logic of their thoughts and any available evidence regarding their validity. In couple therapy, the therapist needs to exercise caution when drawing an individual's attention to possible illogical or extreme aspects of their thoughts in front of their partner, as one or both members may interpret the therapist's comments as suggesting that the individual's negative thoughts are invalid, and that the other partner's views are more realistic. This may create an opening for the person's partner to criticize the person as being irrational. Therapists must emphasize that they assume all people need to be cautious about negative thoughts they have about themselves and other people, and people routinely need to check whether there may be other possible reasons for upsetting events. One should not assume that any negative thought is inappropriate, but it is important to examine the evidence. Thus, as long as Steve and Carissa's attributions about each other's behavior result in them viewing each other as uncaring adversaries, they are likely to feel anxiety, anger, and sadness, and to behave negatively with each other.

A variety of interventions can be used in **Socratic questioning**. The therapist can teach the couple about stream-of-consciousness "automatic thoughts," as well as common types of biased information processing such as all-or-nothing thinking, selective abstraction, and overgeneralization (Beck, 2020; Leahy, 2017), and can guide them in identifying instances when they engage in these themselves. For example, Carissa may express an overgeneralization, exclaiming, "Steve, you always choose your friends over me," which immediately elicits a defensive response from Steve, "That's so untrue! I have turned down invitations from them a number of times to spend time with you." Therapists can give the couple a handout (Epstein & Falconier, 2024) that lists and describes common "cognitive distortions" to facilitate their identifying instances in their own responses to each other.

A second type of intervention in Socratic questioning is guiding each individual in evaluating the logic that supports or is inconsistent with their thoughts. It involves generating alternative ways of thinking about the partner, self, or their relationship. For example, when Steve has attributed Carissa's insistence on continuing infertility treatment to a negative motive (e.g., "She doesn't care about my unhappiness and its negative effects on our finances and intimacy."), the therapist can reply, "That might be the reason she behaved that way, Steve, and if it is, then we have some important issues to discuss about mutual empathy in our sessions. However, in case there may have been other reasons for her wanting to keep going, what other possible explanations can you think of?" If Steve has difficulty generating alternative attributions, the therapist can guide him in asking

Carissa to tell him more about her motivation and in providing her with empathic listening. If the therapist notices that the couple has overlooked another possible cause (e.g., hints from Carissa that she views herself as a failure as a woman if she cannot conceive a child), the therapist can introduce those hints and encourage her to disclose them, with Steve providing supportive empathy.

Regarding personal standards that are unrealistic in one's relationship, a therapist can guide the individuals in considering a revised standard that still captures their values but is more appropriate for their circumstances. For example, Steve and Carissa may hold different standards for how an individual should demonstrate their love and commitment to their partner. This is consistent with the popularization of the concept of different "love languages" (Chapman, 2015), in which individuals have strong preferences for ways in which they and their partner should express love for each other (verbal expression of loving feelings and affirmation, time spent together, actions to help the other, gift giving, physical touch), and devalue differences in their partner's standards. In CBCT, the therapist normalizes diverse ways of expressing and experiencing caring, and focuses on partners validating each other's preferences and making efforts to behave in ways that will feel good to each other.

Couple therapists often need to intervene with partners' different standards regarding other aspects of a relationship, such as preferred ways of interacting with extended family members, ways to manage finances, how to make decisions together when they disagree, etc. (Epstein & Baucom, 2002). Discriminatory behavior on the part of Steve's father has created issues for the couple's interactions with his family, so the therapist can explore their beliefs about an appropriate way to deal with the situation and guide them in resolving any difference in their standards. It appears that by the time the couple entered therapy, they had a history of avoiding in-depth, collaborative discussions of their differences, and their polarized negative views of each other resulted in what seemed to them to be petty arguments. Their therapist can help them understand that their conflicts touch on themes of beliefs that hold significant meaning to them (e.g., caring, respect, sharing of power), which truly need mutual empathy for each other.

Socratic questioning also can involve asking each individual to think about the advantages and disadvantages of adhering to a particular cognition such as a standard, based on their view that the advantages outweigh the disadvantages. For example, the therapist might explore Steve's resistance to complying with Carissa's preference that he spend less time with his friends. Perhaps Steve would reveal that he attributes her requests as due to her desire to control his behavior, based on observations of his parents' severe conflicts, and his belief that a man should not let his partner dominate him. First, the therapist may use Socratic questioning to guide Steve in considering other possible causes of Carissa's requests regarding his friends (e.g., that they are based on her enjoying his company and feeling somewhat insecure about his level of caring for her). Next, even if the more benign causes of her requests still result in her efforts to change his behavior, the therapist could explore with Steve the advantages and disadvantages of adhering to his belief that "as a man," he should avoid complying. He might list advantages such as "It will show her that I am a strong and decisive person" and "My friends will respect me more for not giving in." The therapist would express understanding of those advantages, but then ask Steve to think of possible disadvantages of following his belief. Steve might conclude that "It escalates a tug-of-war and more distance between Carissa and me," "It gives her the impression that my friends are more interesting to me than she is," "I might be living up to my father's prediction that our interracial marriage won't last," and "Being obstinate isn't really a positive quality of a man, as my father demonstrates."

Guided discovery: In contrast to Socratic questioning that focuses on logical analysis of one's cognitions, in **guided discovery**, the therapist creates experiential exercises and homework that produce information for the partners regarding the logic or validity of their cognitions. For example, based on their family-of-origin experiences in which members either had aversive confrontations or avoided communication about significant issues, both partners may have developed a general expectancy that it is futile to discuss and try to resolve their differences. The therapist can express empathy with their fears, but emphasize that whenever someone avoids things that they fear they may miss out on opportunities for a better outcome. Guided discovery then may involve encouraging the couple to use expressive and empathic listening skills to discuss a hierarchy of topics that begin with ones they agree are benign. As they experience success with this behavioral experiment, it moves on to more uncomfortable topics, including those identified as most threatening. Direct experience of a positive process and outcome reduces their negative thoughts about communicating.

Another approach to guided discovery experiences involves focusing the couple on information from past interactions with each other that contradict their cognitions. Regarding Carissa and Steve's shared negative expectancy that discussing their differences will backfire, the therapist can ask them to recall any past instances in which they were at least partly successful in having such discussions. This is consistent with a CBCT focus on identifying conditions that have been conducive to more positive couple interactions (Epstein & Baucom, 2002; Epstein & Falconier, 2024), as well as a solution-focused therapy identification of exceptions to a problem (see Chapter 11).

Finally, a therapist can draw a couple's attention to a circular pattern in which they influence each other's negative responses, to increase their circular causal thinking (Epstein & Baucom, 2002) and see opportunities to change the dyadic pattern by responding differently to their partner. This experience can increase optimism that one can influence what appeared to be an unchangeable relationship.

Interventions for Emotion

Intimate relationships have the potential to be a source of very positive emotional experiences but also can elicit intense emotional distress. A CBCT model concurs with Greenberg and Goldman's (2008) emotionally focused therapy (EFT) premise that partners co-regulate each other's positive and negative emotional states, and for distressed couples, interventions are needed that can modify the co-regulation. Some interventions for emotions focus on each partner's individual internal processes (in the tradition of Beck's cognitive therapy) whereas others address dyadic processes. CBCT authors (e.g., Baucom & Epstein, 1990; Baucom et al., 2023; Baucom et al., 2020; Epstein & Baucom, 2002; Epstein & Falconier, 2024) have differentiated between two major goals of interventions for emotion: those intended to increase awareness and expression of inhibited emotions and those intended to moderate the experience and expression of poorly regulated emotions.

Both types of intervention begin with psychoeducation regarding emotions and factors that influence them: their partner's actions, their thoughts about the meaning of those actions, and their ability to regulate the intensity of the emotional responses. The therapist also can note that emotional responses are normal and alert an individual that something important is affecting their life, often regarding degrees to which their personal needs are being met. Positive emotions commonly signify that needs such as attachment, control over one's life, security, and validation from others are being met, whereas negative emotions likely indicate that important needs currently are unmet. The therapist can propose that the couple has discussions to uncover what each partner's emotional responses suggest about their needs, and changes that could be made to address unmet needs better.

A variety of factors that can interfere with awareness and outward expression of emotions can be addressed with CBCT interventions. Some cognitions such as expectancies (e.g., that expressing one's feelings to one's partner will be met with indifference or criticism; that allowing oneself to feel even a mild emotion will lead to a breakdown in self-control) and standards (e.g., that feeling and expressing emotions constitutes personal weakness) can lead to inattention to cues of one's feelings, or a failure to tell others about them. Behavioral and cognitive avoidance (learned ways of steering one's attention away from situations that elicit emotions) also can operate automatically, without a person planning them. Furthermore, some individuals tend to "somaticize" their negative emotions, feeling them as physical symptoms (e.g., nausea, fatigue, body aches), sometimes based on cultural traditions that foster that mode of emotional expression. Finally, members of some couples exhibit difficulty experiencing and expressing positive emotions regarding their relationships. Planalp et al. (2018) stress the need to help those couples develop strategies to enhance shared positive emotional experiences in daily life.

In contrast to inhibition of emotions, individuals may have difficulty moderating their experience and outward expression of strong emotions such as anger and anxiety, and clinical assessment and treatment of emotion dysregulation has become prominent in mental health fields (e.g., Linehan, 2015). In couple therapy, individual partners each can learn ways that work best for them for moderating their emotional responses, but therapists also must intervene with the co-regulation process (Greenberg & Goldman, 2008) by attuning the couple to the patterns whereby they reciprocate and amplify each other's negative emotional states. They then can practice ways to collaborate on interrupting such cycles. The affective component of Carissa and Steve's argument over cat litter is an example of specific experiences they and their therapist can use to practice **de-escalation co-regulation processes** (e.g., pointing out signs that their emotional intensity is rising and agreeing to implement strategies such as a brief "time out" to separate and cool down, and joint self-soothing activities such as muscle relaxation, taking a quiet walk together, etc.). It also can be helpful for the couple to communicate about a partner's experience that led to a negative emotion, with the upset person using constructive expression skills and the other person using empathic listening to demonstrate caring and respect for their partner's feelings.

Case Transcript

In CBCT, the first joint session with a couple is primarily to establish a positive therapeutic alliance, provide them with information about typical processes that occur in CBCT sessions, answer questions they may have about the therapy or therapist, gather information about the history and current functioning of their relationship, and begin to set treatment goals to address their presenting concerns. Although some preliminary interventions often occur, that session is not representative of typical CBCT sessions that emphasize interventions. The initial assessment also includes an individual session with each partner to collect information about their individual history (family of origin, peer relations, academic performance, job history, prior romantic relationships, psychological functioning and any prior therapy, physical health), current individual functioning, and any concerns about risks regarding pursuing conjoint therapy (e.g., partner aggression). It is assumed that assessment is an ongoing process, as a couple may reveal new information as they become more comfortable with the therapist, and the therapist might notice an aspect of their interactions that had not been obvious previously.

Because assessment sessions are different from ongoing therapy sessions, this case description begins with a brief description of the therapist's interactions with Carissa and Steve during the couple assessment and then transitions to a detailed description of a subsequent intervention session.

Initial Joint Assessment Session

For the sake of describing topics covered in the couple assessment interview concisely, they are listed in bullet-point format. More detailed descriptions can be found in books such as Epstein & Baucom (2002) and Epstein & Falconier (2024).

- Review of the informed consent form previously sent to each partner and returned to the therapist
- Therapist's overview of the CBCT model, goals, and common interventions, therapist's professional background and qualifications
- Open-ended questions about concerns that brought them to couple therapy for which they would like assistance
- Questions about the history of the relationship, from how they met, what attracted them to each other, the process of becoming seriously involved, events that affected their relationship either positively or negatively, similarities and differences in partners' social identities (race, ethnicity, immigration/citizenship, gender, sexual orientation, religion, ability, socioeconomic status [SES], etc.), activities they share in life and those they pursue individually, when and how they first noticed they were having difficulties, and how they tried to deal with their concerns
- Identification of initial goals for couple therapy, with preferences of both partners represented (with the option for the therapist to suggest other possible goals based on information the couple presented during the assessment)

This assessment would have uncovered information about the individual histories of Carissa and Steve including family-of-origin relationships, academic and employment histories, social relationships, the development of their relationship (including differences in their racial backgrounds and interactions with each partner's family), conflict over Steve's relationships with his friends, the impact of infertility and its treatment on their relationship, their communication and problem-solving patterns, and each person's goals for therapy. At the end of the session, the therapist would summarize what was learned during the assessment and propose that for homework (a typical component of CBCT) the couple review the goals and think of any they would like to modify or add. This couple agreed on the following goals:

1 Reduce the frequency and intensity of their arguments.
2 Improve their communication for expressing thoughts and emotions and for listening in a respectful manner to gain deep understanding of each other's experiences, preferences and goals.
3 Improve their problem-solving skills and dyadic coping skills for working as a team to resolve issues between them and stressful experiences from outside their relationship.
4 Improve their overall intimacy.

Subsequent CBCT Intervention Session

Therapist: Hi Carissa and Steve. I would like to begin our session by agreeing on what we'll try to cover, including topics I have in mind and things you'd like to discuss. I find that setting an agenda helps reduce the chance that we'd get to the end of a session and realize that we didn't discuss something important. I'd like to begin with both of you giving me a brief update on how things have been between the two of you since our last session. That kind of update is something I'd like to continue in all our sessions. I'd also like to review the goals that you proposed for our couple therapy, see if you want to revise them, and decide together where to begin. I'd also like to hear if there's anything else you'd like to spend time on.

Setting a session agenda is a common component of cognitive-behavioral therapies, as it creates some structure for using the time well. It is a flexible guide, and therapists make decisions to stray from the agenda based on the ongoing process (e.g., if a member of a couple becomes very upset, or partners become entrenched in opposing goals or perceptions, more time would be spent addressing those processes). Topics that are not addressed can be postponed to a subsequent session.

Carissa: The week was mixed for me. I felt good that we both acknowledged we have problems and want to do something about it. Knowing we agreed on that resulted in minimal arguing this week, which was a relief. The part that upset me is when we discussed goals that we discussed with you, we have different priorities. Steve wants less pressure from me about important issues such as infertility treatment and how much we share time, while I want a closer connection in which we are best friends and share values and goals. As soon as we started talking about our goals, it got tense. I could see him stiffen up and avoid eye contact, and my anxiety shot up about whether we want the same things. We never did finish the discussion about shared goals.

Therapist: Thanks for giving me your impressions, Carissa. Steve, I'd like to hear from you about how the week seemed to go, and how you felt about your discussion with Carissa regarding goals for therapy. If you agree with aspects of how she described it, do mention those, as well as any different views you have.

Steve: Sure. I agree with Carissa that we both know we've developed some problems and are less happy together than we were earlier, and we both care about each other and our relationship. What frustrates me is that it feels like her goal is to get me to want our relationship to be the way she prefers. It's not like "My way or the highway," but I don't see much flexibility on her part. For example, when I've felt stressed and kind of burned out about the huge expenses and efforts of trying to have a baby, she makes it seem like she's the only one who really cares about having a family. This tense atmosphere really gets to me, and she's right that I find it so upsetting and feel so helpless that I just shut down. I don't want to be one of those couples who fight and fight for years, or who have a nasty divorce. I understand why you asked us to discuss the goals so we could be ready to settle on some with you, but it did not go well.

Therapist: Thanks Steve. It's important for both of you to express not only how you behaved with each other, but how you were thinking and feeling about it. I can see your relationship is important to both of you and the shift from happier times in the past to the present conflict is unsettling. This seems especially upsetting to both of you because you have the impression that you are in a stalemate about what you want in your relationship. I'm hearing from both of you that you feel helpless to get unstuck when your discussions deteriorate. That escalation of conflict and logjam in discussing areas of conflict seem to have occurred again this past week when you did your homework of reviewing goals for therapy. Have I gotten the right impression?

Both partners nod in agreement. It is important for the therapist to model empathic listening so they feel heard, and to communicate a desire for feedback from the couple about the therapist's perceptions of their relationship. If the couple reply that a therapist's observations seem off the mark, the therapist invites them to describe their own observations. In addition, the therapist tries to find a general goal the partners can share, in spite of the differences they described.

Therapist (continuing): Based on our discussions so far, it seems that the two of you have been experiencing two types of difficulties. The first type is that you have some conflicting preferences about how to handle aspects of your relationship, including time together versus with friends and what to do about your infertility problems. The conflict about friends has existed for a long time, whereas the conflict about infertility treatment is more recent but has become more intense due to the stress it has placed on your daily life and finances. You've mentioned some other challenges such as how to interact with Steve's dad or how to cope with some other racially-oriented discrimination experiences you've had as a couple, but the first two are the ones that have stood out in our discussions so far. Does that seem to be true to you, or do you see it differently?

Both partners express agreement with the therapist's formulation.

Therapist: OK. Because those are very stressful issues in your relationship, you share a goal of finding ways of resolving them—overcoming the stalemates. Is that so?

Both partners nod in agreement.

Therapist: I know it has been difficult for you to discuss those two issues, so I am wondering whether you have any concerns about us spending time on them in couple therapy, such as that talking about them here will make things worse if more of the same upsetting interactions take place.

Steve: That's exactly what my concern is—will this just get us more upset with each other and hopeless?

Carissa: I know we need to do something about those issues, because they aren't just going away, but I do worry whether sessions here will be more of the same.

Therapist: That's a very natural and reasonable concern, because this is so painful for both of you, and at this point, it may be hard to imagine being able to discuss and improve your conflicts. I see my role as guiding you in being able to talk about issues here in ways that feel positive and hopeful, and to quickly jump in and interrupt negative interactions. It will be important for you to feel comfortable giving me feedback at any point if what we are doing is making you very uncomfortable, so we can do something about it. Does that help at all with your concerns? I imagine you won't fully believe that until you see it happen in our sessions.

The partners both laugh a bit and say that they do want to proceed and hope the therapist is correct.

Therapist (continuing): The second type of difficulty you seem to be having, which is related to your concerns that we just discussed, is that your ways of communicating and trying to solve those problems have been ineffective and actually have increased the tension and frustration between you. That's why in our couple assessment interview you set goals of improving your abilities to communicate and do joint problem-solving that will feel much more supportive of each other and more effective. Our sessions together can focus on developing those ways of discussing challenging issues that will not only make you feel better about your relationship, but also make progress in dealing with the challenges. I'd like to hear what each of you thinks about a plan like that.

In CBCT, a therapist's level of talking varies considerably, based on the stage of therapy. Early on, as in this example, the therapist has collected a good deal of information about the couple's presenting concerns and interaction patterns through empathic listening and observations of the couple during sessions. The therapist then provides feedback, including psychoeducation about sources of "primary distress" they described (e.g., conflict between their preferences for time together versus independent activities) and sources of "secondary distress" (e.g., mutual criticism, withdrawal) when they discuss those areas of conflict, which fail to resolve the conflicts and instead exacerbate their negative perceptions of their relationship (Epstein & Baucom, 2002). Asking the couple about their thoughts regarding this educational information makes this a collaborative exchange in which the partners need not agree with the therapist's observations, but they become actively engaged in observing their interactions, identifying patterns that are interfering with resolving problems, and begin to consider new options. It involves broadening their cognitions about each other and their relationship, paves the way for the therapist to suggest trying some different actions toward each other, and has potential to reduce their hopelessness about their relationship.

Carissa:	I do think that makes sense, that it is the way we communicate when we disagree about something that makes it a lot worse, even with small issues like the cat litter. When it's a really big deal, like what we're going to do about becoming parents, either failing to talk or just bickering gets me even more upset.
Steve:	I agree. But when Carissa keeps insisting that we talk more about those issues, it feels like she wants to pressure me into accepting her way of doing things, and I get frustrated and want to avoid her.
Carissa:	Oh, that's just great, Steve! Blame it all on me and paint me as a bully. I wouldn't keep trying to start discussions with you if we even got anywhere before you took off!
Therapist:	Excuse me, but I feel a need to interrupt this—something I try to do tactfully but firmly if it looks like things are deteriorating and there's an opportunity for the three of us to look at what's happening and see if it can go in a more positive direction.

It does not take much for one member's remark to start an adversarial exchange if the other member perceives it as critical and blaming, whether or not the speaker intended it to be so. The therapist uses it in an experiential way to draw the couple's attention to the rapid shift in their way of viewing each other, the resulting emotional responses, and an escalation of negative behavior. The emphasis of the therapist's input is on the partners' mutual influences on each other's negative cognitions, emotions, and behavior, interrupting that process, and redirecting the couple toward more constructive communication.

Therapist (continuing):	Carissa, you seemed to have a strong reaction to Steve mentioning that he perceives your trying to initiate conversations about issues as you pressuring him to view it your way, and when he interprets it that way, he has an urge to withdraw. Please describe what it was about his comment that upset you. We are going to focus more in this session on developing your skills as a couple to express your thoughts and emotions to each other and to be good listeners, but first this looks to me like a good opportunity for the two of you to step back a little and become aware of what happens that quickly shifts you from talking in a relaxed way to being upset with each other and interacting negatively, as just happened. So, Carissa, what went through your mind when Steve said that, and what emotions did you feel suddenly?
Carissa:	I felt angry that he blames me for our trouble communicating about issues, describing me as a bully and him as an innocent victim, like

	he has no part in it. You may remember that when I brought up the issue of the cat litter, he made it clear that he didn't care about how unpleasant the smell is for me.
Steve:	Wait a minute, just because…
Therapist (interrupting Steve):	Just a minute, Steve. I understand that you may disagree with Carissa's description of your intentions and behavior. However, in our sessions I would like to stop the two of you from quickly escalating an argument, as I think was beginning to happen just now. The needs, intentions, emotions, and behavior of both of you are very important, but if you quickly deteriorate into an argument, none of those get the attention they deserve. I see my role early in our therapy as being to interrupt the usual arguments that you both said you want to eliminate, slow down the process, look closely together at the sequence between you, and try some different ways of responding to each other that lead to mutual understanding. Early on, I may need to stop the action between you somewhat often, but after a while, you'll be able to stop the arguments yourselves and shift into good communication that we'll practice. How do you each feel about me taking that role?
Steve:	Sounds OK to me. I'm sick of the bickering.
Therapist:	OK, Steve, but since Carissa got the impression a few minutes ago that you were saying her behavior is the whole problem, can you clarify if by "bickering" you mean only her talking negatively to you, or that both of you communicate in ways that seem to pour fuel on the fire?
Steve:	No, it's not just her. I can get pretty cold and unsympathetic when we argue, so I'm part of it too.
Therapist:	OK. Willingness on both your parts to look at contributions you can make personally to communicate better will go a long way toward building a partnership in improving your relationship. Carissa, how are you feeling about my approach to doing a little coaching to shift the two of you away from getting set off by each other and toward communicating how you'd like your relationship to look? That would apply to small disagreements such as how to manage cat litter and large issues such as balancing time apart with time together and how to proceed from here regarding efforts to have a child? That will involve looking at how each of you expresses what you'd like from each other in a way that is sensitive to the other's feelings too.
Carissa:	It's clear that we do need a mediator at this point, because our discussions fall apart fast, which we both find really frustrating and demoralizing. Sure, that's a good plan.
Therapist:	So, thinking back to what just happened between you, how would the two of you describe specific aspects of your own thoughts, emotions, and behavior that influenced the eruption of an argument? You can mention particular actions of the other person, but let's avoid making assumptions about the other person's thoughts and emotions that you couldn't see. It would be fine to say something like "My partner said X, and that led me to get angry because I interpreted that

statement as a sign that my partner didn't care about my feelings." That statement describes your observation of the other person's behavior and *your own* interpretation and associated emotion. However, it acknowledges that you are making an assumption about your partner's intentions that needs to be checked for accuracy. Your partner will then have an opportunity to tell you about the reasons for their behavior.

The therapist's goal is to encourage the partners to take an active role as "participant observers" of their couple interactions, and to distinguish between an observation of a partner's actions and one's own subjective interpretation of those actions. The therapist uses opportunities during sessions to guide the couple in noticing circular interaction processes between them as well as each person's cognitions and emotional responses that mediate between one person's action and the other's behavioral response to it. The goal is to shift partners' tendencies to think in linear causal terms ("My partner's pursuing me to discuss issues makes me withdraw") to circular causal thinking ("We are locked in a pattern in which the more my partner pursues me for discussion, the more I cope by withdrawing, and the more I withdraw, the more my partner copes by trying to get me to talk."). In CBCT, the therapist also is likely to describe stream-of-consciousness "automatic thoughts" that naturally enter people's minds, and that serve as their reality in the moment unless evidence disconfirms them.

Carissa: What I noticed is that when you asked about our communication patterns, I started by saying we have difficulty as a couple, but Steve's response focused on complaining about my part in pursuing him and suggesting that I want to control him. It reminded me of how when I have asked him to spend more time with me because I'd like to feel more connection between us, he also said that I want to control him. At this point I have little tolerance for him accusing me of being controlling, when I feel lonely and just long for more closeness with my husband. I got angry and criticized him for blaming me and for suggesting I have such ugly motives. Usually at that point we give up trying to talk.

Steve: I agree I'm very sensitive to Carissa's pursuing me to talk about issues. I immediately become tense and irritated and want to get away from her, and I can see that my response comes across as disrespectful or uncaring. When I say that she wants to control me, it's because she has strong opinions about what we should do and interrupts and debates me rather than listening to my ideas and feelings. She's very smart and can out-talk me any day.

Therapist: Steve, I appreciate that you are paying attention to the reactions you have to Carissa's communication style and how they lead you to want to withdraw. I also think it was helpful that you stated that you tend to feel out-talked by her, because if in general you feel at a disadvantage in your discussions, it's not surprising that you have an urge to withdraw. I think it will be useful for us to explore further your perception about that and where your view of being at a disadvantage may have come from. So, from what both of you have described, the way you communicate about issues ends up making both of you feel like the other person isn't trying to understand your point of view. I think it would be very helpful if we spend some time in our sessions practicing communication skills for expressing your thoughts and emotions clearly while your partner listens closely to understand your experience, and reflects back that empathy. I find that when couples communicate that way, they feel understood and respected by each other, even if at times they still disagree. Nobody talks like that all the time, but being able to use those skills when discussing a tough topic can feel very good. Demonstrating understanding and respect for each other's perspective makes it easier to discuss ways to solve a problem such as balancing togetherness and independence. How do you both feel about spending time in our sessions focusing on communicating in that way?

Both partners acknowledge that their current communication pattern is frustrating and unproductive, and they would like the therapist to guide them in improving their communication skills.

Therapist: I want to mention another topic that both of you described during our assessment interviews, that may have influenced your communication patterns, and that's your personal histories, especially growing up in your families. I got the impression that neither of your sets of parents provided a model of open and constructive communication. Steve, your parents had severe conflict that led to divorce, and Carissa, although your parents re-united after separation, you never saw any evidence of how they resolved the problems between them. In addition, your own experiences of arguing a lot over even small issues may have added to your concern about the potential for understanding each other and solving problems. It may be a relief to you to see that you actually can develop positive ways of communicating with each other.

Both partners nod in agreement and comment on the poor communication they witnessed, and that those experiences left them uneasy about the potential for a couple to resolve painful issues. They also agree that their own history of frustrating discussions has resulted in their pessimism about their relationship.

Therapist: I'm mentioning this because practicing expressive and listening skills in our sessions and applying them at home is very valuable, but may take you a bit out of your comfort zone. I'd like both of you to be aware of your feelings as we work on communication and to share them so we can help you deal with them. In the approach to couple therapy that I emphasize, paying attention to one's emotions and thoughts is very valuable, because our emotions and thoughts influence us a lot, including making communication uncomfortable.

I want to note to the reader that as the therapist, I am thinking that another factor that may be influencing the tension regarding their communication was reflected in Steve's comment that Carissa is very smart and can out-talk him, which I mentioned to Steve. I am thinking that his perception of a difference in intelligence and communication ability between them also may have been shaped by their different levels of academic and career success. At this point, I choose to place these hypotheses "on the back burner" rather than potentially overloading the couple with issues in this session and potentially triggering Steve's shaky self-concept. This material can be introduced in a later session, especially when the couple has had success communicating and both partners have felt empathy from the other. I also have developed a hypothesis that Carissa and Steve are upset about their conflict regarding the amount of time Steve spends with his friends, but for different reasons associated with underlying schemas or beliefs tied to core needs. Steve tends to interpret Carissa's efforts to motivate him to spend more time with her as power plays, which seem partly associated with his belief that she has a power advantage over him. In contrast, Carissa tends to interpret Steve's involvement with his friends as indicating his limited emotional availability to her, perhaps associated with her having either a general pre-existing insecure attachment schema (working model) or insecurity specific to their relationship that developed as he withdrew from her repeatedly. At this early point, I would not focus on these potential underlying factors but would probe for power and attachment themes (and associated emotional responses such as anger and anxiety) when the partners express thoughts that they experience as they communicate during sessions. This probing can involve a cognitive therapy technique such as the "downward arrow." For example:

"Carissa, when Steve informs you that he planned an activity with his friends without checking your schedule, what meaning does that have for you?" "It means he's more interested in spending time with them than with me." "And if that is true, what would that mean to you?" "It means that I'm alone in this world, with no one who loves me and who I can count on.".

Carissa: At this point, and maybe I'm speaking for both of us, I'm very uneasy about trying to discuss the issues in our relationship and I think we need a third party like you to monitor and guide us. (*Steve nods in agreement*)

Therapist: That's fine. Many couples I have worked with have felt uneasy at the beginning about trying to have discussions without a mediator, and my goal is by providing some feedback and guidance to help them develop confidence that they can monitor and control their interactions on their own. The three of us can watch your skills and ability to communicate well without input from me improve over time.

Another process the therapist must monitor is the couple's ability to regulate negative emotions such as anger, and intervene to improve anger management as needed. At this point, the therapist has heard about the argument regarding cat litter, which seemed to involve mild to moderate anger, and has also observed the couple exhibiting cues of fairly mild anger in their exchange regarding Steve's focus on what he viewed as Carissa's intention to control him. Thus, anger management skills would be included in some CBCT sessions. However, at this point, the therapist is likely only to mention that there were some cues of anger on both members' parts, ask them how intense the emotion was (e.g., on a 0 to 10 scale), and also ask them how intense the anger has been when they have argued at home. The decision about when to include anger management in sessions would be based on an evaluation of the current risk for levels of anger that could interfere with constructive communication and even elicit partner aggression (Epstein & Falconier, 2024).

Therapist: Both of you told me about some uncomfortable experiences with racial discrimination in our earlier interviews. Some couples who experience discrimination find that it puts stress on them as individuals and as a couple, but I'm not assuming that's a significant issue for you. Because your focus has been on how well you got along as a couple and not on concerns about other people, I'm not sure if it would be helpful for us to spend some time on it, but we certainly can.

Carissa: Growing up as a Black person in a vastly White area and going to predominantly White schools, I had lots of good relationships with White people, but definitely experienced discrimination, especially what people refer to as micro-aggressions. It's never all that far from my consciousness, but I do try to focus on having a good life, and Steve and I have taken that approach too. I see value in discussing ways to make sure others' negativity doesn't affect us. What do you think about it, Steve?

Steve: I can get pretty angry when I see people expressing their prejudices, and when someone like my dad basically says we can't be successful, it eats at me. That does cross my mind when we are arguing. Maybe there are some negative voices in my head that make me want to withdraw.

Therapist: It sounds like both of you think putting that on our agenda during some sessions could be helpful. However, just like I asked about your other goals, I want to check on any concerns either of you have about pursuing it.

Steve: My main concern is getting through all of this. Like when I feel upset about reactions from people like my dad, I haven't wanted to tell you about it, Carissa, because I fear it'll just get you upset.

Carissa: I know what you mean, but maybe we can gain strength as a couple in developing ways to face those stresses together rather than each having private feelings about them but not talking about it.

Therapist: I like the way you just discussed this challenging topic together. If you choose to include it as a goal, we can make sure we focus on how to support each other and face stressful experiences as a team. Would you like me to add it to our goals list or hold off for now?

Carissa: Adding it sounds good to me.

Steve: Me too.

Therapist: OK. I'll add it to our list, and we can figure out when to spend time on it. For now, I'd like to go over communication guidelines for expressing thoughts and emotions, and for being a good listener. I have some handouts that list the guidelines, and after we discuss them, we can spend some time during the rest of this session starting to practice them. I prefer starting with discussions of topics that are not stressful or about areas of conflict before moving on to the more challenging ones you face, so you can develop confidence in your skills. We certainly will get to talking about your core issues before long. How does that sound?

The therapist has noted that the couple described some discrimination experiences, including a prediction of failure from Steve's father, so it was appropriate to propose it as another goal for couple therapy, as research has indicated that discrimination on the basis of race, sexual orientation, religion, and many other characteristics can have harmful effects on couple relationships (Pittman et al., 2024). In CBCT, the therapist emphasizes collaboration among the therapist and two partners by making a suggestion and exploring the couple's preferences, concerns, etc. The therapist then gives Steve and Carissa handouts with communication guidelines (see Baucom et al., 2020; Epstein & Baucom, 2002; Epstein & Falconier, 2024), explains each expresser and listener guideline and models them for the couple, and answers any questions the partners have about them. Next, each member of the couple selects a benign topic to tell the other about when in the role of expresser (generally that topic does not involve their relationship, such as an issue at one's job) and the therapist coaches the expresser and listener as they practice their roles.

Therapist: It's about time to wrap up today's session. I like to end by summarizing what we covered and get your feedback about what was helpful as well as anything that was not. We'll then decide on something you can do together as homework, to transfer what we've been doing into your daily life.

The therapist then summarized the topics discussed, including therapy goals, a close look at the process that occurs when the couple engages in an argument (their internal thoughts and emotions as well as their behavior toward each other), and finally an introduction to using communication skills. Carissa and Steve both said the session seemed productive in that the goals are central to their life together, and the focus on identifying how their nonproductive arguments develop and how they can substitute positive communication gave them hope that they could overcome their problems. They agreed to review the goals and communication guidelines as homework. The therapist asked them not to try using the communication guidelines on their own yet, allowing for more coaching by the therapist during the next session. If a couple exhibits a good level of ability with the skills during the next session, the therapist will agree to at-home practice with low-conflict topics. Subsequent sessions will include time devoted to communication (and then problem-solving and dyadic coping skills), especially applied to the core issues in the couple's relationship. Partners' individual issues such as family history, self-concept, core conflicts regarding power and attachment, etc., are brought into the therapy process when relevant.

In reviewing this sample session, this writer has some concern that readers may conclude that CBCT clinicians talk a lot more than their clients and are consistently directive rather than observing couple processes and listening to the clients. Therapists do talk a lot during early sessions, due to a focus on psychoeducation about the CBCT model, but also in drawing partners' attention to their interaction patterns, as well as issues in their individual histories that have sensitized them to particular relationship dynamics, and then introducing them to communication skills. The early emphasis on interrupting negative dyadic cycles to reduce stress in the relationship and instill hope for change is typical of CBCT, and it does involve a good deal of therapist activity. However, a core goal is to steadily turn over the initiative to the couple, building their abilities and confidence to have productive and satisfying interactions to resolve relationship issues and increase intimacy.

References

Anderson, H. (2007). The heart and spirit of collaborative therapy: The philosophical stance "A way of being" in relationship and conversation. In H. Anderson & D. Gehart (Eds.), *Collaborative therapy: Relationships and conversations that make a difference* (pp. 43–61). Routledge.

Bandura, A. (1977). *Social learning theory.* Prentice Hall.

Baucom, D. H., & Epstein, N. (1990). *Cognitive-behavioral marital therapy.* Brunner/Mazel.

Baucom, D. H., Epstein, N. B., Fischer, M. S., Kirby, J. S., & LaTaillade, J. J. (2023). Cognitive behavioral couple therapy. In J. L. Lebow & D. K. Snyder (Eds.), *Clinical handbook of couple therapy* (6th ed., pp. 53–78). Guilford Press.

Baucom, D. H., Epstein, N., Rankin, L. A., & Burnett, C. K. (1996). Assessing relationship standards: The Inventory of Specific Relationship Standards. *Journal of Family Psychology, 10,* 72–88.

Baucom, D. H., Fischer, M. S., Corrie, S., Worrell, M., & Boeding, S. E. (2020). *Treating relationship distress and psychopathology in couples: A cognitive-behavioural approach.* Routledge.

Beck, A. T. (1976). *Cognitive therapy and the emotional disorders.* International Universities Press.

Beck, A. T. (1988). *Love is never enough.* Harper and Row.

Beck, J. S. (2020). *Cognitive behavior therapy: Basics and beyond* (3rd ed.). Guilford Press.

Bodenmann, G. (2005). Dyadic coping and its significance for marital functioning. In T. Revenson, K. Kayser, & G. Bodenmann (Eds.), *Couples coping with stress: Emerging perspectives on dyadic coping* (pp. 33–50). American Psychological Association.

Bodenmann, G., Randall, A. K., & Falconier, M. K. (2016). Coping in couples: The systemic transactional model (STM). In M. K. Falconier, A. K. Randall, & G. Bodenmann (Eds.), *Couples coping with stress: A cross-cultural perspective* (pp. 5–22). Routledge.

Bronfenbrenner, U. (1979). *The ecology of human development: Experiments by nature and design.* Harvard University Press.

Chapman, G. D. (2015). *The 5 love languages: The secret to love that lasts.* Northfield Publishing.

Christensen, A., Dimidjian, S., Martell, C. R., & Doss, B. D. (2023). Integrative behavioral couple therapy. In J. L. Lebow & D. K. Snyder (Eds.), *Clinical handbook of couple therapy* (6th ed., pp. 79–103). Guilford Press.

Dattilio, F. M., & Padesky, C. A. (1990). *Cognitive therapy with couples.* Professional Resource Exchange.

Dobson, K. S., Poole, J. C., & Beck, J. S. (2018). The fundamental cognitive model. In R. L. Leahy (Ed.), *Science and practice in cognitive therapy: Foundations, mechanisms, and applications* (pp. 29–47). Guilford Press.

Eidelson, R. J., & Epstein, N. (1982). Cognition and relationship maladjustment: Development of a measure of dysfunctional relationship beliefs. *Journal of Consulting and Clinical Psychology, 50,* 715–720.

Ellis. A. (1962). *Reason and emotion in psychotherapy*. Lyle Stuart.

Ellis, A., Sichel, J. L., Yeager, R. J., DiMattia, D. J., & DiGiuseppe, R. (1989). *Rational-emotive couples therapy.* Pergamon.

Epstein, N. (1982). Cognitive therapy with couples. *American Journal of Family Therapy, 10*(1), 5–16.

Epstein, N., Schlesinger, S. E., & Dryden, W. (Eds.). (1988). *Cognitive-behavioral therapy with families.* Brunner/Mazel.

Epstein, N. B., & Baucom, D. H. (2002). *Enhanced cognitive-behavioral therapy for couples*: A contextual approach. American Psychological Association.

Epstein, N. B., Berger, A. T., Fang, J. J., Messina, L., Smith, J. R., Lloyd, T. D., Fang, X. Y., & Liu, Q. X. (2012). Applying Western-developed family therapy models in China. *Journal of Family Psychotherapy, 23,* 217–237.

Epstein, N. B., Dattilio, F. M., & Baucom, D. H. (2016). Cognitive-behavior couple therapy. In T.L. Sexton, & J. Lebow (Eds.), *Handbook of family therapy* (4th ed., pp. 361–386). Routledge.

Epstein, N. B., & Falconier, M. K. (2024). *Treatment plans and interventions in couple therapy: A cognitive-behavioral approach*. Guilford Press.

Epstein, N. B., Falconier, M. K., & Dattilio, F. M. (2020). Cultural factors in the practice of couple and family therapy. In W. K. Halford, & F. J. R. van de Vijver (Eds.), *Cross-cultural family research and practice* (pp. 479–521). Elsevier.

Epstein, N. B., LaTaillade, J. J., & Werlinich, C. A. (2023). Couple therapy for partner aggression. In J. L. Lebow, & D. K. Snyder (Eds.), *Clinical handbook of couple therapy* (6th ed., pp. 391–412). Guilford Press.Falconier, M. K., Randall, A. K., & Bodenmann, G. (2016). Cultural considerations in understanding dyadic coping across cultures. In M. K. Falconier, A. K., Randall, & G. Bodenmann (Eds.), *Couples coping with stress: A cross-cultural perspective* (pp. 23–35). Routledge.

Fischer, M. S., Baucom, D. H., & Cohen, M. J. (2016). Cognitive-behavioral couple therapies: Review of the evidence for the treatment of relationship distress, psychopathology, and chronic health conditions. *Family Process, 55,* 423–442.

Gottman, J. M. (1979). *Marital interaction: Experimental investigations*. Academic Press.

Gottman, J. M., Notarius, C., Markman, H., Bank, S., Yoppi, B., & Rubin, M. E., (1976). Behavior exchange theory and marital decision making. *Journal of Personality and Social Psychology, 34(1),* 14–23.

Greenberg, L. S., & Goldman, R. N. (2008). *Emotion-focused couples therapy: The dynamics of emotion, love, and power*. American Psychological Association.

Guerney, B. G. (1977). *Relationship enhancement: Skill-training programs for therapy, problem prevention, and enrichment*. Wiley.

Gurman, A. S., & Kniskern, D. P. (1978). Research on marital and family therapy: Progress, perspective, and prospect. In S. L. Garfield & A. E. Bergin (Eds.), *Handbook of psychotherapy and behavior change (*2nd ed., pp. 817–901). Wiley.

Jacobson, N. S., & Christensen, A. (1996). *Integrative couple therapy: Promoting acceptance and change*. Norton.

Jacobson, N. S., & Margolin, G. (1979). *Marital therapy: Strategies based on social learning and behavior exchange principles.* Brunner/Mazel.

Johnson, S.M., Wiebe, S. A., & Allan, R. (2023). Emotionally focused couple therapy. In, J. L. Lebow, & D. K. Snyder (Eds.), *Clinical handbook of couple therapy* (6th ed., pp. 127–150). Guilford Press.

Leahy, R. L. (2015). *Emotional schema therapy*. Guilford Press.

Leahy, R. L. (2017). *Cognitive therapy techniques: A practitioner's guide* (2nd ed.). Guilford Press.

Lebow, J., & Snyder, D. K. (2022). Couple therapy in the 2020s: Current status and emerging developments. *Family Process, 61,* 1359–1385.

Linehan, M. M. (2015). *DBT skills training handouts and worksheets* (2nd ed.). Guilford Press.

Meichenbaum, D. (1977). *Cognitive-behavior modification.* Plenum.

Meichenbaum, D. (1985). *Stress inoculation training*. Pergamon Press.

Nezu, A. M., Nezu, C. M., & Hays, A. M. (2019). Emotion-centered problem-solving therapy. In K. S. Dobson & D. J. A. Dozois (Eds.), *Handbook of cognitive-behavioral therapies* (4th ed., pp. 171–190). Guilford Press.

Northey, W. F. (2002). Characteristics and clinical practices of marriage and family therapists: A national survey. *Journal of Marital and Family Therapy, 28*, 487–494.

Pittman, P. S., Kamp Dush, C., Pratt, K. J., & Wong, J. D. (2024). Interracial couples at risk: Discrimination, well-being, and health. Journal of Family Issues, *45*(2), 303–325.

Planalp, S., Fitness, J., & Fehr, B. A. (2018). The roles of emotion in relationships. In A. L. Vangelisti & D. Perlman (Eds.), *The Cambridge handbook of personal relationships* (2nd ed., pp. 256–267). Cambridge University Press.

Price, S. J., Price, C. A., & McKenry, P. C. (2010). Families coping with change: A conceptual overview. In S. J. Price, C. A. Price, & P. C. McKenry (Eds.), *Families & change: Coping with stressful events and transitions* (4th ed., pp. 1–23). Sage.

Rathus, J. H., & Sanderson, W. C. (1999). *Marital distress: Cognitive behavioral interventions for couples.* Jason Aronson.

Revenstorf, D., Hahlweg, K., Schindler, L., & Vogel, B. (1984). Interaction analysis of marital conflict. In K. Hahlweg & N. S. Jacobson (Eds.), *Marital interaction: Analysis and modification* (pp. 159–181). Guilford Press.

Rizvi, S. L., & King, A. M. (2019). Dialectical behavior therapy. In K. S. Dobson & D. J. A. Dozois (Eds.), *Handbook of cognitive-behavioral therapies* (4th ed., pp. 297–317). Guilford Press.

Skinner, B. F. (1953). *Science and human behavior.* Macmillan.

Skinner, B. F. (1971). *Beyond freedom and dignity.* Knopf.

Sprenkle, D. H., Davis, S. D., & Lebow, J. L. (2009). *Common factors in couple and family therapy.* Guilford Press.

Stuart, R. B. (1980). *Helping couples change: A social learning approach to marital therapy.* Guilford Press.

Sue, D. W., & Sue, D. (2003). *Counseling the culturally diverse: Theory and practice* (4th ed.). Wiley.

Thibaut, J. W., & Kelley, H. H. (1959). *The social psychology of groups.* Wiley.

Weiss, R. L., Hops, H., & Patterson, G. R. (1973). A framework for conceptualizing marital conflict, a technology for altering it, some data for evaluating it. In L. A. Hamerlynck, L. C. Handy, & E. J. Mash (Eds.), *Behavior change: Methodology, concepts and practice* (pp. 309–342). Research Press.

7 Structural Couple Therapy

Michael D. Reiter

History of the Model

Structural family therapy was developed by Salvador Minuchin, and colleagues, in the 1960s and 1970s, with continued growth and adaptation of the model until the present. This theory of therapy primarily highlights how the whole family system functions, with the couple being but one subsystem. Thus, structural couple therapy is not a clear couple's modality, as it was derived from structural family therapy (Simon, 2015). However, the main tenets of the model work quite well when engaging just the couple subsystem. So, what makes couple therapy structural? Couple therapy can be called structural when it focuses on the dynamics occurring between the couple members as well as shifting the boundaries between and around them (Nichols & Minuchin, 1999).

Salvador Minuchin was born into a Jewish family in a rural village in Argentina during a time when there was high antisemitism. This led to many physical fights with other children regarding his Jewishness, leaving him experiencing the impact of being a member of a minority and challenging the unfairness that can occur from it (Minuchin & Nichols, 1993). This challenging identity was firmed when he participated in the student uprisings against the Argentinian dictator, General Juan Perón (Minuchin et al., 2021). He was jailed for three months and expelled from the university he was attending. Because of this, he had to complete his medical schooling in Uruguay.

When Israel was recognized as a nation in 1948, Minuchin moved there and became a medical officer in the Israeli Army. After Israel's War of Independence, he moved to New York City to specialize in child psychiatry. He was a stranger in a strange land, having a minority experience in this new country. During his first year in the United States, he met Pat, a child psychologist, whom he married and who became very influential in his understanding of children, child-rearing, and working with child agencies (Minuchin et al., 1998).

Minuchin was then hired at the Wiltwyck School for Boys in the 1960s. Here, he and his team worked with adolescent males who were involved in the judicial system (Minuchin et al., 2021). Most of these youth were African American or Hispanic boys from Harlem, and all came from families on welfare. The school was several hours away from New York City. Over the course of a year or so the boys made significant improvements in their behavior. However, upon returning home, many of them went back to engaging in their previous problematic behavior. This led to Minuchin and his colleagues switching to the emerging family therapy practice of the time (Minuchin et al., 1967). Minuchin traveled the country and met with the leaders of this emerging field. On one such trip to Palo Alto, California, to talk with the therapists at the Mental Research Institute, he met Jay Haley (founder of Strategic therapy), who later joined him at the Philadelphia Child Guidance Clinic (PCGC). The two collaborated for about 10 years and for a time people talked about the integration of these two models as structural-strategic family therapy.

In the mid-1960s Minuchin became Director of the PCGC. The beginning of his leadership was a bit rocky as he challenged the standing expectations and processes, a common theme in

DOI: 10.4324/9781003369097-7

Minuchin's life that became the hallmark of structural therapy. A few years later, the PCGC became the most significant institution for the dissemination of family therapy. Many of the field's most influential family therapists, such as Carl Whitaker, Murray Bowen, and Virginia Satir, spent time visiting and training at the PCGC. During this time, Minuchin published his most groundbreaking book, *Families and Family Therapy* (Minuchin, 1974/2012) and then the follow-up book, *Family Therapy Techniques* (Minuchin & Fishman, 1981). These two books each sold over 500,000 copies and were, for many new family therapists, their first exposure to the field. Minuchin stepped down as Director of the PCGC in 1976 and left in 1981 when he started the Family Studies Institute, and provided training and consultation. When Minuchin eventually retired, the Family Studies Institute was renamed The Minuchin Center for the Family, which is still providing training in structural therapy.

The structural model has maintained its foundation but has grown and expanded in a variety of ways, influencing models such as ecosystemic structural family therapy (Lindblad-Goldberg & Northey, 2013), intensive structural therapy (Fishman, 1993) and brief strategic family therapy (Szapocznik & Hervis, 2020), which uses structural therapy as its foundation to work with adolescents experiencing substance abuse and problem behaviors. In 2007, the model was expanded to include a structural exploration of the past, which expanded the temporal landscape the structural therapist used to understand people's current ways of relating to one another (Minuchin et al., 2007).

Structural theory, as applied to couples, has the advantageous factor of maintaining an understanding of an ecosystemic perspective (Aponte & DiCesare, 2000). That is, it understands not just an individual or just the couple. It factors into its assessment each person, the couple as a dyad, and the couple's social context. The structural therapist attempts to understand how each of these pieces comes together to form the organization of the couple at present.

Conceptualization of Problem Formation

People tend to have a very individualistic view of behaviors, which leads them to come to therapy with a perception of *who* is the problem rather than *how people come together* being the problem (Minuchin et al., 2021). In a couple, one will think things would be better if the other just stopped doing something they think is problematic or did something more that they think will be beneficial. Steve thinks that if Carissa just laid off of him on things like when to scoop the litter or calmed down about having a child, their relationship would be just fine. Carissa thinks that if Steve spent less time with his friends and more time with her and was more motivated to conceive a child, their relationship would be better.

In relationships, one of the reasons that problems maintain themselves is that people do not accept or recognize their own role in the pattern but rather continue to blame someone else (Minuchin & Nichols, 1998). They fail to look at what happens between people. That is, they operate from a position of cause-and-effect where the other person does something that leads them to react. Carissa yells at Steve and Steve feels attacked. Steve goes out with his friends on Saturday and Carissa feels betrayed. Neither is fully able to see the **mutuality** that occurs between them. They tend to see the "I" and the "You," but not the "We"—the mutual constraints that they put on each other (Minuchin, 1974/2012).

The way that people come together in relationships is viewed as its **structure**. Minuchin (1974/2012) explained, "Family members relate according to certain arrangements, which govern their transactions. These arrangements, though usually not explicitly stated or even recognized, form a whole—the structure of the family" (p. 68). These patterns then become predictable and recurrent (Minuchin et al., 1998). This structure stays fairly constant because it is supported by people's actions. People know how to be in a relationship based on the variety of overt and covert rules of interaction. Thus, a couple's structure is held together through the connection between members who hold spots in one or more subsystems that have connection and separation from one another. How this plays out leads to a certain hierarchy that leads people to develop certain relational identities over the course of the family life cycle.

Subsystems

Families are comprised of multiple **subsystems**, with the spousal, parental, and sibling subsystems being of the utmost importance (Minuchin & Fishman, 1981). The couple is but one of a variety of subsystems in a family system. When they have children, the two people will likely comprise the spousal and the parental subsystems. However, they are also connected to each person's family-of-origin, leaving them to be a subsystem of at least two larger systems.

Many couples have difficulty when there is too much closeness between one member and another member in their larger family. For instance, Carissa has been spending a lot of time with her family, engaging in potential triangulation between herself, Steve, and her mother. Steve, on the other hand, has tried to place more rigid boundaries between himself, Carissa, and his father.

Thus, the couple (and any subsystem) must find ways to be able to be autonomous while staying in connection to the other subsystems of that family as well as various systems outside of the direct family (e.g., school, work, extended family, church, etc.). Minuchin and Fishman (1981) stated, "One of the spouse subsystem's most vital tasks is the development of boundaries that protect the spouses, giving them an area for the satisfaction of their own psychological needs without the intrusion of in-laws, children, and others" (p. 17). Many times, problems develop in a couple because there is too much overlap between the couple subsystem and another subsystem in their relational field. For a lot of couples, this comes from having a very close relationship between one partner and their parent and/or sibling. This leaves the other partner to have an experience of being intruded upon. Further, the couple then does not fully learn how to have individuation as a unit. While parents or siblings tend to be the primary outside units that may impinge on the couple subsystem, friends, work, substance abuse, etc., may also play a role. For the Hogarths, Carissa's family is one larger system that has a significant impact on the couple subsystem. However, Steve's friends are another larger system that is having a serious influence on the couple's functioning.

Boundaries

The way to maintain a subsystem is through the designation of boundaries. These **boundaries** are based on rules of who can participate in that subsystem and how (Minuchin, 1974/2012). These rules allow that subsystem to complete whatever functions it needs to. This can present difficulties when other people/subsystems make demands on it. Minuchin (1974/2012) explained that "the capacity for complementary accommodation between spouses requires freedom from interference by in-laws and children, and sometimes by the extrafamilial" (p. 40). This is the first task that a couple must successfully accomplish; the development of a boundary that protects them from too much influence of outside systems (Nichols & Minuchin, 1999).

There are three potential boundaries that are connected across a continuum where functioning at the extreme poles can lead to interpersonal difficulties (Minuchin, 1974/2012). These boundaries are rigid, clear, and diffuse. **Rigid boundaries** do not let a lot of information flow back-and-forth and thus these relationships are described as **disengaged**. In couples, this may take the form of not communicating much or having little emotional connection or involvement with one another. Between the couple and other systems, this might manifest in not disclosing too much information about what is happening within the couple. For the Hogarths, there are two main ways that rigid boundaries are occurring. First, Steve and Carissa do not tell Steve's family much of what is happening in their relationship. They are likely to hold back information and divert attempts at interference and influence. Second, there is growing disengagement between Steve and Carissa. While they might be around each other in the house, they are finding that their emotional connection to one another is lessening, and they are finding it difficult to have open conversations with one another about this.

On the other side of the continuum, **diffuse boundaries** blur the distinctions between people/ subsystems. Information is readily given and influence between people is high. Diffuse boundaries lead to a relationship of closeness, which is called **enmeshment**. In these relationships, people know each other's business and look to each other for ideas, suggestions, and advice. In enmeshed relationships, there is usually a lack of personal space and autonomy. Carissa's relationship with her family is more on the diffuse end of the spectrum.

For the most part, boundaries at either end tend to be problematic since the subsystem is either too isolated from connection with or the influence of others (rigid boundaries) or is too connected and not separate enough (diffuse boundaries). However, there may be times when one or the other is useful for the family's current functioning. For instance, parents who have very young children will likely need more rigid boundaries between the parent and child subsystem to ensure the child is safe and healthy. The parents would set the rules (e.g., bedtime, eating, bathing). However, as the child grows, more flexible boundaries help the child learn how to accommodate to outside larger systems. They are able to develop more autonomy, such as being asked for their ideas of what they would like to be picked up at the grocery store for one or more of the meals for that week.

In the middle of rigid and diffuse boundaries are **clear boundaries**, which provide some type of structure with flexibility. Take, for instance, a family with a teenager where the parents set certain rules (such as a curfew), but those rules can be negotiated for certain events (such as staying out a little later to attend the prom). For the Hogarths, there are a variety of clear boundaries, such as those between Steve and his mother and brother. Several years ago, Steve and Carissa seemed to have a clear boundary where they were able to engage in more negotiation of needs and wants between them. This clear boundary has been shifting to become more rigid, which is one of the reasons leading this couple to therapy.

For a new couple, one of the primary boundaries that can become problematic is that between the couple and one or both family-of-origins. Minuchin (1974/2012) stated, "The couple also faces the task of separating from each family of origin and negotiating a different relationship with parents, siblings, and in-laws. Loyalties must shift, for the new spouses' primary commitments are to their marriage" (p. 13). For Steve, this wasn't much of an issue. He had moved away from his family and set boundaries on the more rigid side. He also has some friction with his father, especially with his father's racial beliefs. To protect his relationship with Carissa, he keeps his distance and doesn't share much information or intimacy with his father, which maintains a rigid and disengaged relationship. Carissa, on the other hand, wants to be quite close to her family. She had to learn how to shift from the closeness with her sister and mother to more intimacy with Steve. Thus, she had to move from relationships more on the diffuse/enmeshed side to shift those boundaries to be clearer. However, as she is not experiencing the desired intimacy she wants with Steve, she is finding that she is loosening those boundaries and talking with her family about the issues she is having with Steve. When couples are experiencing disengagement there is usually some type of enmeshment between one member and someone outside of the dyad (Nichols & Minuchin, 1999). This usually happens because the disengaged couple is not addressing the conflict happening between them.

In conducting a structural therapy assessment of the couple, the therapist won't just see the couple as enmeshed or disengaged since couples tend to have more than one interactional style (Wilk & Storm, 1991). These styles may change based on the particular developmental task that the couple is currently facing. Some of these tasks include negotiating new relationships with each member's family-of-origin, their own unique balance of togetherness and separateness, intimacy with one another, compromising with one another, responsibility and authority, and personal roles. Couples may interact flexibly regarding one of these tasks, be disengaged for another, and enmeshed for a third. Steve and Carissa seem to utilize a more disengaged transactional style for several developmental tasks; compromising with one another, togetherness and separateness, and personal roles. Steve uses a more disengaged style with his family while Carissa uses a more enmeshed style with her family.

Complementarity

Each member of the couple has an equal role in the structure of their relationship; however, these roles are usually complementary (Simon, 2016). Many couples may tell stories about how they "fit" together in that they had similar values and interests but also that the other person completed them. **Complementarity** is the notion that people function as a unit rather than an individual. They are tied together, and one person's behaviors are directly tied to the other person. Minuchin and Nichols (1998) stated, "The first thing to understand about how couples are structured is that some measure of complementarity is the defining principle of every relationship" (p. 108). Minuchin would often talk about this in terms of the yin/yang where one can't change without changing the other's shape and vice versa. This prevents one member from being viewed as the cause of the problem (what we call in systemic therapy the identified patient).

By viewing a couple through the lens of complementarity, the structural therapist can see how each member creates the other. One person's behavior comes under the other's influence (Minuchin & Fishman, 1981). A person cannot have power unless the other gives up some power. One person cannot overfunction unless the other person underfunctions. Steve doesn't have to worry about scooping the litter because Carissa will do it. Carissa must focus more on how they might have a child since Steve doesn't focus on that area. Steve seeks outside connection because Carissa seeks a lot of connection from him. None of these behaviors happens in isolation. Steve and Carissa are tied to each other; however, they are not likely to see how their behaviors mutually influence one another. That is one of the processes that will be uncovered during couple therapy.

Complementarity happens as the couple moves from being two separate individuals to two people who function mutually with one another. Minuchin (1974/2012) explained,

> In this process of mutual accommodation, the couple develops a set of patterned transactions— ways in which each spouse triggers and monitors the behavior of the other and is in turn influenced by the previous behavioral sequence. These transactional patterns form an invisible web of complementary demands that regulate many family situations.
>
> (Minuchin, 1974/2012, p. 13)

That is, life for a couple tends to become known and predictable. Steve doesn't have to be concerned about when to go food shopping or what to buy because he knows that Carissa will do it. Carissa knows that Steve won't go shopping on his own, so she takes ownership of that responsibility. Each person finds the various ways in which they function to maintain the status quo of the relationship. However, this doesn't mean that they like what the status quo is. It is just that breaking habitual patterns is difficult because we are so tied to the other person. It takes steady and repetitive attempts to change these developed ingrained ways of being with one another.

Life Cycle

Couples go through a developmental process from first meeting, becoming a couple, potentially having children, raising children, being empty nesters, and then being together in later life.

Many of the problems that couples have are in response to life-cycle demands (Todd, 1986) as their current ways of being are not useful to the new life situation (Minuchin et al., 1998). The couple has developed patterns to assist in succeeding in a particular life-cycle stage. The issue comes when there are transitions between these stages. Problems are likely to occur when the couple maintains their functioning from the previous stage after they have moved to a new developmental stage. For the Hogarths, this can be seen in patterns of functioning that worked well enough in the new couple stage, yet are not as conducive to harmony in the potential couple with child stage.

When two people come together to form a couple, they gain, but they also lose pieces of themselves (Minuchin & Fishman, 1981). This new system includes some loss of individuality while also gaining a sense of belongingness. Steve is likely experiencing the potential loss of his individuality so that he is now making attempts to assert it (e.g., hanging out with friends) over the shared sense of belonging. However, each partner may not always be aware that there are patterns that are developing; they just may be taken for granted. If both partners come from a patriarchal family-of-origin, they will just assume that this is how their relationship should be. It is rare for couples to talk about how they are engaging one another and the role each of them is taking in their continued growth as a couple. It is much easier just to blame the partner for their actions or inactions.

At the beginning of the couple's relationship, they will need to learn how to deal with conflict (Minuchin & Fishman, 1981). This is because conflict is an inevitable aspect of relationships. For the Hogarths, this included how much time to spend together, where they would live after graduation, and now whether to continue trying to have a child. Any couple needs to develop interactional patterns that allow them to express and resolve whatever conflict they experience. This requires clear boundaries so that they don't think they need to agree with one another or not talk with one another about the issue to avoid conflict. Either of these conflict resolution styles will lead to enmeshment or disengagement, respectively. Both will be problematic as this will likely become the habitual reaction surrounding conflict—avoidance of the conflict (or blaming of one another which is also likely not to lead to the resolution of the conflict). Rather, the couple needs to develop clear boundaries with one another so that they can have open conversations to be able to resolve the current conflict as well as potential future conflicts.

Besides life-cycle transitions such as the birth or launching of a child, acute stressors are also significant times in which a problematic structure for the couple may develop (Simon, 2015). Simon explained the difficulty in knowing why one couple would show problems while another didn't:

> The structure exhibited by any given couple subsystem at any given point in its development is the product of the complex and largely idiosyncratic interplay of numerous factors, including the family-of-origin histories of the individual partners, the partners' respective biological endowments, the sociocultural environment in which the couple is immersed, chance events that have influenced the couple's life, and (not least) the couple's decisions about how to deal with all of these factors.
>
> (Simon, 2015, p. 361)

Steve comes from a family where there was conflict between his parents, but then this was followed by disengagement. Carissa comes from a family where there was not a lot of overt conflict and where people stayed together. While they do not have to exactly follow the patterns that they were exposed to in their families-of-origin, these ways of being may have become part of their lenses through which to contact another person, especially when there is conflict in the relationship.

These life-cycle stages demonstrate that a couple changes over time. Structural therapy is a strengths-based approach (Minuchin et al., 2021) which holds that people are not predetermined to be a certain way or deficient, but have the competencies and resources to evolve a different structure (Simon, 2015). As Minuchin was wont to say, people are richer than they think they are (Reiter, 2017). Steve and Carissa are stuck in a view of their relationship with a view of limited potentialities. They are not seeing how they might be different beyond what they expect. They are likely viewing each other as having a limited identity. Carissa is beginning to see Steve as a disengaged husband, and Steve is starting to view Carissa as an overbearing wife. The longer that they interact with each other through these identities, the more likely they will retain their disengaged way of being with one another and will jeopardize the long-term viability of the marriage.

Identities

People tend to develop an identity through relationships yet become stuck in those limited identities. Minuchin explained, "One of the certainties that a family brings to therapy is the knowledge that the identity of their members is unique and unchangeable, and this certainty is maintained by years of daily transactions among its members" (Minuchin et al., 2021, p. 32). The family's structure is maintained by people behaving in predictable ways; ways that are tied to their identities. However, these identities are fluid rather than solid.

People's identities tend to be constructed within their families (Minuchin, 1974/2012). This identity has two components: one of belonging and one of separateness. One of Steve's identities is "Carissa's husband," but others are "distant son," or "Frank's friend." Each of these identities leads to inclusion into certain subsystems and exclusion from others. Carissa's identity as "loyal daughter" maintains her as an active member of the subsystem in her family-of-origin and separates her, to some degree, from Steve.

As a couple experiences increased conflict and stress, they increasingly relate to each other from their stereotyped, narrow behaviors (Rait, 2010). The options that seemed to have been available shrink and they lose flexibility in how they might think or act in relation to one another. Their roles and identities become more rigid, and they don't have their possibilities as available to them as they otherwise might. Steve and Carissa now find themselves limited in the view of who they are as a couple and what potential pathways they can take, leading them to come to couples therapy.

Conceptualizing Diversity

Structural therapy was initially developed through work with minority families from lower-income neighborhoods (Minuchin et al., 1967) and continued to be applied to families in a variety of contexts and countries, such as foster-care families (Minuchin et al., 1998), Chinese families (Lee, 2017), Asian and Hispanic families (Navarre, 2009), as well as in a variety of other countries and ethnic/cultural groups. It can be used with any cultural group as the model keeps in mind the social factors that impact families such as culture, race, socioeconomic status, religion, and a variety of diverse family values (Aponte & DiCesare, 2000).

Given Minuchin's experience of being a religious minority member while growing up in Argentina, as well as his experience emigrating to the United States, the model has honored people's ethnic, cultural, and socioeconomic struggles. Structural therapists understand that one's minority status has a significant impact on family functioning, both in terms of harmony as well as problems (Minuchin et al., 2006). One of the knocks on structural therapy is that the therapist has a prescribed view of how the family should be at the outcome of therapy. While structural therapists tend to help couples and families develop clearer boundaries, there is not one set type of clear boundary that needs to be achieved. Rather, it is dependent on the couple/family and their cultural ways of being, as there is diversity in how people approach their problems and in how they heal one another (Minuchin, 1974/2012).

When thinking about diversity, there is also the related concept of connectivity. That is, we are all humans who experience similar situations (e.g., we want to belong, and we want to be an individual) but experience these things uniquely (e.g., some come from families that expect closeness while others come from families that prefer separation). Structural therapists hold that there are universals in families as well as idiosyncrasies. The **universals** include the notion of organization, subsystems, and boundaries. How these are played out is based on the **idiosyncrasies** of that couple, which are based on the many factors of each partner's social location. Minuchin et al. (2006) explained, "Culture contains more than can be captured in laundry lists of concepts that purport to describe the values and worldview of a particular ethnic group" (p. 29). Thus, structural therapists attempt to understand the generalities of a couple's cultural context, but also understand that the couple will have their own unique way of engaging or not engaging those cultural norms and expectations.

So, how should a couple be? Structural therapists do not have a specific way they expect a couple to organize and function. Rather, they understand that throughout history and based on geographic location, societal contexts, and a variety of other factors, couples will have different expectations of formation, behaviors, and maintenance (Minuchin et al., 2006). In various societies, the roles and possibilities of people of any gender have changed and couples come together in a myriad of ways including arranged marriage, online dating, face-to-face dating, as well as the variety of gender possibilities (i.e., male–female; male–male; female–female; or those who don't identify as binary). Further, couples may actually comprise more than two people, such as open relationships or throuples. Regardless of how a couple came to be or the gender of each party, the members are tied together in ways that can be explored and changed so that they find more satisfaction in the relationship.

It is easy for people, therapists included, to view the functioning of a couple as being either functional or dysfunctional. In structural therapy, this can happen through viewing couples as having too rigid or too diffuse boundaries. Yet, structural therapists acknowledge that boundaries are predicated on culture, class, and gender role socialization (Simon, 2015). Instead of imposing the therapist's definition of functional, it is the couple that determines whether their functioning is problematic or not. This helps prevent the therapist from engaging in cultural colonialism (Sciarra & Simon, 2008). It is the couple who lets the therapist know that the way they have come together is not working for them at the current time.

This becomes even more complex since the couple may or may not be of similar cultural backgrounds, which has significant implications for how that couple will organize. A couple's ethnic roots influence the family's power structure (Minuchin et al., 2007). Some couples may be more egalitarian while others are complementary. **Complementarianism** holds that men and women have unique responsibilities in a marriage that are complementary to one another. For instance, one may be expected to be the breadwinner while the other oversees domestic life. It is not the structural therapist saying what the gender roles for the members of the couple should be, but helping them to expand their patterns so that however they want to be is more satisfying to them.

These have been the philosophical underpinnings of the structural therapist's understanding of diversity. The primary way this is operationalized is through the process called **mimesis** (Minuchin, 1974/2012). Instead of trying to get the couple to adapt to the therapist's way of being, the therapist accommodates to the functioning of the couple. They will slow down, speed up, become more casual, more formal, or any number of behavior and affective variations to join with the couple. These modifications of self are designed to flow more with how the clients are, rather than expecting them to be more like the therapist.

Role of the Therapist

The primary role of the structural therapist is as a practitioner of change (Minuchin et al., 2007). This entails a quite active stance by the therapist where they push against the resistance of the family. "Therefore a therapist is a changer with limited options who will be effective only if he or she can disrupt the family norms that maintain their assumptions" (Minuchin et al., 2007, p. 13). That is, the therapist must join with the family to be able to be connected enough in the therapeutic system to get client buy-in, but separate enough to instigate a variety of changes in the couple's standard ways of functioning.

As explained, in order to challenge the couple to change, the therapist has to join. Minuchin liked to say that challenge comes from connection (Minuchin, 1974/2012; Minuchin & Fishman, 1981; Reiter, 2017). Thus, the first role of the therapist is as a connected member of the system. However, the second role is that of challenger. This requires being able to successfully manage the craft of family therapy, which can be quite difficult. Nichols and Minuchin (1999) explained, "The trick is to challenge families bluntly enough to push them past habit and avoidance but sympathetically enough for them to accept the challenge" (p. 131). If the therapist doesn't challenge the couple, the couple will likely retain their current boundaries, structure, and patterns. These ways of being have led them to therapy and thus are not how the couple wants to be with one another. Thus, the therapist must try to get the couple to change their transactions.

The therapist is also the solver of mysteries. Minuchin likened the therapist to a detective uncovering a mystery, describing this process,

> Knowing that the symptom is but one piece of a larger puzzle that, when put into the context of relationships, uncovers the mosaic of the family, the therapist begins with the symptoms but searches underneath for the relational rules in place that maintain the symptom.
> (Minuchin et al., 2021, p. 12)

The problem presented to the therapist at the first session is taken as the symptom of an underlying organizational dilemma that needs to be uncovered. To do this, the therapist becomes a key factor in the therapeutic process.

The therapist as a person may be the most important tool in structural therapy. That is, use of self is the therapist's greatest tool (Minuchin et al., 2021). Minuchin et al. (2006) described the dilemma of having a viewpoint and trying to maintain openness to new information: "While engaging the family, encouraging disclosure, and scanning for problems and possibilities, he [they] associates, tries to fit, probes, modifies assumptions in accordance with the results, and probes again" (p. 75). The therapist becomes the active agent in a therapeutic process designed to understand the couple and see possible areas of change. This comes through the therapist modifying themselves and their engagement to the couple so that they join yet have the freedom to challenge.

Thus, one of the primary roles of the therapist is an active use of self (Aponte & DiCesare, 2000). Given the central position of the therapist, their strategic use of self is extremely important for the therapeutic relationship (Aponte, 1992). This requires the therapist to be personally present in the therapeutic encounter, where they want to engage the client (Aponte, 2016a). They do this through making an internal connection with the client, enabling them to be empathic but also to maintain their separateness. Therapists thus attempt to be aware of who they are and how they are being present in the therapy room based on everything that they bring into the equation. To do this, the therapist needs to be self-aware; of their emotionality, culture, spirituality, personal history, and triggers, as well as how they are intentionally using themselves in the session (Aponte & Carlsen, 2009).

Last, the role of the structural therapist has been compared to that of a director-actor of a play (Simon, 2015). The therapist fulfills the director role by providing guidance in which scene to play and observing the outcome of those enactments. As an actor, the therapist adapts themselves to fit the scene—what Minuchin called mimesis (Minuchin, 1974/2012). There will be times during the session when the therapist is an actor and at other times, they will remove themselves from the drama but direct the members of the couple to act with one another. This will be explained more below when discussing the primary therapeutic intervention of enactments.

Conceptualization of Problem Resolution

Structural couple therapy seeks to help individuals in a couple move away from their automatic patterns that have maintained a destructive and unhappy relationship (Minuchin & Nichols, 1998). This happens by bringing forth each person's individuality, power, and responsibility. However, it is also based on discussing the connection of the two individuals. Rait (2010) explained, "From the structural point of view, the therapeutic task is to help the couple or family move from one stage of family development to a new stage where members' developmental needs are met" (p. 235). That is, the therapist assists the couple in changing their structure and organization that might have been useful in a previous life stage and shifting it to the current stage. For the Hogarths, this would be moving from a dating position to a married position where they can have clear boundaries between each other and between themselves and other systems, such as friends and family.

The structural therapist believes that the change that will happen for one person is yoked to the other family member (Minuchin et al., 2021). As Minuchin explained his position, "I am committed to the idea that people in a family are responsible for each other, and are therefore responsible for healing and protecting each other" (Minuchin et al., 2021, p. 79). Thus, problem resolution happens as the therapist connects with the couple and challenges them to be different with one another. The therapist creates a context for the couple to begin to engage one another in new ways, helping the other to grow and change so that new patterns and couple organization develop.

Joining

The first step in structural therapy is joining. **Joining** is the process of the therapist letting the couple know, through a variety of means, that they understand them and are working with and for them (Minuchin & Fishman, 1981). There is not an exact way of how to join as some people prefer the therapist to be more empathic, more firm, more challenging, more engaging, or less engaging, less confrontational, etc. An exact way of how to join belies the craft of therapy and trying to get in tune with the individual as well as the couple.

While formal joining may begin at the start of the first session, structural therapists view joining as a mindset more than a technique (Minuchin et al., 2021). Joining is the empathic connection the therapist makes with the couple (Nichols & Minuchin, 1999). It provides the foundation of connectedness that will be needed for the eventual challenges to the system the therapist will make. As Minuchin and Fishman (1981) described, "Since the therapist's use of himself [themself] in the therapeutic system is the most powerful tool in the process of changing families, he [they] needs to be knowledgeable about the range of his [their] joining repertory" (p. 32). Here, the therapist will need to understand their own social location and use it in relation to the clients' social locations. For instance, young therapists with a soft demeanor may need to take a "one down" position, rather than firmly challenging as an older more experienced therapist might. It will likely be easier for a therapist who is currently in a serious relationship to work with a couple, as they can join from a position of experience of having to accommodate to their partner, as compared to a therapist who has never been in a long-term romantic relationship. Whatever one's age, gender, race, culture, relationship status, etc., the therapist will need to use themself as the primary tool to join and connect with the couple.

When working with couples, conjoint sessions are used since the goal is to have the couple have a new relational experience with one another, first in the session and then outside in their everyday life (Simon, 2015). The caveat to this would be if there is potential violence and/or abuse. While, for any couple, the therapist may meet individually with its members, it is not advised, as what will be obtained will likely be biased and partial information and may unintentionally encourage the perception of an alliance with one member and not the other (Nichols & Minuchin, 1999). Given that both members are present in the session, the structural therapist is continually engaging in a balancing act between themself and each member of the couple as well as the couple as a whole (Rait, 2010). Thus, there are four relationships that need to be fostered: (1) therapist and one member, (2) therapist and the other member, (3) therapist and the couple, and (4) the two members of the couple. In our case scenario, the therapist will need to join with Carissa, with Steve, with Carissa and Steve, and help Carissa and Steve connect with one another.

An additional aspect of the development of the therapeutic system is **accommodation**, which occurs when the therapist makes minor modifications of self in order to join (Minuchin, 1974/ 2012). Many times, these maneuvers are outside the therapist's awareness. However, the structural therapist goes into an encounter being open to shifting to the client's ways of being. Thus, the structural therapist enters into a therapeutic relationship where they do two things simultaneously; they accommodate to the couple sufficiently to join with them while also maintaining the leadership position of the therapeutic system. This provides enough connection while also having maneuverability to be able to challenge the couple when needed.

Therapist Proximity

Part of that maneuverability is the proximity the therapist decides to take, at that point in the session, to the couple. Structural therapists choose, based on what is happening in the session, to shift their proximity to the action of the session. This provides them with the ability to be involved in the action or to step back and take more of the role of the director. There are three main positions: close, median, and disengaged (Minuchin & Fishman, 1981).

Given that therapists want to join with clients, the **close position** provides an opportunity for affiliation. Here, the therapist is part of the action, confirming the reality of each member of the couple. Confirming happens by pointing out the positives of the person. This can occur when the therapist sees the client acting in a way that supports the new and desired family organization. For instance, "Steve, that was very nice what you just did. Carissa was in distress, and you didn't wait for her to request something of you. You initiated helping her out." Confirming can also happen by pointing out negative characteristics of the person; however, their behavior is tied to someone else. "Carissa, you were just very short and impatient with Steve. How does he snip your fuse?"

The **median position** allows the therapist to be engaged yet neutral. Here, the therapist will usually help the couple tell their story. This process is called **tracking** (Minuchin & Fishman, 1981). By not being so central, the therapist can be a participant-observer, pushing along the flow but also having enough distance to view the couple's process. However, the therapist is aware of self, keeping in tune with whether they are spending too much time talking to one member or the other. This awareness helps the therapist to try to not get drawn into the family's process, but rather be separate from it and recognize it when it occurs.

The **disengaged position** is more that of an expert. This is when the director role of the therapist comes into play (Minuchin & Fishman, 1981). Minuchin and Fishman explained the procedures of a therapist in this position, "Perceiving the patterns of the family dance, the therapist creates scenarios, facilitating the enactment of familiar movements or introducing novelty by forcing family members to engage with each other in unusual transactions" (p. 40). The common technique used in this position is the enactment (see below), where the therapist prompts the couple to engage one another and then sits back to observe the process. Minuchin liked to tell students that when they begin the enactment, they should look at their left foot (Minuchin et al., 2021). When they do so, they send a message to the clients and themself that they are not an actor in that particular drama.

Enactments

The primary therapeutic technique in structural therapy is the **enactment** (Minuchin & Fishman, 1981). Here, the therapist attempts to get the clients to engage in their typical transaction patterns in the therapist's presence which provides a portal into the couple's relational process. Simon (1995) went as far as to say that enactments were the essence of structural therapy.

An enactment allows the therapist to see the couple's problematic interactions in the therapy room rather than just hearing the explanation of the problems. While seeing it happen, the therapist can experience it in the here-and-now (Aponte, 2016b). There are three phases of enactments: initiation, facilitation, and closing (Nichols & Fellenberg, 2000). Perhaps the best way a therapist can initiate an enactment is to have one partner respond to a specific complaint that their partner just made in the session (Nichols & Minuchin, 1999). With the Hogarths, this might be when Carissa mentions she is upset that Steve is spending so much time outside the house, or when Steve says that he would like to stop trying for a baby. These pressure points hold the fodder for the couple's ingrained reactions to one another and provide the therapist with a glimpse into their actual transaction patterns rather than their explanations of what happens.

During enactments, the structural therapist has three main options (Rait, 2010). First, they can just observe the couple's interactional process. They might think to themselves, "How are they negotiating the power in this interchange?" "How well are they listening to one another?" or "They don't seem to be turning to one another." Observation is the preferred option for therapists during the first or second session (Nichols & Minuchin, 1999). The therapist needs to shift back in their seat and not interrupt the couple, maintaining their disengaged position so that they can observe the couple's process (Nichols & Fellenberg, 2000). Second, the therapist can provide support to the couple. This may come in the form of statements, such as, "Wow. That was a really nice way of talking with one another." To increase the intensity, Minuchin would often mark positive behaviors by standing up, walking over to the client, and shaking their hand to congratulate them for engaging with the other in a new and more effective way. Third, the therapist might challenge the clients. Minuchin liked to challenge through what he called the **stroke and kick** (Minuchin et al., 2021). The therapist first says something nice to the couple and then follows that up with something that needs to change. For the Hogarths, this might be, "It is interesting. You two are very bright people. So how is it that you continue to interact with one another in ways that make you each miserable?"

In closing enactments, the therapist summarizes the process of what occurred (Nichols & Fellenberg, 2000). Instead of explaining the content of what one person said, the therapist highlights how the couple interacted. The emphasis is on the couple's dynamic and the need for both people to change as they are connected to and created by one another. If, at the end of an enactment, the therapist says, "Carissa, you wanted Steve around the house more; and Steve, you wanted two days where you could be with your friends. How can you resolve this?" the therapist has put themselves in more of a mediator position and will likely need to mediate the next conflict between the couple. Rather, the therapist might end the enactment by saying, "How does that happen? That when you two discuss this, Carissa moves in and it becomes overwhelming for Steve, and Steve moves out which forces Carissa to move in." In this case, there is no talk about the content of the conversation, but instead the therapist focuses on the process between the two. When they can change the process, they will change their ability to navigate any of the plethora of disagreements that they will have in their relationship.

Intensity

One of the keys to being an effective structural therapist is the ability to function with intensity (Nichols & Minuchin, 1999). **Intensity** is engaging with the clients in a way that they can experience something new (Minuchin & Fishman, 1981). If no new information enters the system, it will remain as is, leading to the continuation of repetitive patterns. The question for the therapist is what level of intensity is needed with this couple at this point in the session. In some situations, subtle messages can have enough intensity to make a difference. Other times, the therapist will need to create significant drama to resonate with the clients. This leads to the therapist needing to be cognizant of the therapeutic process as there are many ways of creating intensity.

One way this can be done is by keeping an enactment going past the point where family members try to end it (Nichols & Minuchin, 1999). In this way, the couple's normal way of handling the situation is shown to be ineffective. The therapist can raise the intensity by stating something like, "The two of you were just talking *at* one another rather than *with* one another. Keep talking so that maybe you can start to really listen to each other."

Another way to increase intensity is through repetition of one's message (Minuchin & Fishman, 1981). The therapist can say a message again, utilizing varying vocalics (how they use their voice) to highlight the point they were trying to make. This marks the message as something different, potentially leading the couple to hear it as they did not before. Visual imagery is a prime area for repetition as it will leave a lasting image in the couple's minds.

Repetition of interpersonal transactions is another means of working with intensity (Minuchin & Fishman, 1981). Given that a couple's process is the culmination of many repeated transactions, a single intervention is not likely to change it. Couples and families tend to maintain their homeostasis, leading to the necessity for the therapist to continue to push for change. "Therapy is a matter of repetition, in which desired structural changes are pursued in many different ways" (Minuchin & Fishman, 1981, p. 123). Carissa and Steve have developed their current way of being over several years of repetitive ways of viewing themselves and interacting with one another. The therapist working with them will likely need to hit a few points several times to start making inroads in their process.

Challenging/Restructuring

The couple will likely come to therapy with a clear and firm view of what the problem is. This view tends to hold that one person of the couple is the problem and if they just changed, things would be hunky-dory. The therapist's job is to challenge their certainty since the more they hold their viewpoint, the less open they are to seeing things differently and thus changing (Minuchin et al., 2021).

One of the primary challenges the therapist will use with the couple is **restructuring**, which are the interventions the therapist uses that lead to therapeutic change (Minuchin, 1974/2012). A standard restructuring maneuver is **boundary making**. Boundary making with a couple helps them to restore structural integrity by enhancing the couple subsystem's functional boundaries with other people, subsystems, or situations (such as pets, addiction, employment, etc.) (Ford et al., 2012). In family sessions, this may come through having people switch seats, "Koji, change seats with your mother so that she and your father can talk about parent issues." Boundary making might also happen during enactments through techniques such as blocking, where the therapist serves as a traffic cop, directing who can go and who has to stop. As an example, the therapist might say, "Shavonda, hold on a second. Philip and Sylvia are having a perfectly fine conversation. Sit back and let's see how they talk to one another." Boundary making helps to shift rigid or diffuse boundaries, making them become clearer.

Unbalancing

All couples argue. That is a universal of relationships. What they argue about and the severity of the arguments are particular to that couple. When conflict between the couple becomes chronic or conversely is prematurely terminated or avoided, the couple loses potential resources in their relationship (Simon, 2016). Those couples with chronic conflict tend to have a relational structure that hinders their ability to incorporate their differences. On the other hand, couples who avoid conflict have developed a relational structure that inhibits the members' ability to have and embrace their differences. For those couples who avoid conflict or prematurely end it, unbalancing can be a useful technique (Simon, 2015, 2016).

Unbalancing is when the therapist joins one member of the couple in a coalition and acts as if that person's behaviors/position is right and the other member's position is wrong. This coalition is temporary yet significant. By taking one party's side, the therapist destabilizes the conflict-avoiding pattern the couple has developed (Simon, 2016). That is, the therapist will support one member while creating stress for the other member (Minuchin et al., 2021).

To engage in unbalancing, the therapist will usually first initiate an enactment, particularly around a conflict area the couple is likely to try to avoid. Once the enactment begins, the therapist will intervene and join one person's side before the couple can enter into their typical conflict-avoidance cycle. The therapist encourages one member to advocate for themselves. For instance, the Hogarths' therapist might initiate an enactment about whether to have a child and then temporarily join Steve. Unbalancing would happen when the therapist said, "Steve, Carissa is telling you what should be rather than listening to you and appreciating your position. You were just about to shut down. Don't. Tell her where you are coming from." Once done, the therapist would take a less central position to allow the next enactment to occur; this will hopefully have a new interactional process occur that avoids conflict-avoidance. Depending on how quickly the members engage each other differently, the therapist may need to have several rounds of unbalancing.

Reframing

Clients come in with a story of how they understand how and why things are as they are. This story is usually quite narrow, providing a limited view of each person's identity and the pathways that are available to them. The structural therapist attempts to widen their story, unwrapping family member identities and increasing people's sense of potentialities. One means of doing this is through reframing.

Reframing is providing an alternate explanation of events. It is one of the most common therapeutic techniques, not just for structural therapy, but for any modality. Minuchin believed that the family was wrong (Minuchin et al., 2021). That is, they entered therapy with a story of what the problem is (i.e., the identified patient) and thought the therapist was going to go along with them and try to change that individual. Minuchin and Fishman (1981) held that this is one of the therapist's first tasks; to shift the client's reality to the therapeutic reality (one which focuses on relationships instead of individuals).

Regardless of what technique a therapist utilizes, the goal is to help the couple have a new relational experience (Simon, 2015). When one member behaves differently toward their partner, the other partner will likely change as well. As with all systems theories, one change in the system leads to system-wide change. Thus, the therapist attempts to get at least one of the members to change their way of engaging with the other. However, when both can change, both partners find a new relational experience with the other.

Therapeutic Goal

The ultimate goal of structural couple therapy is to alleviate the couple's presenting problem (Simon, 2015). Therapy can be viewed as successful when the couple says they are satisfied that their problematic situation has been resolved. In general, this will happen when the identified patient is relieved of being the symptom bearer, there is a reduction in stress and conflict, and the couple has learned new ways of coping (Minuchin & Fishman, 1981).

Change is not likely to be seen in one fell swoop. Rather, it occurs in successive steps, each progressive step moving closer to a new couple structure that provides greater options for how people can view themselves and engage their partner (Rait, 2010). Through realigning and restructuring the organization of the couple, the therapist helps to increase the couple's closeness and intimacy so it becomes the structure which will reinforce these new patterns (Ford et al., 2012).

One of the key components of a structural case conceptualization is that of possibilities (Reiter, 2016). This is where the therapist has introduced novelty into the system. Minuchin and Nichols (1993) explained, "The basic quest of family therapy is to release unused possibilities" (p. 45). These possibilities may lie in how people view a situation, expand their identities, engage in new relational patterns, and/or realize that there are many more pathways available for them than previously.

There are many pathways and processes that can occur in a structural session. One of the fairly new ways is a four-step model of family assessment (Minuchin et al., 2007). The first step, which most structural therapists do regardless of their pathways is opening up the presenting complaint. In this step, the therapist usually begins to deconstruct the symptom (Minuchin et al., 2021). Couples and families come to therapy with an identified patient. The longer they maintain this view, the longer they will continue to sit within their troubles. This leads into step two, highlighting problem-maintaining interactions. The therapist helps family members realize how their own involvement with each other keeps the problem in place. This may be through the use of unwrapping identities, which shows how one person's identity is tied to someone else (Minuchin et al., 2021). Step three is a departure from typical structural therapy sessions since it focuses on the past, whereas most structural therapy has focused on the present. In this step, one family member is interviewed while the others listen. The therapist elicits what the person is bringing with them—their lenses—that influence their current engagement with others. In a couple, this process would then be repeated with the other partner. The fourth stage, and the last part of any structural therapy process, is an exploration of alternative ways of interacting. Many structural therapists might not engage in step three as it was not a foundational part of the model. However, it is presented here to explain more possible pathways to achieve change with a couple.

Case Transcript

Therapist: Hello. It is good to meet you both. Would one of you like to start and tell me how I can be of help to you.

The therapist opens the session by attempting to gain an understanding of what brings the couple to therapy. This is the primary agenda of a first session in structural couple therapy (Simon, 2015). It is an open-ended inquiry so that the therapist can start, right from the beginning of the session, to assess the couple's process. Who begins? Who takes over? How do they negotiate the situation? This is the first step of a structural family assessment.

Carissa: We are going through quite a rough patch right now.
Therapist: Tell me about it.
Carissa: We are trying to get pregnant as I really want to be a mother and things just, for some reason, haven't worked in our favor. We have gone to a fertility clinic, but they couldn't find anything. Steve wants to give up and now is spending a lot of time outside of the house.
Therapist: That sounds very tough for you that you want to be a mother, but conception is not coming easy. Steve, she is starting to take your voice. What is your position?

The therapist quickly ascertains that Carissa is trying to make Steve the identified patient. One of the first tasks of the structural therapist is to deconstruct the symptom (Minuchin et al., 2007; Minuchin et al., 2021). One means of doing this is giving the identified patient a bigger voice. There is also a stroke and a kick where the therapist joins Carissa in her pain of unfulfilled motherhood while also challenging her to speak only for herself.

Steve: It's not that I want to give up, but it doesn't seem to be happening right now and it's taking its toll on us. It will be very expensive if we try more fertility procedures. So, I suggested we put a pause on it.
Therapist: Okay. So, it is not that you don't ever want to try, but right now you want to take a pause. How do you convey that to Carissa?

The therapist acknowledges the content and then moves the conversation to process.

Steve: I've told her that it's a lot on us. A lot of pressure. A lot of money.
Therapist: This is a very important topic for you both. Talk with each other about this.

This is the beginning of an enactment so the therapist can take a more distant position and observe the couple's process. The therapist initiates an enactment and then backs out of the dynamics, looking at their left foot instead. However, they are fully aware of the process happening between the couple but are shifting their position from central to distant. Nichols and Minuchin (1999) explained, "One of the biggest mistakes therapists make is getting caught up in the content of a couple's problems and losing sight of the process and structure that supports such problems" (p. 132). Enactments allow the therapist to view the process of the couple and give clues as to where next to intervene to develop a more functional structure.

Steve: You know, we have talked with the doctors, and they don't know what's going on.
Carissa: Yes, which is why we can't stop trying. But you've given up. On me getting pregnant. And making our relationship work. You need to change your priorities and prioritize me and your marriage. You focus too much on your friends. On doing things with them.
Steve: No, I'm not.
Carissa: Yes, you are. It's like you're married to them and not me. You have responsibilities at home. Cooking. Cleaning. And being a husband.
Therapist: Steve, I was just observing this conversation the two of you were having. For a moment or two there, it seemed that you were no longer husband and wife, but rather mother and son. Have you ever had that experience with Carissa?

The therapist begins to engage in unbalancing, joining in a coalition with Steve to support him to step up in the relationship. This is also beginning to play around with unwrapping their identities.

Steve: Yes. More and more lately she tries to tell me what to do.
Therapist: How do you keep her on you like that?

Couples find their process and patterns based on mutuality and complementarity. This challenge to Steve highlights that neither partner is the problem. How they have come to be at this moment is based on both of their actions. This is the second step in a structural family assessment—exploring how family members' behaviors maintain the problem.

Steve: I don't know what you mean.
Therapist: Steve, talk with Carissa about this. However, when you do, do so as her husband rather than her son. Don't give up. That is what a child might do. Have her understand your position.

Once the therapist has joined with one member of the couple, they then initiate an enactment to shift the standard pattern of Carissa taking on more of a leadership/parental role and for the two spousal members to experience one another more equally.

Steve: I still don't know why you think I'm not doing what I'm supposed to be doing. I work. I contribute a lot of money to our household. I try to do things with you.
Carissa: What you want. When you want. And if you think you're doing what you're supposed to be doing you have another thing to think about.
Therapist: Steve, even more. How can you interact with her so that she can be your wife rather than your mother?

The therapist is highlighting the complementarity of the couple, helping to restructure their relationship and unwrap their identities.

Steve: Please stop telling me what to do or not to do.
Carissa: I only tell you what I need. Not what you need to do.
Steve: It sure feels like you're telling me what to do. Maybe if you tell me what you want, and I tell you what I want.
Carissa: I want you to want this marriage. I want to feel valued and loved and heard and prioritized.
Steve: What you're saying is you want me to do what you want.
Therapist: Carissa, I don't think Steve heard you right then. Can you tell him again, but this time in a way that he listens?

Here, the therapist uses repetition of the client's statement to increase the intensity of the process that is happening between the couple.

Carissa: No. I am telling you what I want. That I want to feel appreciated. I don't right now. I want a husband. Someone who puts this marriage first in their life. What do you want?
Steve: I want this marriage. I want you, as my wife.
Therapist: That was very nice. Right then, you both were husband and wife. That is the opening for you to have a new way of being with one another. Spouses change each other. I have been married for 20 years and I know my spouse has changed me a lot. And I have

changed them. Some couples, even without the formal and legal process, divorce each other but stay married. When they don't think they can change their partner anymore, they are at that point divorced. That doesn't seem to be the case here. Steve, I want to talk with you for just a bit while Carissa listens. I was impressed by your willingness in letting Carissa parent you. I'd like to talk about you before you met Carissa. Where do you think you learned to approach someone close to you from a position of trying to avoid conflict?

The therapist highlights the strengths and competencies of this couple. They just had an interaction that shifted their previous dynamics of Carissa being above Steve in their couple hierarchy. Instead of being his mother, she became his wife. Steve stood up for himself and didn't put Carissa into a mothering position and became her husband. The therapist then begins step three of a structural assessment—an exploration of the past.

Steve: I don't know. In my family, my parents didn't seem to get along. They had fights that we heard, and it didn't work out for them. With guys, no issue. I can be competitive with them.

Therapist: Yes. But competition and conflict aren't quite the same. Conflict is more personal and intimate. What did you learn about intimacy in your family?

Steve: Maybe not much. We weren't that close of a family. Like now. With my sister. Maybe I talk to her a few times a year. For birthdays or holidays. My brother and I get along but probably not the in-depth types of conversations I think you are alluding to.

Therapist: What about you, Carissa? What did you learn about intimacy from your family?

This is a very condensed version of a structural session. Typically, more time would be spent, first in joining, and then in all areas bringing out new information to help the therapist with their assessment of the couple's structure. The point here is that each member of the couple is recognizing their part in their current transactions. It is not only the other person. They also have ways of being that they brought into this relationship. However, these ways are not set. They are lenses of glasses that tend to be worn. Similar to the person who wears glasses and then sees the world differently once they get a new prescription, this process helps people to become aware of the restricted view they may have of themselves and their partner.

Carissa: We were a pretty close family. We still are. It's weird for me seeing how disengaged Steve is with his family. Especially his father. In my family, I was very close with my sister. We probably told each other most everything.

Therapist: What was that like for you? Being that close?

Carissa: It felt good. I didn't have a ton of friends growing up. My sister was really my best friend.

Therapist: Okay. So, here we have one person that learned to get along by keeping things calm and distant and another who learned that there is benefit in connection and intimacy. How does that play out in your current relationship?

This is a move to continue to deconstruct the symptom. Neither party is in the wrong. They just learned two different ways to engage with the world and, at this point in time, these two ways are not fully working for them. Therapy will help them to find a rhythm with one another.

Carissa: I hadn't really thought of it like that. I know that I want to spend more time together. Talk about our day. Open up to one another. And Steve tends to just be more okay with existing with one another.

Therapist: Steve, what's your perspective on that?

The therapist ensures that one person's perspective is not taken as the end of the conversation. This is a push for them each to bring their ideas into the conversation. That way, they might do so more often when they are out of the therapist's office.

Steve: I hadn't realized I'm a bit avoidant of conflict. I don't like it when we start to argue or even if she starts nagging me about things. I tend to go where I know things are more fun, like hanging with my friends.
Carissa: So I'm not fun?
Steve: No, it's not that. You and I can have fun. We do. Lately, though, not so much.
Therapist: Continue talking with each other about this.

When the therapist initiates enough enactments, clients will do so on their own to continue the therapeutic process (although some couples will come in and initiate enactments without any prompting by the therapist. However, usually, these are moments where they are blaming and attacking one another.) At this point in the session, Carissa and Steve have opened up the possibility of being different with one another and having more intimate conversations that are talking about what they want rather than who is at fault.

Steve: I want to have fun with you. And be with you, in lots of different ways. I know I am not as determined to have children. I can go either way. But I recognize that's important for you.
Carissa: Thank you. It's important for me to know you understand that and want our relationship to keep moving forward.
Therapist: Steve, if Carissa was a sculpture, how would you carve her so she is more as you want?

The therapist then pushed for alternatives. This is the fourth step of a structural family assessment (Minuchin et al., 2007).

Steve: She is as I want.
Therapist: You were able just before to take a step forward and be more intimate with her. How might you take one more step? Our partners are never exactly how we want them to be. That is the beauty of relationships like these. We are always learning something new about our partner. And about ourselves. And about our relationships.

This is a challenge to Steve to really be different in the relationship. He is used to avoiding conflict. The therapist is not trying to have them fight, although at times the structural therapist is very comfortable having that happen to see the couple's process. That has already happened. Now is the point of the session to see how they might be different with one another. Here, the therapist supports Steve in his ability to withstand the tension of tension and trust Carissa that she can engage him without it leading to fireworks.

Steve: Perhaps she can calm down just a little on things.
Therapist: She does seem wound a little tight. What can you do to loosen her, so she doesn't have to be in charge so much?
Steve: I tell her all the time to just chill out.
Therapist: Right, but that won't help. That will just be you trying to be in the foreman position. Rather than what you can *say* to her, what can you *do* differently so she can relax?

This is the use of intensity, repeating a message so it is heard. It also unwraps identities and plays around with metaphors that highlight mutuality and complementarity. When Steve can be more proactive in the relationship, Carissa will not have to be the primary person to ensure things get done.

Steve: I guess I can write a list of things that need to be done around the house and have it mapped out when I will do things.

Therapist: Carissa, what would that do for you?

Rather than ask, "How would that make you feel," which is a generic therapy mainstay, this question implies that Steve and Carissa are tied together, like the yin and yang. When yin changes, so does yang.

Carissa: That would be a good start.

Steve: I could also make sure I ask her out for a date night every week.

Carissa: That would be a better start.

Therapist: Okay. So Steve will, instead of tending to hold back and avoid contact, will initiate getting things done and interactions. And Carissa can relax a bit. She's used to intimacy through close connection. Steve, the more that you initiate with her the less she will go to her family for that sense of connection.

This attempt at boundary making begins to shift the diffuse boundaries between Carissa and her family to a greater affiliation between the couple rather than the somewhat rigid boundary that has been growing over the last year or two.

Therapist: This is probably a good place to end this session. This seemed like a nice start for therapy that is focused on how to get you both to be a couple instead of two individuals. We will see how you each change the other person this week.

The therapist ends the session continuing to deconstruct the symptom. It is neither Steve nor Carissa that is the problem and the only one to change. Rather, their relationship is the focus of intervention. The therapist challenges them to change the other person with the paradoxical understanding that to change the other person you have first to change yourself.

Termination

Termination happens when the couple believes that they have met their goals. This usually happens when the couple views themselves in new and more complex ways, with more possibilities available to them in how they feel, think, behave, and how they choose to be with one another (Rait, 2010). In essence, the couple believes that they can continue on without the therapist (Aponte & DiCesare, 2000). They are likely to accept responsibility for their own behavior in the dyad, have balanced the dilemma of togetherness and separateness, and learned how to work together in new ways.

References

Aponte, H. J. (1992). Training the person of the therapist in structural Family therapy. *Journal of Marital and Family Therapy, 18*(3), 269–281.

Aponte, H. J. (2016a). Joining: From the perspective of the use of self. In G. R. Weeks, S. T. Fife, & C. M. Peterson (Eds.), *Techniques for the couple therapist: Essential interventions from the experts* (pp. 12–14). Routledge.

Aponte, H. J. (2016b). Enactment from the perspective of the use of self. In G. R. Weeks, S. T. Fife, & C. M. Peterson (Eds.), *Techniques for the couple therapist: Essential interventions from the experts* (pp. 33–36). Routledge.

Aponte, H. J., & Carlsen, J. C. (2009). An instrument for person-of-the-therapist supervision. *Journal of Marital and Family Therapy, 35*(4), 395–405.

Aponte, H. J., & DiCesare, E. J. (2000). Structural theory. In F. M. Dattilio & L. J. Bevilacqua (Eds.), *Comparative treatments for relationship dysfunction* (pp. 45–57). Springer.

Fishman, H. C. (1993). *Intensive structural therapy: Treating families in their social context.* Basic.

Ford, J. J., Durtshi, J. A., & Franklin, D. L. (2012). Structural therapy with a couple battling pornography addiction. *The American Journal of Family Therapy, 40,* 336–348.

Lee, W-Y. (2017). An unexplored subsystem—Young children as healers: Dialogue with Sal Minuchin. *Journal of Systemic Therapies, 36*(4), 35–45.

Lindblad-Goldberg, M., & Northey Jr., W. F. (2013). Ecosystemic structural family therapy: Theoretical and clinical foundations. *Contemporary Family Therapy, 35*(1), 147–160.

Minuchin, P., Colapinto, J., & Minuchin, S. (1998). *Working with families of the poor.* Guilford.

Minuchin, S. (2012). *Families and family therapy.* Routledge. (Original work published 1974.)

Minuchin, S., & Fishman, H. C. (1981). *Family therapy techniques.* Harvard University Press.

Minuchin, S., Lee, W-Y., & Simon, G. M. (2006). *Mastering family therapy: Journeys of growth and transformation* (2nd ed.). Wiley.

Minuchin, S., Montalvo, B., Guerney, B. G., Rosman, B. L., & Schumer, F. (1967). *Families of the slums: An exploration of their structure and treatment.* Basic Books.

Minuchin, S., & Nichols, M. P. (1993). *Family healing.* The Free Press.

Minuchin, S., & Nichols, M. P. (1998). Structural family therapy. In F. M. Dattilio (Ed.), *Case studies in couple and family therapy* (pp. 108–131), Guilford.

Minuchin, S., Nichols, M. P., & Lee, W-Y. (2007). *Assessing families and couples: From symptom to system.* Allyn & Bacon.

Minuchin, S., Reiter, M. D., & Borda, C. (2021). *The craft of family therapy* (2nd ed.). Routledge.

Navarre, S. E. (2009). Salvador Minuchin's structural family therapy and its application to multicultural family systems. *Issues in Mental Health Nursing, 19*(6), 557–570.

Nichols, M. P., & Fellenberg, S. (2000). The effective use of enactments in family therapy: A discovery-oriented process study. *Journal of Marital and Family Therapy, 26*(2), 143–152.

Nichols, M. P., & Minuchin, S. (1999). Short-term structural family therapy with couples. In J. M. Donovan (Ed.), *Short-term couple therapy* (pp. 124–143). Guilford.

Rait, D. S. (2010). Opening steps: A structural approach to working with couples. In A. S. Gurman (Ed.), *Clinical casebook of couple therapy* (pp. 232–254). Guilford.

Reiter, M. D. (2016). A quick guide to case conceptualization in Structural family therapy. *Journal of Systemic Therapies, 35*(2), 25–37.

Reiter, M. D. (2017). 10 things I learned from Dr. Salvador Minuchin. *Journal of Systemic Therapies, 36*(4), 46–56.

Sciarra, D. T., & Simon, G. M. (2008). Assessment of diverse family systems. In L. A. Suzuki & J. G. Ponterotto (Eds.), *Handbook of multicultural assessment: Clinical, psychological, and educational applications* (3rd ed., pp. 247–272). Jossey-Bass.

Simon, G. M. (1995). A revisionist rendering of structural family therapy. *Journal of Marital and Family Therapy, 21,* 17–26.

Simon, G. M. (2015). Structural couple therapy. In A. S. Gurman (Ed.), *Clinical handbook of couple therapy* (4th. ed., pp. 358–384). Guilford.

Simon, G. M. (2016). Unbalancing. In G. R. Weeks, S. T. Fife, & C. M. Peterson (Eds.), *Techniques for the couple therapist: Essential interventions from the experts* (pp. 115–118). Routledge.

Szapocznik, J., & Hervis, O. (2020). *Brief strategic family therapy.* American Psychological Association.

Todd, T. C. (1986). Structural-strategic marital therapy. In N. S. Jacobson, & A. S. Gurman (Eds.), *Clinical handbook of marital therapy* (pp. 71–105). Guilford.

Wilk, D. M., & Storm, C. L. (1991). Structural marital therapy: Assessment of pas de deux families. *The American Journal of Family Therapy, 19*(3), 257–265.

8 Gottman Method Couples Therapy

Vagdevi Meunier

History of the Model

John Gottman is a world-renowned relationship researcher with possibly the most comprehensive and thorough understanding of the development and dissolution of intimate committed relationships and marriages of any relationship researcher in the world. From the early 1970s, Gottman was interested in studying relationships, first children's friendships and then adult relationships. In his first position as assistant professor at Indiana University, Gottman set up some simple research studies with the help of graduate students to see if they could teach couples more effective communication techniques. Initially, the couples in their research relapsed within a year. Dr. Gottman then began a collaboration with a psychophysiological researcher, Dr. Robert Levenson, in 1976, which resulted in a four-decade period of joint research that led to multiple significant longitudinal scientific studies of healthy and unhealthy relationships, many of which are the most often cited and referenced articles and books on marriage. See Gottman (2014) and Gottman and Gottman (2018) for a detailed description of the history of the research.

Gottman's collaboration with Levenson was based on the hope that studying emotion and physiology might yield some understanding of internal subjective experiences that would provide more predictive power to their observational research (Gottman, 2014; Gottman & Gottman, 2015). In the first few trials of this collaboration, Gottman and Levenson knew very little about what to look for and what they were going to find, so much of that early research was just observing couples in a variety of contexts and looking for patterns. Gottman writes about being inspired by a 1969 paper by Goldfried and D'Zurilla that suggested observing how "masters" solve a problem that "disasters" (i.e., the clinical population) have not yet solved. This became the basis of their research approach and Gottman and his colleagues designed multimethod multidimensional studies that systematically analyzed the differences between happy stable couples (**The Masters of Marriage**) and unhappy failing couples (**The Disasters of Marriage**) as well as unhappy stable couples (the married and miserable group). Gottman and Levenson systematically observed, coded, and documented the repeating patterns in the development and demise of more than 3500 couple relationships across spans of 20 years or more and replicated their results across 12 studies, seven of which were the primary nonintervention longitudinal studies that followed groups of couples from newlyweds to couples in their late 60s (Gottman, 1999; Gottman & Navarra, 2011). The seven foundational studies both replicated their initial findings and taught them how to predict with over 90% accuracy whether a married couple would be together six years later or be divorced (Gottman & Silver, 2015). See John Gottman's book, *The Marriage Clinic* (1999), for a description of the primary seven longitudinal studies and their findings.

At the University of Washington, Gottman was offered an apartment lab that came to be known as "**the Love Lab**," where couples were invited to come and spend a whole day with each other while being observed. Couples participating in the research were observed interacting casually with

DOI: 10.4324/9781003369097-8

each other or were asked to have specific conversations of a positive or negative nature (Gottman, 1999, 2014; Gottman & Gottman, 2018). While the couples interacted, the researchers tracked their physiology and videotaped their conversations to track and rate their facial expressions, tone, and quality of interaction. Along with observation and direct measures of their interactions and physiology, couples were also interviewed using a research protocol that traced the trajectory of their relationship, evaluated their perceptions and experiences of several variables in the relationships, and completed surveys on marital satisfaction, psychological distress, and other self-report measures. In later studies, couples were asked to watch their own discussions, and using a rating dial, rate their perceptions of the conversation as negative or positive on a scale of 10 (Gottman & Gottman, 2018; Gottman & Silver, 2015). Many of these measures were synchronized to the video recording so analyses of emotion, physiology, or perception could be tied to specific events in the discussion. The wealth of data that was collected for over 40 years provided a unique glimpse into the inner and outer experiences of couples in happy as well as unhappy relationships and gave the researchers the power to successfully predict the outcome of a relationship with over 90% accuracy from a 15-minute conflict conversation (Gottman et al., 1998). At present, the Love Lab has been expanded and updated with new technology and research methods and work is underway on a clinical outcomes study as well as studies on infidelity recovery and marathon couples therapy (Gottman et al., 2019).

Gottman's background in mathematics was prominent in the research as he explored how to conduct time series, repeated measures, and covariant analyses. His first book, *Marital Interactions: Experimental Investigations*, published in 1979, was a primer on how to conduct statistically sound research on couples using coding systems for affect, behavior, and physiology. The research findings from the primary studies on heterosexual married couples were finally made available to the public through his first book for the general public titled, *Why Marriages Succeed or Fail* (1995) where he outlined the significant results from the seven primary studies. It was not until 1999 that his book, *The Marriage Clinic*, gave students and researchers, as well as clinicians, a glimpse into the methodology, measures, and techniques that were developed not only to observe couples but also to redirect or prevent distress.

In 1994, Gottman began collaborating with his wife, Julie Schwartz Gottman, a psychologist with many years of clinical experience working with trauma survivors and other complex populations. She helped John and his team translate his research into theory and then the theory into practice. John quips that as a researcher he was fascinated with simply observing couples deteriorate in front of his eyes, while Julie wanted to do something about it (Gottman & Gottman, 2015). Through this husband–wife collaboration, as well as working with other expert researchers in the fields of emotion, couples, psychophysiology, and psychotherapy such as Robert Levenson, Neil Jacobsen, Paul Ekman, Howard Markman, Paul Peluso, Julia Babcock, and others, the Gottmans were able to learn from and influence the direction of many research studies on relationships up to the present.

Four decades of systematic observational and empirical research later, they had two checklists of successful and unsuccessful behaviors that distinguished the Masters from the Disasters of relationship (Gottman, 1999). The Gottmans realized they needed a framework, or a theory that would help provide a causal explanation or a blueprint for how couples developed and maintained successful relationships as well as what goes awry in relationships that don't succeed. Julie Gottman's contributions spearheaded the dissemination of the Gottman research to the public with the development of the Sound Relationship House theory. This then led to the development of a clinical intervention program, a training program for clinicians, and also a two-day seminar for couples called The Art and Science of Love Workshop (Gottman & Gottman, 2015).

The seven observational studies that discovered and then replicated the key findings were based on regional representative samples of cisgendered heterosexual married couples, some of whom were in happy stable relationships and others in distressed relationships that were headed towards dissolution. Later, a 12-year study was conducted on same-sex relationships where many of the findings from the earlier research were found to apply with some key exceptions (Gottman & Gottman, 2016; Gottman et al., 2003). For example, same-sex couples began arguments with more positivity, were able to receive feedback more calmly, and had a more egalitarian perspective with regard to power and affect. More recent research from around the world has expanded this model to other special populations (Gottman et al., 2019; Rajaei et al., 2019; Rajendrakumar et al., 2023).

Primary Findings from the Gottman Studies

The 5 to 1 Ratio of Positive to Negative Interactions

As a mathematician, Gottman was interested in developing simple heuristics or formulas to distinguish the Masters from the Disasters of relationship. Contrary to previous literature on couples therapy, Gottman and Levenson (Gottman & Silver, 2015) found that Master couples were much gentler and softer in their approach to conflict. Master couples demonstrated a consistent pattern during conflict discussions of a 5:1 ratio of positive to negative moments when coded by trained observers. Distressed couples had a .8 to 1.0 ratio when they were fighting. This ratio was present regardless of whether the conflict management style of the couple was conflict-minimizing or volatile.

   The ratio of positive to negative moments is important because it suggests that healthy relationships have a very high level of positive interactions. In fact, when a Master couple was observed simply spending time with each other in the apartment lab, in other words in a non-conflict context, their ratio was closer to 20:1. While the 20:1 ratio may be difficult to achieve in real life, it is clear that lasting satisfying relationships are a rich environment of fun, easy, and light-hearted interactions, and positive expressions of appreciation and admiration.

Perpetual, Gridlocked, and Solvable Problems

Not all conflicts are the same. Some conflicts trigger underlying existential agendas or "dreams" such as what it means to be a husband or wife, what a home means, what parenting means, emotional or attachment needs for connection or autonomy, etc. The research showed that across all couples, 69% of the problems were perpetual and unsolvable (Gottman, 1995). These problems usually represented differences in personality styles, preferred ways of doing things, or values that each partner was fighting to maintain in the relationship. The topics and issues the couple were arguing about were remarkably stable after three years. Perpetual problems are not predictive of distress if the couple can maintain a dialogue on the issue and both feel heard and understood by the other. If 69% of all problems are perpetual, then the focus of couples therapy needs to be on helping a couple manage and minimize harm from differences rather than trying to solve or eliminate arguments.

   Gridlocked perpetual problems (about 16% of all problems) were characterized by several aspects that made them entrenched and distressing impasses in a relationship (Gottman, 1995). Conflict discussions that become gridlocked have certain similar qualities:

1 Each partner in the relationship feels rejected.
2 They have the same fight multiple times without making progress.
3 Both partners dig in and become more stubborn and/or polarized in their positions on the issue.
4 At some point, one or both of them begin to vilify their partner's perspective on the issue and label or judge their partner's actions as selfish, cold, unreasonable, or worse.
5 After repeated failures at discussing the issue, both partners feel flooded or physiologically activated each time they discuss the topic and begin to avoid talking about it.

The Master couples knew how to stay in dialogue, have a low threshold for negativity and prevent escalation, and really understand each other's position. John Gottman states that in the midst of the worst conflict is the possibility for the greatest closeness (Gottman & Gottman, 2018). When a couple is in a productive dialogue, they demonstrate a gentler approach to conflict, respond less defensively, harness a sense of humor or compassion for each other, and can postpone persuasion until they understand each other's perspectives at a deeper level which is where the possibility of feeling close to each other exists.

What Predicts Divorce?

The Gottmans found that the Masters of relationship engaged in certain behaviors that increased the likelihood of preserving their connection such as a strong friendship, high levels of positivity, absence of contempt, and successful repair during and after conflict; while the Disasters of relationship had certain deficits of friendship, emotion regulation, and conflict management that drove them to the brink (Gottman, 1999). Conflict was found to be inevitable in all relationships because being in an intimate environment will inevitably bring to the surface the ways in which each partner moves through time and space differently. So managing these predictable misattunements, solving what can be solved, and creating temporary or partial compromises and agreements to handle gridlocked perpetual issues becomes the pathway to health.

Couples in stable relationships were able to express their feelings or needs, even with emotion, and not damage the bond if they were able to keep the conversation at a low threshold of negativity and the 5:1 positive to negative ratio was present. When the intensity or negativity in the conversation or the relationship starts to escalate, distressed couples resort to four behaviors the Gottmans call the **Four Horsemen of the Apocalypse** which are Criticism, Defensiveness, Contempt, and Stonewalling (Gottman, 1999, 2014). These four behaviors were found to be highly predictive of conversations that deteriorated, and when repeated often, predicted relationships that were headed towards dissolution. The four horsemen concept became the cornerstone of the Gottmans' predictions about which relationships would last and which would not, especially Contempt, which was found to be the number one predictor for conversations and relationships that derail.

The Four Horsemen and Their Antidotes

Some of the early research (Gottman et al., 1976) had already shown that distressed couples tend to misinterpret communication as more negative than intended. In further studies, it was found that criticism and defensiveness were common behaviors found during disagreements between partners, and even Master couples were found to fall into them (Gottman & Silver, 2015). **Criticism** was defined as an attack or blaming statement when a problem that exists in the relationship was blamed on one partner's personality or habitual patterns. In essence, one partner was saying, "We have this problem in the relationship because something is wrong with you." The antidote to criticism was to learn to complain with a gentle startup. A **gentle startup** would include an "I" statement, a statement of feeling, a neutral description of a problem, and a positive request. **Defensiveness** was defined as a rebound or countering statement that was characterized by a sense of righteous indignation or innocent victimhood. In both cases, defensiveness was marked by an absence of taking responsibility for even a small part of the problem. The antidote to defensiveness was to help the partner find something in their partner's complaint that they can take responsibility for or agree with. Criticism and defensiveness tended to occur together such that when one partner was critical, the other partner became defensive and offered a counter-criticism. When two people were both using these tactics, the argument became stuck in an "attack-defend" mode.

Contempt was the most toxic of the four horsemen and was the single best predictor of deterioration in the conversation or relationship. Contempt was defined as any statement or behavior that communicates superiority or involves one person talking down to another. Examples of contempt included name-calling, swearing, correcting the partner's grammar or facts, or non-verbal facial expressions like a sneer along with an eye-roll. When contempt was present repeatedly in the first 15 minutes of a conversation, not only did this predict the end of the relationship, but it also correlated with the number of infectious illnesses in the recipient over the next four years. Gottman (1999) refers to contempt as "the sulphuric acid of love" (p. 129). The antidote to contempt is more complex. In Master couples, contempt was almost never used during arguments and if one of them said something hurtful or cruel, they realized it right away and took it back. Gottman believed that contempt was absent in Master couples because they had a rich climate of fondness and appreciation; that is, "The masters seemed to have a habit of mind in which they scanned their social environments for things to appreciate" (Gottman, 2015, p. 21). In the clinical setting, the antidote to contempt was defined as helping the contemptuous partner reframe their statement in terms of their own feelings and needs and avoid describing their partner. In a more general sense, however, contempt is organically eliminated when fondness and admiration, gratitude, and cherishing of each partner are found at high levels.

The fourth horseman was **Stonewalling** which was defined as non-verbal behaviors which communicated that the partner had stopped participating in the conversation and had in effect become like a stone wall. The recipient of stonewalling may experience this as a deliberate attempt to shut them out or as the partner becoming non-responsive on purpose. However, Gottman found that stonewallers were usually physiologically flooded and were engaged in suppressing their responses in an ineffective attempt to avoid making things worse. In the samples studied, 85% of the stonewallers were men. However, stonewalling was also present in lesbian relationships. The antidote to stonewalling, then, is for the flooded partner to ask for a break to help them return their physiology to baseline before re-engaging in the conversation.

It is important to note that one or two instances of using a four horsemen strategy was not necessarily a sign of relationship demise. Typically, these four horsemen were part of a larger framework of an isolation and distance cascade (described later) and would show up repeatedly and early in conflict conversations. In the case of Steve and Carissa, we know they came to therapy after tension began to build between them and they noted they had regular fights. We get to witness one such fight during which Carissa's complaint about Steve not scooping the cat litter begins to sound critical, especially when she says: "Do you want our house to smell like cat shit? What is wrong with you?" This fits the research definition for criticism because she is taking a problem in the relationship and blaming it on Steve (i.e., what is wrong with you?). Steve, on the other hand, is more defensive rather than critical. Early in this interchange, when Carissa is upset that he has not scooped the cat litter more often, Steve has an opportunity to diffuse the tension by taking some responsibility, such as admitting he has fallen behind or that he did not scoop it as often as she wanted. Instead, he argues that he has been doing it enough and then tells Carissa to do it herself. This is fairly typical of how tension can lead to bickering and arguing about small things. The final straw came when Steve was quite critical of Carissa, telling her she needed therapy. We don't know what else transpired in that argument, but perhaps this was when one or both of them resorted to using contempt (i.e., talking down to each other), and that became the last straw that brought them into therapy.

Physiological Arousal

Couples engaged in a conflict discussion showed physiological activation very similar to soldiers in a combat zone (Gottman, 1994, 1999). Inside their bodies, the sympathetic nervous system was activated, causing Diffuse Physiological Arousal (DPA) as if the organism was in danger, which included increased heart rate, rising blood velocity, narrowing of the visual field to reduce distraction from the periphery, narrowing of the auditory spectrum, and the movement of blood away from the extremities to the core to prepare the body to take action to escape the danger. These physiological changes are critical if we are trying to escape a physical danger, but in a verbal argument with a spouse, DPA can result if there is escalating negativity and one or both partners begin to feel unsafe. DPA during an argument can predispose the partner to take actions that escalate the argument, shut down the argument, or typically engage in the four horsemen strategies which are verbal analogues to fight, flight, or freeze.

A convenient measure of DPA is an elevated heart rate which can be measured manually or with a pulse oximeter. When the heart rate goes above 100 beats a minute, it is assumed the person in DPA cannot hear things accurately, cannot see things completely, and is likely to use escalating coping strategies such as fight, flight, or freeze to escape the situation. It was found that a high heart rate predicted stonewalling within 10 seconds.

Successful Repair

Gottman (2014) found that Master couples had more successful repair both during as well as after a fight or regrettable incident which was important to maintain the friendship and goodwill in the relationship. Master couples were found to be sensitive to signals of escalation and used repair attempts to diffuse or lower the negativity. **Repair attempts** were any gestures, words, or non-verbal signals from one partner to another that invited or suggested an apology, an acknowledgement, or a redirection.

Distressed couples had a higher threshold for negativity, did not repair often or effectively (typically they brushed unresolved arguments under the rug and tried to move on), and even when they attempted to repair, the partner did not accept their repair. If there was a general sense of tension and lack of safety, partners often misinterpreted even neutral signals as more negative than intended, a state called **Negative Sentiment Override** (NSO). If NSO was present, the person's ability to be open to repair and to be generous and forgiving when they received a repair from their partner was often lacking. **Positive Sentiment Override** (PSO) was present when partners were able to receive even what appeared to be negative feedback with generosity and compassion towards each other.

A Scientific Model for Healthy Relationships

The **Sound Relationship House** (SRH) is the theoretical model developed by the Gottmans based on their decades of longitudinal studies, clinical experience, and knowledge expertise. The model was developed as a way of translating their research into an explanatory system that showed how healthy relationships functioned in an integrated fashion, and how the three dimensions of a relationship—Friendship, Conflict Management, and Shared Meaning—interact with each other. More recently, the SRH model was modified to include trust and commitment as a result of ongoing research and publications on trust and betrayal that offered a new understanding of how problems developed and became entrenched in distressed relationships (Gottman, 2011).

The Sound Relationship House model (see Figure 8.1) has seven levels and two walls. The seven levels were the basis for John Gottman's bestselling book, *The Seven Principles for Making Marriage Work* (Gottman & Silver, 2015). The seven levels can be classified into three dimensions; namely, the friendship, conflict, and shared meaning dimensions. These three dimensions form the basis for the assessment as well as the treatment plan in Gottman method couples therapy.

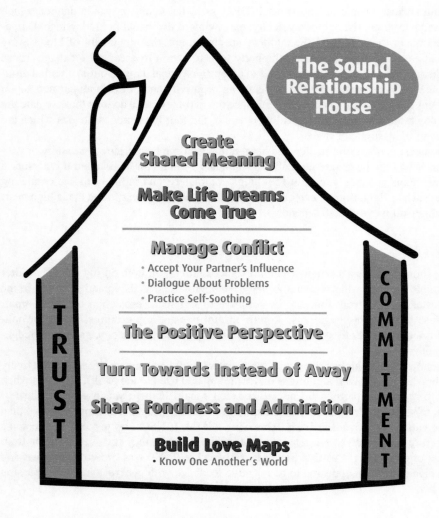

Figure 8.1 The Sound Relationship House.

Source: Reprinted with Permission from The Gottman Institute, Copyright 2015.

Friendship Dimension

Friendship is seen as the foundation of the relationship in the beginning. The components of friendship are the first three levels of the SRH. **Love Maps** refer to the mental map each partner has of their partner's world including preferences, interests, childhood experiences, priorities, stressors, and dreams. In healthy relationships, each partner makes an effort to keep these love maps updated as the relationship grows and life experiences impact each person. **Fondness** and **Admiration** refer to the amount of gratitude and appreciation that is shown and expressed between the partners. When appreciation is expressed on a regular and frequent basis, especially for meaningful traits and behaviors, the relationship is enveloped in a rich culture of positivity and gratitude. The third level is **Turning Towards**, which stands for the frequency with which partners in a couple respond to each other's bids for attention with positive and supportive gestures. Jani Driver, an associate of John Gottman, discovered this critical difference while observing couples spending time together in the lab between tasks (Gottman, 2014). She defined the fundamental unit of intimacy as the bid and the turn where the **bid** is a gesture or statement inviting the partner's attention, and the **turn** is the response from the partner. In response to a bid, the partner can turn towards or respond positively, turn away or ignore the bid, or turn against or respond harshly to the bid. Turning towards increased intimacy and safety, turning away increased distance and loneliness, while turning against increased resentment and anger. In the newlyweds' study (Gottman, 1995), couples in stable relationships were turning towards each other 86% of the time, while couples headed for separation were turning towards each other 33% of the time. The turning towards functioned as an emotional bank account that served as a bridge between the friendship and conflict dimensions of the relationship. A relationship rich with deposits into the emotional bank account through expressions of appreciation, turning towards, and attention to each other could weather hard moments with ease and humor.

The Positive Perspective

The fourth level of the SRH is the **Positive Perspective** and is adapted from Robert Weiss's work on Positive or Negative Sentiment Override (Hawkins et al., 2002). Couples in PSO had a general sense of trust and positivity in the relationship and were likely to interpret ambiguous signals with positive intent. Couples in NSO were likely to interpret neutral or ambiguous signals with negative intent. Negative perspective suggested that the overall feeling or weather of the relationship felt tense and uncertain, so interactions were viewed with suspicion and taken as personal affronts; while positive perspective meant the partners gave each other the benefit of the doubt or did not take gestures and statements as personal attacks. The perspective of the relationship cannot be changed directly because it is an outgrowth of a positive friendship foundation, but it had a significant impact on how conflict was managed in the relationship and whether partners were able to repair and recover from negative experiences.

The Conflict Dimension

The fifth level of the SRH is the **Conflict Dimension**. Gottman found conflict was inevitable in all couples and reciprocal anger was not predictive of ailing relationships (Gottman, 1999, 2014). When conflict included escalating negativity, the presence of the four horsemen, and failures in repair, the negativity impacted the functioning of the relationship at a high level. Distressed couples were likely to fall into negative arguments easily, struggle to solve even the simplest of problems, and did not have exit strategies from negative interactions. Major disagreements were likely to end in gridlocked impasses where each partner felt vilified, rejected, and reactive to each other. Satisfied couples, on the other hand, had a gentle approach to conflict, a low threshold for negativity, frequent repair and recovery from arguments, and a sense of humor that created the positive to negative ratio of 5:1 during disagreements.

Shared Meaning Dimension

The final two levels of the SRH comprise the shared meaning dimension. The sixth level, **Making Life Dreams Come True**, is both about supporting each other's existential agendas and attachment needs during conflict as well as more generally supporting each other's life dreams. In intimate relationships, some conflicts have a hidden agenda, often relating to one or both partners' emotional needs, values, or deeply felt longings, that can make simple solutions challenging. The research showed that 69% of all conflicts across satisfied and distressed couples were perpetual which meant that the couple argued about these issues for many years without ever solving them (Gottman, 1999). Master couples seemed to understand that in perpetual conflict, maintaining dialogue and seeking partial or temporary compromises that supported each other's existential or attachment needs were important. Unhappy couples often tried to win or persuade their partner to give up their agendas and created gridlocked conflict that became the source of great distress in the relationship. Similarly, when couples experienced the relationship as supporting their life dreams, they were more willing to sacrifice for each other and built a sense of family with each other.

The last level, **Creating Shared Meaning**, refers to the fact that couples enter into intimate attachment relationships to experience a bond that goes beyond roommates and friends. The adult romantic bond is about creating shared experiences, new values, and life dreams, and building memories of special events and experiences with each other. This is often referred to as the "attic" of the SRH where couples create a sense of purpose, home, family, and shared culture and memories with each other through repeated events and activities that have special meaning in their lives. The couple builds rituals of connection, where they have repeated activities or experiences they can count on. The key to shared meaning is that small things often make a big difference. So small gestures, rituals, habits, or events done on a regular and frequent basis can change the trajectory of the relationship.

Conceptualization of Problem Formation

It is important to reiterate that the Gottman research was phenomenological and was based on observations of couples interacting without therapeutic intervention. The Sound Relationship House theory (SRH) is an explanatory model that describes the main ingredients of a healthy relationship. In order to understand how problems develop in relationships, we need to first understand how romantic relationships evolve.

In his book, *Principia Amoris*, Gottman (2014) describes the three stages of falling in love.

Phase 1: Limerence

The first stage is characterized by **limerence** which has been described as the intoxication caused by a cocktail of hormones and neurotransmitters that surge through the body when one person is attracted to another. Steve and Carissa's story begins with such an experience of limerence: meeting at a club and ending up in bed together the same night. The cascade of falling in love is based on a highly selective and complex interaction between mate selection parameters, physiology, and emotional variables that signal a match between two people. The interplay of these variables creates a sense of rightness or good fit between two particular people who feel physically attracted to each other. During this phase, it seems effortless to dream about a future together, to want to know everything about the other person, and to happily take risks (for example, sexually) or give our trust and heart to the other person.

This first phase is strengthened when the couple engages in building love maps and expressing fondness and admiration for each other in frequent and meaningful ways. As the adrenaline and excitement start to lessen, other hormones and chemicals such as oxytocin help build a sense of comfort, bonding, attachment, receptivity, pleasure, and a motivation to deepen the relationship. Friendship, safety, intimacy, and eroticism function together to create a foundation for the love the couple feels for each other. As phase one is navigated, the couple is drawn into a more intimate and personal relationship with each other. One can imagine Steve and Carissa building love maps and feeding their physical and emotional attraction with each other as they spent almost every evening in Steve's apartment. The intensity of the bond that is created by so much contact right away can sometimes make one or both partners a little blind to each other's faults and quirks. The excitement of being in their first interracial relationship might have fueled a sense of novelty and excitement that increased the rapid attachment they felt for each other.

Phase 2: Building Trust

Early in the relationship, excitement and adrenaline override common sense, and trust can be given easily with small gestures and verbal declarations of love. Trust in the first phase may be more gifted than earned. In the second stage, the chemicals have faded, and the reality of the complexity or rough edges of the relationship may begin to surface. Steve and Carissa did not seem to experience the doubt, fear, or disappointment that disperses the rosy glow for many couples. Traits and behaviors that seemed charming may become sources of irritation or annoyance. Gottman (2014) found that most fights occurred in the first two years of a relationship because of this disillusionment experience. Steve and Carissa's relationship did not face this challenge because they were actively dating and engaged in gaining trust and credibility with each other through lots of intimate couple time.

Trust is built through small and large experiences in the relationship where each partner demonstrates that they value the other, prioritize the other's needs or interests, and will work towards building intimacy and commitment. Each partner in the relationship looks for evidence that their partner will be there for them, especially during emotionally significant moments, and will care enough to "have their back." Carissa and Steve showed care and consideration in how they told their parents about this intercultural relationship and how they helped each other to become a part of their family and friends' circles.

Attunement during moments of turning towards each other or during emotionally significant experiences helps strengthen the feeling of having the partner's support and empathy (Gottman, 2014). Building trust at this stage is about setting aside one's self-interest and holding the partner's best interest in heart and mind. When this occurs, each partner experiences fairness and justice in relationship negotiations or decisions. Interracial relationships often require a greater degree of fairness and justice to overcome societal judgment and discrimination. Steve and Carissa were building this solid foundation by navigating all the stressors of being in an interracial relationship while they were dating and later living together after marriage.

Trust building, attunement, fairness, and being there for each other are essential in establishing a foundation of intimacy as well as building a container of positivity that generates the PSO in the relationship. Steve and Carissa invested a lot of their time and energy in the relationship, especially when Steve took the job in Orlando and spent a lot of time with Carissa and her family in Bushnell, building closeness and emotional safety with all of them. In this positive context, Steve and Carissa managed conflict easily, were able to have dialogues rather than gridlock about their perpetual issues; they accepted each other's influence, humor and appreciation were high, and repair was both easy and successful.

Through consistent interactions demonstrating mutual support and engagement with each other's interests, Steve and Carissa seemed to experience the relationship as having a foundation of trust leading to long-term investment in each other. When trust and commitment are present, the relationship progresses from dating to engagement and then to exchanging vows in a marriage or commitment ceremony.

Phase 3: Building Commitment and Loyalty

Gottman's contribution to the understanding of trust and betrayal is unique and very useful for clinical practice with couples. Building and losing trust in a relationship is not the same as betrayal and many couples therapy approaches have a misunderstanding of this difference (Gottman, 2011). The process of building trust versus mistrust happens in all relationships. **Trust** is gained when partners are attuned and emotionally present for each other. **Mistrust** is created when mis-attunement or turning away takes place, which is actually quite common, but trust is restored through the repair process. In Steve and Carissa's story, one sees how much they invested in knowing each other and each other's families in the early years by spending almost every weekend together, both while dating and married. One can imagine that because of this positive investment, both were able to build trust, repair mistrust, and overcome the challenges they faced. One can see how this would have contributed to a relatively happy and peaceful few years at the start of their marriage.

Betrayal, on the other hand, is related to failures in investment, true commitment, and loyalty. Once set in motion, betrayal becomes a downhill cascade. Betrayal comes in all forms, not just infidelity, and provides evidence that one or both partners are taking care of their own needs and interests at the expense of the other person. In Carissa and Steve's case, betrayal began in small ways when Steve made friends at work and began to spend a lot of time with them playing disc golf, softball, or watching football. While Carissa initially accepted Steve's friendships and time away from her, it soon became a source of conflict between them when she graduated and wanted more time alone with Steve.

Gottman found that during this third phase of building commitment and loyalty, the couple is faced with significant choices. The first choice is to nourish gratitude and cherish the partner, focusing on what they have gained in being with their partner. The second choice is to nourish resentment and focus on what they have lost or sacrificed in the relationship. If the couple focuses on cherishing their relationship and being grateful, they work together towards a lifetime commitment and deep loyalty. One can see this slow build-up towards resentment and trashing each other (in their heads) and finding fault in each other in Carissa and Steve's situation. Carissa begins to spend more time at her mother's house and expresses her ambivalence about her commitment. Steve begins to think Carissa is out of control and blames or criticizes her way of functioning. These internal narratives put both partners on the cascade towards betrayal or divorce with increasing feelings of loneliness, ambivalence, and judgment towards each other.

Distance and Isolation Cascade

The Gottmans found that the first two years after commitment or marriage tend to be critical in establishing patterns of creating and maintaining positivity as well as negativity (Gottman, 2014). They believe that buyer's remorse usually sets in within the first two years after two people have begun cohabiting. In a relationship headed towards distress and possibly dissolution, the couple does not manage these initial conflicts very well and their arguments become escalated; they each get flooded, or they brush the conflict under the rug and avoid discussing challenging topics leading to more disconnection and less psychological safety. Avoiding conflict is usually not possible for long periods, so the couple will engage in a conflict discussion at some point and when they do, the act of suppressing past arguments means they have unresolved hurts or resentments that get carried forward into the new argument. This increases the chance that subsequent fights become more intense, negative, or overwhelming, leading to more withdrawal and resentment which in turn leads to less intimacy, self-disclosure, and friendship. With repeated cycles of fighting, withdrawal, and avoidance set in motion, the partners begin to live parallel lives and turn away from each other or meet their needs elsewhere. This becomes a sort of emotional divorce which then increases the chance of one or both taking the step of a physical divorce.

Trust and Commitment: The Walls of the Sound Relationship House

Trust and commitment as two important variables in a healthy relationship were added to the SRH model in recent years because of observing that teaching couples the skills associated with the seven levels of the model did not guarantee that all couples could have a happy stable relationship (Gottman, 2011, 2014). The key elements seemed to rest in how trust was built and preserved in the relationship through the three phases of love and how much each partner was invested in the relationship (Gottman, 2011). Gottman (2011) describes a 24-step cascade towards betrayal that begins with repeated experiences of one partner reaching for the other during moments of pain or need and the responding partner turning away with negative internal thoughts such as "Who needs this negativity or this demand? I can do better." Gottman called this internal dialogue "**negative comparisons**" or "**negative comps**" and found that this sets the relationship on the course towards disconnection and dissatisfaction. We hear echoes of these negative comps in Steve's judgment of Carissa as being out of control, or in Carissa's doubts about the viability of the marriage and her coping by turning away from Steve (for example, by leaving and staying with her mom). However, the couple has only been experiencing this tension and negativity for a couple of years, and it is situationally connected to their frustrations around Carissa getting pregnant, so the prognosis for treatment is still positive.

In the relationship that is building loyalty, both partners are cherishing each other, accepting the positive aspects of the relationship they have, sacrificing self-interest for mutual benefit, and creating a culture of gratitude and appreciation that reinforces itself. In relationships where resentment and self-interest are being nurtured and reinforced, partners may mentally or verbally trash each other and develop resentment and disrespect for each other. Depending on circumstances, cultural values, or other factors, the relationship may enter the distance and isolation cascade or the 24-step cascade towards betrayal. Steve and Carissa are not yet very far on this cascade. They have experienced the first few steps where fights have escalated and become gridlocked, one or both have used criticism or defensiveness in their arguments, and one or both have turned away from each other. However, we don't see the later stages of the cascade such as living parallel lives and being emotionally disengaged to the point of being in an emotional divorce.

When the couple enters therapy, the Gottman trained therapist carefully evaluates the strengths and challenges of the relationship using the Sound Relationship House model and judges whether the distance and isolation cascade or the cascade towards betrayal is in play in the relationship to create a treatment plan that addresses the specific causes of the distress and reverses the negative trajectory.

Conceptualizing Diversity

There is a growing trend for diverse couples to be seeking professional help, and this has put diversity considerations front and center in couples work in a way it has not been in previous decades (Lebow & Snyder, 2022). Diversity considerations live at both the surface level in terms of differences in attitudes, values, world views, and behaviors, but also at the internal level in terms of internalized -isms related to race, gender, religion, social class, and other intersectional identities. We cannot separate interpersonal struggles in a relationship from the identity struggles that each individual brings to the table.Increasingly, therefore, couple therapists are being asked to demonstrate greater comfort and competence in navigating complex interpersonal dynamics in couples that go beyond the theoretical models being used and incorporate complex identity politics and implicit bias or oppressive experiences as they are being played out in the couple relationship. Working with diverse couples means working with the subtle and explicit differences in identity and culture as experienced by each partner, and understanding that when one partner is a member of a minority culture or has an oppressed or marginalized identity, they're coming into the therapy room already anticipating that they're going to feel "othered" and they're going to feel different from everybody in the room and that their concerns may or may not be addressed. The therapist has to know how to raise the issue of key intersectional identities in the room without problematizing them. They must provide a comfort level and a skill in inviting rich and complex dialogue without triggering shame, guilt, or fear and help the partners have safe honest dialogue about these topics. The basic premise is that diversity makes us stronger. Diversity is additive and enriching and goes beyond simply accepting, tolerating, and living with differences. Diversity is about affirming and welcoming the complexity of different cultural, ethnic, religious, or class backgrounds and seeing it as a potential for the couple to have a more nuanced, rich, and fulfilling relationship.

In many of the early articles on his research, Gottman and his research collaborators noted the lack of racial and ethnic representation in their research samples (Carstensen et al., 1995; Driver & Gottman, 2004; Gottman, 1994). All the initial studies were conducted with married cisgendered heterosexual adults in traditional relationships and the findings were cautiously extrapolated to all relationships (Gottman, 1994). Efforts were made to achieve representative samples based on the local or regional context which was a midwestern small city or a large west coast city. Subsequent research and clinical scholarship have confirmed that the Gottmans' research and theory apply to diverse identities and populations in most Western cultures and also some non-Western cultures (Rajaei et al., 2019; Rajendrakumar et al., 2023). Concepts such as contempt, repair, harsh startup (discussed later), and accepting influence can be found universally, even though their expression or mannerisms might be culturally mediated.

Just as the Sound Relationship House (SRH) theory and model informs every aspect of Gottman couples therapy from assessment to treatment planning to intervention, it can also be used as the template to understand how to integrate diversity considerations into Gottman couples therapy. We can look at how to help each couple work through each level of the SRH using a diversity sensitivity lens.

1 Love Maps means knowing and acknowledging one's self-narrative in terms of what one tells people about oneself, and what one's partner should know about one's internalized beliefs, -isms, stigmas, and view of self in the world from a social identity perspective. This might include self-disclosing not only past experiences with culturally different ways of being in the world, but also disclosing experiences with oppression and discrimination, how marginalization has affected one's view of self, and how one navigates and manage intersectional identities in terms of salience, context, and safety.

2 Fondness and admiration is about affirming, celebrating, and honoring each other's whole identity. This is where one's intimate partner needs to go beyond cultural tourism or surface-level understandings of their partner's values, behaviors, and mores, but learn what it means to celebrate and honor their partner's contribution to the multicultural home life the two partners are creating.

3 Turning towards becomes important in interactional spaces and when navigating subgroup or intergroup experiences. For example, one partner being able to take your partner to a family reunion where they may be the only non-White person and making sure you're turning towards your partner, checking in with them, attuning to them, and being conscious of their experience. Turning towards is also about recognizing how your partner bids for attention and what lands for them in terms of a response. In this context, the non-White partner may not be able to give explicit signals or set boundaries with the White partner's relatives (for example, Steve's aunt who repeatedly touches Carissa's hair, claiming she wants to know what Black hair feels like). Steve has to be really sensitive to this and possibly talk ahead of time with Carissa about how they are going to signal each other when she needs him to turn towards her.

4 Trust is defined in terms of three concepts: (1) Fairness, (2) Do you have my back? and (3) Will you be there for me when I need you, especially in emotional moments? In an intercultural relationship, we need to bring a social justice sensitivity that includes acceptance and repair of microaggressions that inevitably happen. Many interracial/intercultural couples fail to explore and negotiate how to acknowledge and repair microaggressions both within the relationship as well as when they are interacting with the outside world. The Gottman therapist maintains this awareness and helps the couple have a dialogue about these topics.

5   Commitment in a diverse relationship is not just about committing to each other, but goes beyond the dyad to the level of commitment each partner has to fully integrate each other into their lives. The Gottman therapist helps the couple explore how to interact with and build a sense of belonging to both sets of relatives or negotiating how to handle a parent or relative who might not be diversity-friendly. In Steve's case, he was lucky to be welcomed and integrated into Carissa's family as they grew to know him. However, his father has indicated his discomfort and judgment about their interracial marriage so Steve may need to be collaborative in how much Carissa is asked to interact with her father-in-law, especially if Steve notices that his father does not soften towards Carissa as he gets to know her. Some interracial couples will keep their family and friends separate and not work towards integration because of discomfort or lack of skill. The Gottman therapist would help the couple engage in dialogue about this process in order to help each partner learn how to be a more sensitive, attuned, and comfortable person to bring to the diverse contexts.

6   Conflict management looks at the emotional and conflict cycle between the partners and explores the parallel process between intergroup or subgroup tensions in society that may be getting played out in the home. Many interracial couples ignore or avoid these conversations, but it affects their safety, intimacy, and comfort in bringing their family or friends to the house. The therapist's role in this situation is to help the couple develop some skills in communicating without using the four horsemen behaviors of criticism, defensiveness, contempt, and stonewalling. The therapist also helps the couple develop ground rules, boundaries, or learn cultural humility so they can acknowledge their blind spots or discomfort and work towards becoming allies and having a united front.

    Conflict management in the context of diversity is about teaching people how to repair mistakes and misunderstandings. The therapist normalizes and validates that we are all products of our circumstances and that mis-attunements and microaggressions may happen, but teaches the partners how to repair, to have a low threshold for negativity, to turn towards each other and tolerate negative affect when we upset our partner, and to learn how to do preemptive and early repair so that trust, closeness, and psychological safety within the relationship are maintained and improved over time.

7   Shared meaning is about supporting each other's life dreams as well as building shared meaning, values, and an integrated bi- or multicultural household. The goal is to make the world inside the home an authentic integrated ecology that feels like a truly multicultural world. A world where people are educated, informed, sensitive, mindful, aware, able to talk in a courageous manner about differences without judging or problematizing them. In terms of shared meaning values, the diverse couple needs to have more explicit and collaborative conversations about what aspects of their background and upbringing they want to bring forward into their relationship. Shared meaning becomes a process of creating "just" partnerships where fairness, equity, and belonging are all treated as important and worked on.

There's always an aspect of cultural difference, superiority/inferiority, and social status for people in a relationship who are from different religions, cultures, ethnicities, or races. There will be an experience of one culture that is/may be regarded as less than the other. Thus, there will be a subjugated culture and one that is the dominant culture. And it's very important for the therapist to know and be aware of this.

The Role of the Therapist

There are several assumptions underlying the Gottman method of couples therapy that all therapists who receive formal training in this method are asked to embody in their clinical approach. The key assumptions that relate to the therapist's role or approach in Gottman couples therapy are highlighted here (see Figure 8.2 below).

1 **Couples therapy should be primarily dyadic**: The therapist's job is to help the couple talk more to each other, navigate conversations with each other, and experience better communication in the room with each other than with the therapist.

2 **Couples therapy should be emotion focused:** All emotions are considered adaptive and acceptable. Emotions function as signals for therapeutic content that is important, meaningful, or historically significant, and the Gottman couples therapist guides and coaches the couple to become more "emotion coaching" or accepting of emotions in their interactions with each other.

3 **State dependent learning**: The best learning in couples therapy takes place when new skills or strategies are learned in the emotional or mental state in which they will be required outside the therapy office. Learning to pause and reflect while being angry or sad will equip the partner to remember and use that strategy at a future time when they are feeling angry or sad.

4 **Diffuse Physiological Arousal (DPA)**: When one or both partners are physiologically activated such that their sympathetic nervous system goes into the stress-coping response of fight or flight and simultaneously their adrenal axis is activated with the experience of fear, hopelessness, helplessness, or threat of danger, their bodies go into DPA. In a state of DPA, the heart rate is elevated, the hearing and vision change, and the partner is no longer able to process information and communication accurately. The couples therapist has to watch for these signs and help both partners take a break and self-soothe before continuing the conversation.

5 **The therapist's role is not to soothe:** A Gottman therapist recognizes when one or both partners are in DPA or in an intense emotional state that prevents them from listening or speaking coherently and invites the partners to take a pause. In the pause or break, the therapist helps the couple learn how to soothe themselves or each other so they learn this skill to use outside of the therapy session and they do not become dependent on the therapist to help them downregulate emotion dysregulation.

6 **Couples therapy should have low psychological costs:** Interventions should feel simple, easy to do, and not require a large expenditure of time or energy. One of the main critiques of couples therapy is the high relapse rate. Couples relapse because interventions they learn in therapy are either too different from who they are, take a large investment of time or energy, and/or seem complicated and artificial. Couples may make heroic efforts to adopt these new behaviors, but they will eventually slip back into old habits. The Gottman therapy motto is "Small Things Often" which represents the belief that small incremental changes that are overlearned (repeated to ensure learning) are more likely to stick.

7 **Couples therapy should be a primarily positive experience:** The Gottman couples therapist maintains an awareness that couples are in distress and tries to look for opportunities to reframe problems in positive or relational and systemic terms so neither partner feels blamed. Framing problems as "dreams in conflict" suggests that two people are both longing for or fighting for different things and the couple can learn to compromise or honor both dreams. Gottman therapists also believe that increasing positivity when not in conflict will help couples reduce tension and increase closeness at home, and within that context, conflict management will become easier and more successful.

8 **Gottman couples therapy is not idealistic about relationships and their potential:** Happy couples do not have the best or ideal relationships. They tend to have relationships where both people basically like each other, enjoy spending time with each other, and represent good environments in which they can grow and raise kids. Since relationships are formed from a variety of circumstances and from diverse backgrounds and cultures, a universal definition of a healthy relationship is difficult. Working towards a good enough relationship that is satisfying to both partners seems much more achievable and worthy as the goal of couples therapy.

Figure 8.2 The key assumptions of Gottman couples therapy relating to the role of the therapist.

The Gottman therapist's role in the sessions, based on the above assumptions, becomes one of coach, facilitator, and "emotion coaching" guide (Gottman & Gottman, 2018) who helps the couple have the deep, connecting, and emotionally vulnerable conversations they long for. After the assessment sessions, in a typical Gottman therapy intervention session, the therapist begins with a check-in and learns what issue or topic is on the front burner for the couple. The therapist always begins with the issue most relevant or active for the couple and guides the couple in a dialogue about the issue using the appropriate Gottman intervention or skill. If the couple does not have a topic or issue to offer, the Gottman therapist will refer to the assessment results and suggest a gridlocked perpetual issue that was highlighted during the assessment.

To embody the principle of small things often, the Gottman therapist helps break down complex large issues into bite-sized segments that can be explored, addressed, and transformed, and the homework from each session becomes practicing the skill or discussing the issue at home on their own. At the beginning and/or end of the session, the Gottman therapist also highlights and invites the couple to express positivity in the form of appreciations, insights, and positive strengths they both bring to the relationship or the problem they are tackling. In this way, the therapist makes sure that couples therapy leaves the couple feeling more positive and connected with each other, and consolidates gains after each session through debriefs or reviews between the couple of the insights and benefits they got from the session, and homework exercises that expand and establish new ways of moving through time with each other at home.

Conceptualization of Problem Resolution

In Gottman method couples therapy the targets of change are three aspects of the relationship: (1) to increase positivity when the couple is not fighting; (2) to reduce negativity during fights; and (3) to increase positivity during fights (Gottman et al., 2002). Changing positivity during the non-conflict context takes place through small positive behaviors repeated on a daily basis and thus is the easiest aspect to improve. Positive affect that creates a general atmosphere of fondness and admiration reduces negativity during fights and also contributes to successful repair. The hardest goal to achieve through therapy is the third goal of increasing positivity during fights, because when NSO is present, it is difficult to convince partners to see the good in their relationship or to practice compassion and generosity. However, if a couple can make improvements in the first goal of increasing positivity outside of disagreements, the likelihood of achieving the second and third goals is greatly increased. Typically, the Gottman therapist addresses communication and conflict management goals in therapy sessions while helping the couple practice friendship and shared meaning activities at home to produce an isomorphic process of improvement on both fronts.

The Assessment of the Couple

Gottman method couples therapy begins with a three-session assessment process based on the research protocol, which is used to identify the strengths and challenges of the couple in therapy by mapping their relationship onto the Sound Relationship House (Gottman & Silver, 2015).

In the first session, which usually lasts 90 minutes, the therapist conducts a semi-structured clinical interview that includes understanding the couple's narrative and reasons for seeking therapy, followed by an oral history interview where the trajectory of the relationship is traced from the very first moment of meeting each other to the critical moments and transitions in the relationship, adjustment to each other after commitment or marriage, and adjusting to life challenges such as becoming parents, health challenges, or outside influences (Gottman, 1999). Based on the research protocol, the oral history interview includes specific questions that can be used to evaluate the couple's friendship, their conflict management style and experiences, their shared meaning, and their experiences of trust and commitment. In the case of Steve and Carissa, the therapist would explore some of the reasons they were attracted to each other and what led them to decide to be sexual with each other so quickly. The sexual encounter so early in the first stage of falling in love (i.e., limerence) might have disrupted the organic process of building a friendship, finding out about each other, and deciding to date each other based on personal qualities and values rather than physical attraction alone. During the first two questions on the oral history interview, the therapist also explores and addresses the racial and ethnic differences between Steve and Carissa. Part of this exploration might include their past relationship history and why they were attracted to each other, and how they handled dating and doing activities in public with the possibility of judgment and prejudice being directed at them.

Towards the end of the first session, the couple is invited to discuss a conflictual topic while the therapist observes and codes the conflict dimensions that have predictive power such as the presence of the four horsemen, especially contempt, physiological arousal (by measuring the heart rate), escalating negativity, low positive to negative ratio, and the failure of repair. While it is not possible in the clinical context to predict the outcome of a single relationship, the research provides a framework for evaluating the danger signals that could lead to the end of the relationship. When Steve and Carissa have their conflict discussion, it will be critical for the therapist to observe and make a note of the power and control dynamics in the relationship. This is particularly important in intercultural relationships where privilege, entitlement, microaggressions, or subtle vertical hierarchies of gender and race might be enacted (Bustamante et al., 2011).

The second 90 minute-session is split into two individual sessions of 45 minutes each and each partner is interviewed about their wishes for the therapy, their complaints about the relationship, and their commitment level. The individual session also allows the therapist to ask questions about domestic violence, secrets, betrayals, and other aspects of the relationship that may not be disclosed in a joint session, with the caveat that whatever is shared in the individual session becomes part of the couples therapy process. In some cases, the therapist may need to hold a secret or confidential information temporarily while helping the partner develop the courage or find the right moment to disclose it. However, the message is that couples therapy is intended to increase honesty and transparency in the relationship, so the therapist cannot undermine that goal by encouraging secret-keeping.

The couple is invited to complete the online questionnaires on the Gottman Connect website which allows each of them to separately rate the strengths and challenges in the relationship. The questionnaires are analyzed, and a report is sent to the therapist which is then combined with the clinical interviews to form a detailed profile of the couple's wishes and dreams, the relationship strengths and growth edges, and the priorities for treatment.

The Gottman Treatment Plan

Once the therapist has gathered the information from the assessment interviews and questionnaires, the treatment plan is developed with specific goals identified in collaboration with the couple in the three dimensions of friendship, conflict, and shared meaning (Gottman & Gottman, 2015). Since the interviews and questionnaires help the therapist map the couple's relationship onto the Sound Relationship House model, the treatment plan is fairly straightforward to create and share with the couple using the model as a template. When comorbidities such as violence, betrayal, addictions, or individual psychological disorders are present, the treatment plan considers not only how the couples therapy plan and techniques need to be adapted to address the comorbidities, but also what adjunct services and treatments need to be in place to provide additional support for each individual in the couple.

A typical treatment plan will include helping the couple establish skills for managing conflict, rebuilding the friendship and shared meaning systems, and strengthening trust and commitment by building a couple system with responsiveness, attunement, and cherishing each other. Couples learn the Sound Relationship House model and how couples therapy will reinforce their strengths and transform their challenges. Couples are encouraged to put time and energy into their relationship at home with a focus on friendship and shared meaning. The pacing of sessions follows the massed sessions with a fading model found to have the lowest relapse rates (Boegner & Zielenbach-Coenen, 1984, as cited in Gottman et al., 2002), which means that early sessions are longer or closer together, and once the relationship is stabilized, the focus turns to maintenance and relapse prevention as sessions are placed farther apart and the couple's ability to stay high functioning between sessions is evaluated.

Conflict management is the primary focus of early therapy sessions to reduce and diffuse the escalating negativity, stabilize the relationship, reinvest in each other, and build hope and optimism for the future. Friendship and shared meaning are brought into the therapy sessions as examples of homework and the couple is encouraged to focus their efforts at home on building positivity outside the conflict context. The **conflict blueprint** provides a four-step framework for understanding and managing conflict discussions, which helps the couple see in a visual form the process of therapy. Steps one and two are about building understanding, exploring each partner's position, experience, or needs on an issue, and laying the groundwork for a compromise or agreement on how they will navigate conflictual topics.

Step one is a communication exercise that includes listening, validation, acceptance of two subjective realities, and building understanding through postponing persuasion. In these first sessions, all techniques are set aside if the four horsemen behaviors of criticism, defensiveness, contempt, or stonewalling enter the discussion or if one of the partners becomes physiologically activated. The couple is coached to implement the antidotes to the four horsemen, take a break if one or both are in DPA, and learn how to take a break or redirect a conversation away from gridlock and escalation. As the safety and stability in the couple increases, step two in conflict management helps a couple engage in dialogue about perpetual problems by understanding each partner's inner world, dreams, values, needs, and longings, and building empathy for each partner's position on the major problems in the relationship. The **Dreams within Conflict** technique is the foundational exercise in Gottman couples therapy because it embodies the spirit and structure of the existential, relational, and narrative focus of the Gottman approach. Couples learn to not only understand, but also begin to nurture admiration for and cherish each other's contribution to the richness of the relationship, and understand how their inner dreams as well as childhood experiences impact and inform their coping strategies during emotional moments. Step three is the **compromise process** where couples learn to focus their compromise efforts on understanding each other's core and non-negotiable needs and finding ways to honor those, while negotiating on their areas of flexibility. If the first three steps are successful, couples will learn that there is a possibility for the greatest intimacy and bonding underlying the most gridlocked perpetual problems. If there are past injuries or unprocessed negative events, step four includes a **structured repair exercise** that takes the couple through five steps for having a recovery conversation and clearing the air so they can let go of resentment or heal attachment injuries from the past. The five steps comprise (1) listening and understanding each other's emotions during the injurious incident, (2) sharing each other's subjective realities and validating some part of each reality, (3) exploring triggers that escalated or caused the hurt and how the triggers relate to childhood or past relationship experiences, (4) understanding how each of them contributed to the regrettable incident, and finally (5) what each of them would like their partner and themself to do differently if a similar incident were to occur. Sometimes step four has to be done first to clear unfinished hurts and resentments from previous incidents before a clean conversation about the issue can be successful in the present.

Friendship and shared meaning techniques include creative and playful techniques for helping couples update their love maps, build fondness and admiration, and create shared meaning, through rituals of connection, for example. To build the emotional bank account and increase their bids and turning towards system, couples are helped to become more mindful, learn their partner's wishes and needs for particular ways to turn towards them, and work towards establishing a rich culture of appreciation so they can achieve the 5:1 ratio during conflict conversations. Many of these creative and easy techniques include small things repeated often so they are relatively easy to introduce at the beginning or end of a session and then take outside the session as homework assignments. The extent to which a couple commits and puts effort into the friendship and shared meaning homework activities often impacts the success of their conflict management process.

Relapse Prevention

Couples therapy cannot be considered successful or completed without some consideration of relapse prevention. Couples tend to relapse to pre-intervention levels of distress within two years if there is no ongoing effort to maintain gains (Gottman et al., 2002). Relapse prevention is addressed in the Gottman approach in several ways. First, the couple is coached to expect relapse and to learn what triggers or variables put them on the road to relapse. These triggers and variables are explored in session and agreements are made about how they will address them with each other. Second, the couples therapy is faded over time, with increasing gaps between sessions to help the couple transfer the gains to their home life and practice the skills on their own to ensure that they are changing their habits and behavior rather than just knowing what needs to change. Third, relapse is addressed through specific guidelines for weekly activities and time together that will maintain a focus on the health of the relationship. The Gottman **"Magic Five Hours"** handout provides the couple with a structured template for daily rituals of connection, weekly state of the union meetings, techniques to buffer their relationship from outside stress, and ways to preserve or strengthen the positivity, friendship, sex, romance, and intimacy in the relationship (Gottman, 1999). Finally, the couple is encouraged to continue building their relationship through periodic booster sessions of therapy, couples retreats and workshops, or establishing joint interests and activities such as dancing, outdoor activities, or community efforts that will bring them together as a team.

Case Transcript

Therapist: Hello, thank you for coming in today. This first session is an opportunity for us to meet each other and for me to learn what you would like to get out of couples therapy and for us to see if I am a good fit for you as a couples therapist. Let's start with the two of you telling me what brings you to couples therapy today, whoever wants to go first.

This is the standard opening question in Gottman therapy. The therapist is providing an opportunity for the couple to tell the story of what brings them to couples therapy without imposing a structure on it. By making this question general and not directed at one person, the therapist can observe not only what the couple says, but also how the story is told, how the two partners interact with each other, who dominates the conversation, the quality of intimacy and friendship in the couple, and the emotional tone of their narrative.

Steve: We have been fighting a lot. And it's gotten to be too much.
Carissa: I agree. Both of us are exhausted and don't know how to change what is happening.
Therapist: Tell me about these fights you are having. How they start, what they are typically about, and how they end.

The therapist is trying to build rapport with both partners and stay in exploration mode. The therapist asks the question of both partners to see who answers, who dominates, and how they navigate the question as a couple.

Steve: I don't know what the fights are about. One minute we're making dinner and the next we're fighting. I just get so frustrated that I usually shut down or storm out.

Steve is describing a dynamic of conflict dysregulation between them that includes a rapid escalation and intense negative reciprocity. Gottman (1999) found that the early divorcing profile tended to have these components—frequent arguments about lots of things (which the couple describe as trivial or not huge issues), but the arguments escalate rapidly into an impasse that is solved by one person leaving.

Therapist: Can you describe what is happening during this escalation and how bad things have gotten between you? If I was a fly on the wall, and you were having a really bad fight, what are some things I would see?

Steve: We don't yell and scream at each other or call each other names, thankfully. But we both get very stubborn, argumentative, and neither of us gives an inch. Carissa gets upset about something I said and won't back down. She misrepresents what I said so I try to defend myself but that just seems to fuel the fire more.

Therapist: Carissa, what is your side of this experience? How do you see the fights between you starting and ending and what is your take on the escalation?

While the therapist was witnessing who answered questions first and who dominated the narrative, at some point the therapist steps in to invite the silent partner to comment on the topic. This shows the couple that the therapist is tracking the flow of the conversation and that both people's voices are heard.

Carissa: I agree that our fights escalate very quickly and that at some point Steve gets angry and storms out. What he is not telling you is why our fights escalate. Steve hates conflict or emotions and I am very emotionally expressive. He is so White in his way of dealing with things—he won't talk to me, he hides his emotions except anger, he tries to fix my feelings and if he doesn't succeed, he gets really angry with me. He's right that we don't swear at each other, but Steve tells me regularly that our arguments are my fault, that I am too emotional or talking too loudly, or that I carry a grudge or resentment and won't let go. I'm really tired of being blamed for all the problems we have between us.

Therapist: Sounds like you both agree that your fights are increasing in frequency and intensity and that you both don't want this to continue. I think you made the right decision to begin couples therapy. It must be painful for both of you to feel this level of conflict and disconnection from each other.

The therapist validates and highlights the strengths of the couple. When a couple agrees that something is not going well or can both agree on a negative aspect of the relationship, that is actually a positive sign that can be used to instill hope. Both partners need to agree on why they are in therapy and what they would like to get out of it.

Therapist: Carissa, I also hear that you and Steve have different ways of handling emotions and conflict. From your perspective, Steve is conflict minimizing, doesn't like expressing emotions, and leaves as a way of ending a fight when it becomes too hot. Steve, is there anything Carissa is saying that you agree with?

Steve: Carissa's right that I don't like conflicts. In my family, when someone got angry, they left and never came back. That's what my father did. So when Carissa gets really angry and raises her voice, I assume she's ready to leave. I don't want to lose Carissa or this marriage, so I just go silent.

Therapist: I appreciate your non-defensive response, Steve. To acknowledge Carissa's experience is a form of validation and this is actually a way to lower the heat on the conversation. I understand what you mean by going silent because you don't know what to do. Sounds like you didn't witness your family healthily resolving conflicts, so perhaps that is something we might target for our work together.

The therapist is building an alliance with Steve, validating his concerns as well as giving him a compliment for being able to admit that he doesn't help in conflict discussions by going silent.

Therapist: Carissa, I also heard you say that you feel blamed and that your way of handling emotions is criticized. How do you react at home when that is what you are taking from what Steve is saying?

Carissa: It only makes me angrier. Just because he grew up in an uptight White family where no one talked about their feelings doesn't mean that is right. In my family we expressed our disagreements and dislikes, we fought, we yelled, and then we made up and resolved things. None of us stormed out, went silent, or gave each other the cold shoulder. It was considered rude to stop talking to a family member and engage in a cold war. I just cannot stand it when Steve does that. I just want to end this relationship.

Carissa is articulating the cultural and family-of-origin differences here. It is the therapist's job, as the one in the room with the most power and authority, to name the cultural differences and direct the conversation towards that exploration. The therapist cannot assume that clients will raise these issues on their own.

Therapist: I hear that it feels unfair because what might be culturally mediated differences are being judged as negative. The two of you come from different cultural backgrounds. Steve, you are from a Caucasian Christian family and grew up around mostly other White folks. Carissa, you came from a more rural and poorer community. Perhaps part of what you are both naming here is one of the stressors that comes from being in an intercultural relationship where your cultural backgrounds taught you very different emotional styles and philosophies of emotion? We call that meta-emotion: how you feel about feelings. From what I am hearing from the two of you, we might call Steve "emotion dismissing." This means he feels uncomfortable, uneasy, and maybe even a bit fearful when emotions get too hot because of his past experiences. Steve, I wonder if you also feel like emotions get in the way of rational thinking and dialogue. On the other hand, Carissa sounds like she is "emotion coaching" which means she tends to express feelings while talking and feels comfortable getting emotional. In fact, emotion coaching folks can sometimes find that their emotions help them have insights about why something is upsetting to them. They not only feel comfortable in their bodies having and showing emotions, but they don't see it as distracting them from thinking.

Steve: Exactly. I can't help it. I don't understand why anyone has to yell to make their point.

Carissa: Duh, Steve, that's because you don't listen. You come into every conversation already convinced that you're right and I'm wrong. You are constantly finding fault with everything I do!

Therapist: I think we're talking about two different things here. One is the racial and cultural differences between you that has taught you different meta-emotion philosophies. That is understandable and probably something you will have to navigate for as long as you are married to each other. But I'm also hearing Carissa express a complaint that she experiences Steve as criticizing and blaming her for the problems in the relationship. Criticism is one of the behaviors that John Gottman called "the four horsemen of apocalypse," four behaviors during conflict that derail conversations, and if repeated often, can derail a relationship as well. The other three horsemen are defensiveness, contempt, and stonewalling. It's not unusual in a couple that has escalating arguments for the four horsemen behaviors to creep into your conflict management. We'll come back to this in a later session and work on learning and applying the antidotes for each of these horsemen.

Since this is still the first session and the assessment phase, the therapist doesn't intervene with the four horsemen or teach the couple the antidotes just yet. If Steve and Carissa were a high-conflict volatile couple that couldn't listen and talk to the therapist in this session, then intervening more directly with the four horsemen and engaging some diffusion and de-escalation strategies might be called for here.

Therapist: I know there's more, but I feel like I have a sense of what precipitated the two of you asking to start couples therapy. You each have some valid points about why your fights are becoming intolerable. Let's move into the past. How long has it been that these fights have been escalating? Was it this way from the beginning or did this get worse more recently?

The therapist is beginning to direct the couple out of their couple narrative (what brought them to therapy) to focus on how these problems developed over time. This is the entry into the structured oral history interview.

Carissa: We've been together for seven years and married for five. The first two years of marriage were easy. We almost had no fights to speak of. We were both working hard and, in the evenings and weekends, we had a lot of fun with each other doing activities, socializing, and just hanging out. In the past two years, Steve has begun to spend more time with his male friends from work and now that I'm also working and have my evenings and weekends free, I don't like being left alone to fend for myself while he's off with his buddies. I bring this up, but it usually ends up in an argument. Now that I've expressed a wish to start a family, I worry about what will happen if I have to work, take care of the house, and raise our children all by myself.

Steve: Well, we don't have to worry about children. I don't think we're going to have any.

Carissa: See, that bothers me too. I want a husband who will respect my wishes and support me even if the journey to have children is not simple or easy.

Therapist: So, what I am hearing is that your couple bond has been fraying for the last two years with Carissa wanting more time with Steve and feeling left alone, and Steve becoming more involved in his social activities. Amid this slow decline in your connection, the question of having children has caused more tension and worry for both of you.

The therapist is reflecting and reframing the issues from a relational systemic framework and validating their concerns without taking sides.

Therapist: Carissa, you mentioned that life felt different in the beginning, so let's go there. Can you both tell me about the first time you met each other, what your first impressions were of each other, what stood out, and what do you remember about that meeting?

The therapist has moved into the oral history interview questions. It is a structured interview that traces the trajectory of the relationship with a specific focus on the quality of their romance, friendship, sexual relationship, and how they navigated the twists and turns of life. The therapist enters this interview seamlessly by looking for an opportunity to take the couple back to the beginning of their relationship. Couples who have fond and nostalgic memories of the beginning have a higher chance of improving their relationship (Gottman, 1999). Couples who have a very negative story have often re-written their origin story with a negative lens based on how they feel in the present and may have a harder time finding the "glue" to stick together.

Steve: We met at a club. I was there with some friends and so was Carissa. I was at the bar buying a drink when I noticed her sitting on the stool to my right and she was looking at me. I turned and looked back at her, and it felt electric. We were instantly drawn to each other.

Carissa: (*Laughs*) Yeah, Steve couldn't take his eyes off me for the next hour, and I could just feel the heat rising in my body every time I turned and saw him looking at me. I kept thinking this is so bizarre because this had never happened to me before. Eventually, I left my friends and walked up to Steve and asked him if he wanted to get a separate table so we could get to know each other.

Steve: And I was like, "Yeah! I definitely would." I just felt so drawn to Carissa that if we had left without connecting that night it would have haunted me.

The therapist notices the reciprocity in the storytelling and the positive sentiments and memories they both have, taking note of how they smile at each other, that humor is a part of the story, and that they are both getting animated as they speak of the attraction. The vibe in the room is that both people instantly evoked the felt sense of the attraction in that first meeting and are feeling it in the therapy session as they retell their story. This is a very positive sign for how much fondness and admiration still exists in this relationship. Couples who have an early divorcing profile (of 5.6 years) may have a lot of negativity and escalation, but they can also have a lot of passion and attraction for each other (Gottman, 1999; Gottman & Gottman, 2015). Reversing the negativity and re-surfacing the passion and attraction through homework or a specific focus on intimacy can bring rapid change in the relationship.

Therapist: What else happened that night? How did that encounter turn into dating?

Carissa: Steve invited me over to his apartment to have a drink. It seems so crazy that I said yes, but I trusted him so much in just an hour of talking. I went to his place, we drank, we talked, and then we had sex. It was amazing, like in the movies.

Steve: That is one of my favorite memories of us, that first night. It was magical!

Therapist: That sounds really special. It sounds like things just moved organically and with speed from the first moment you laid eyes on each other. So how did it progress from there? In your dating period, what were some of the highs and lows? Did you have any moments of conflict and how did you resolve those?

Carissa: I had never dated a White man before, so after that first night I had a moment or two of doubt. But Steve would call me every morning and wish me "Good Morning," and chat with me. It was so loving and sweet. Then he would invite me over to his apartment for dinner or to watch TV and I just melted every time and said yes. I had roommates, but he lived alone, so it just made sense to spend time there because we were both students and didn't have much money to go out and do things. We would cook together, listen to music, dance, watch TV, and it just felt so comfortable and intimate. It was like we had known each other for a hundred years.

Steve: Yeah, we just fit together so well. Carissa is the first Black woman I have dated, and she's so gorgeous that I kept pinching myself wondering how I got so lucky! We had a sense that a White man dating a Black woman was going to be noticed, but we didn't feel any of that tension or awkwardness between us. We felt so comfortable and close, and I cannot remember anything we fought about really.

The style of the oral history interview is to let the couple take center stage and not direct the action too much unless there is negativity or escalation that needs to be managed. By being less directive, the therapist gets a glimpse of how the couple responds more to each other's narrative than to the therapist's questions.

Therapist: I'm hearing that for both of you, dating a person of this different race was a new experience, but it didn't feel difficult or awkward. Inside this relationship, there was a lot of comfort, safety, and closeness even though you both had an awareness that people outside your relationship might have some judgments. How did you introduce each other to your family and friends?

Carissa: I was anxious and a little nervous, but I also knew that my parents would relax if they met Steve and saw how well he treated me. They both want me to be happy so if they saw me happy, that is all they would care about. I introduced Steve to my friends before my parents and most of them were just fine. I think one or two were actually curious about what it felt like to date a White guy because they were sometimes attracted to White men and didn't have the courage to ask them out. It was like we were role models for them.

Therapist: Steve, how was it introducing Carissa to your family and friends?

It is important here for the therapist to carefully choose their words so they don't imply or impose their own expectations or assumptions on the couple. The therapist must be careful not to problematize the interracial relationship by asking questions such as, "How did you handle the difficulties or challenges that come with an interracial relationship?" or "What were your worries about how your parents would take it?" These questions imply that there should be problems or challenges which may or may not be true for this couple.

Steve: I knew my parents were going to be a tough sell, more my father than my mother. We haven't had anyone in our close relatives who dated a Black person. My mom was great, she just said, "Don't let anyone influence you, date the person who makes you happy." My parents are divorced, and my mom has really found herself since the divorce and we get along really well now. My dad was a different story. I waited longer to tell him and predictably he said something negative like, "This is not going to last." I didn't engage him on that because I didn't want to hear his predictions for what could go wrong. My friends really didn't have much of a reaction. We have a lot of interracial couples in our friends' circles so it wasn't such a unique thing.

Therapist: So you dated for a couple of years while Carissa was still in graduate school. Then you decided to get married? Tell me how that evolved. Of all the people in the world, what made you decide this was the person best suited to be your life partner?

Steve: Carissa is the only woman I dated where I felt completely safe. We rarely argued, could hang out for hours and just talk or listen to music and there was no tension or expectations. She's smart, beautiful, and a loving person. Within a few weeks of dating her, I felt so close and attached that I knew very early on that she was going to be the one for me.

Carissa: I didn't have that instant confidence that Steve had. He was the first White man I was dating, I knew his parents were divorced, and I also knew that most of his friends were White and he had gone to predominantly White schools and lived in White-dominant neighborhoods. At first, I wondered how well he would understand my life and my values. But as we dated, I could tell that he wanted to be part of my life. He would come over to my parents' house and it was like we were already married because he would help with the cooking and cleaning. I began to feel more comfortable with the idea of spending the rest of my life with Steve. Then we had a party to celebrate my graduation from the Master's program and right in front of everyone, Steve went down on one knee and proposed to me. I was surprised, but I had an inkling he was going to do something like that because my family was unusually excited that day. I said yes and we started planning the wedding right away.

Therapist: That is a sweet proposal story. So tell me about the wedding and honeymoon. Did anything noteworthy happen? Anything that affected your relationship?

Carissa: It was a small intimate wedding in Orlando. None of us had very much money to have a big celebration. But I loved it and then we did a Caribbean cruise for our honeymoon. It was really nice to just take a week off and hang out with each other on the beach. We were already spending so much time together and had been having sex for a while so this didn't feel like a huge change.

Steve: Yeah, I liked our wedding and honeymoon and we really got along well and enjoyed each other's company. We didn't have any of the tensions or arguments around wedding planning that other couples do. We both wanted so much of the same things. The only thing that annoyed me was my father who barely spoke to anyone at the wedding. I don't know why he even came if he was going to be so rude.

Typically, the Gottman therapist doesn't delve into the specific details of the wedding or honeymoon planning and experience. This is why the question is phrased as "anything noteworthy." In the oral history interview, which usually takes about 30 minutes of the first session, we are attempting to get a broad overview of the relationship trajectory and to identify places where the relationship struggled or events happened that changed the nature of the bond or attachment.

Therapist: Now the wedding and honeymoon are over, you are back to your regular lives and living together as husband and wife. Were there any adjustments or surprises you had to navigate once you were married?

Steve: Not really much. We'd already been pretty much living together in my apartment before the wedding. We were both good at working and playing well together. The first two years we barely fought or argued about anything. The only thing that bothered Carissa was me spending time with my work friends, but I kept trying to balance my friends time and my marriage time to address her concerns. At times it felt like she was happy with me for doing that and then once in a while that discussion would come up again.

Carissa: I agree that our first two years of marriage were smooth. We were both busy during the week, and in the evenings and weekends did things together or socialized together. Indeed, I didn't like Steve spending so much time with his work friends, but I could see he was trying, so I left it alone. Our biggest challenge started about two years ago when I brought up wanting to have children. Steve was reluctant to have children, but agreed because I really wanted that. Neither of us was prepared for how hard this was going to be. We've been trying for three years with no luck. We started the IVF process, but it is so expensive and the first round was not successful. Steve wants to give up, but I don't want to and that is our main source of fights now.

The therapist is tracking the ups and downs in the trajectory of the relationship looking for "moments of brightening" as well as moments of disconnection or when perpetual problems first became obvious.

Steve: Honestly, I think it is a bit out of control. We've already spent so much money and time on this for three years and I think it's time to accept we're not going to have children and move on. It has become such a sore subject that Carissa is spending nights at her parents' house. We have such a good life, and this is putting a strain on us.

Typically, conflict about whether to have children or not can be a deal-breaker issue in couples. This couple appears to have talked about it without breaking up which could be a good sign of the strength of their bond.

Therapist: I think this might be a good place to pause and do something that is important in the Gottman approach to couples therapy. I want to see how the two of you handle a con-flictual topic—in other words, how you communicate and manage conflict. I know this is an artificial setting so you might not act exactly the way you do at home, but I still get a good sense of the dynamics between partners when I watch them have a conflict conversation. So, let's agree on a topic that is not a level 10 on a scale of 10 but more like a 5, and then I am going to ask you both to face each other and just try to resolve this issue right now for about 10 minutes.

This is a good segue to the last part of this first session which is the conflict sample. The Gottman therapist directs the couple to face each other and have a conversation about an issue they don't agree about and to try and solve the problem on the spot. The goal is to observe how this couple handles a point of contention and whether they use dysfunctional conflict strategies such as the four horsemen, get flooded, or derail, or if they can repair, collaborate, and move towards compromise. Typically, we would ask the couple to pick a topic that is not a deal breaker (for example, having children might be a deal-breaker topic for this couple) and choose something more manageable in a 10-minute conversation.

The couple chooses how Steve helps around the house, especially with the cats, and proceed to have their conflict sample conversation.

Carissa: I've been telling you for days now that our apartment smells! And you're ignoring me.

Carissa is using criticism which is a way of blaming Steve for a problem in the relationship.

Steve: What smell are you talking about? I don't smell anything.
Carissa: How could you not smell it? It's so pungent. I think it's the cat litter. Are you scooping it regularly?
Steve: I scooped it last night. I didn't scoop it this morning if that's what you mean.
Carissa: Why not? I've told you that that's your responsibility and that it needs to be scooped twice a day. It's not going to scoop itself.

Carissa's tone sounds sarcastic. While this is not in itself a sign of contempt, sarcasm can sometimes land on the partner as contempt.

Steve: I've been doing it!

Steve sounds defensive. He is not accepting responsibility for even a part of the problem and is not acknowledging that he's not doing it at the level Carissa wants him to.

Carissa: Clearly not enough. When are you doing it?

Carissa's tone may sound harsh although her words aren't. She may be coming across as interrogating Steve which is going to make him defensive.

Steve: Before I go to sleep.
Carissa: It needs to be done more than that! In the morning. In the evening. Maybe even the afternoon.
Steve: If you want it done so often, then you scoop it. I do it before bed.

Another defensive response from Steve. Again, not acknowledging that Carissa's expectations are different from his and that her expectations may be valid even if different from his.

Carissa: You want our house to smell like cat shit? What's wrong with you?

The repeated defensive responses from Steve and his denial of the smell have triggered Carissa who escalates into a criticism: "What is wrong with you?" One of the research definitions of criticism is blaming a problem on your partner in a way that implies they are defective or broken.

This conflict sample demonstrates how Steve and Carissa manage conflict. There are three issues a Gottman therapist might address. The harsh startup is the way a conversation starts and is handled in the first three minutes of a conversation. When the first three minutes feels harsh and includes criticism or contempt, it predicts with over 96% accuracy how the rest of the conversation will go (Gottman & Gottman, 2018). Carissa begins this conversation harshly by accusing Steve of ignoring her. Criticism generally triggers defensiveness, so Steve's response, which is to deny the smell and then argue that he's doing the task adequately, are examples of defensiveness (defined as not taking responsibility for even a small part of the problem). When the couple gets stuck in this pattern of criticism and defensiveness, the conversation is not productive, they get stuck in an "attack-defend loop," and in general, such conversations tend to escalate to more intense blame or accusations. In this sample, we see that repeated defensive responses from Steve make Carissa escalate. The good news is that the couple does not descend into name calling or yelling or swearing. There is no evidence of contempt (talking down to your partner) or stonewalling (shutting down and becoming like a stone wall in the conversation). This conflict management pattern can be reversed by helping the couple learn and apply the appropriate antidotes to their four horsemen behavior.

After the conflict sample, the Gottman therapist wraps up the session with a brief check-in on how the couple is doing and if they need time to cool down from the conflict conversation. Then the therapist invites the couple to take the Gottman questionnaires online by setting up their accounts and asking them to complete the questionnaires individually and before the second session. The therapist then schedules the next two sessions which are the individual sessions with each partner and brings the session to a close.

Following the assessment sessions, the Gottman therapist meets with the couple for a feedback and contracting session. The following questions are typically discussed and agreed upon. What are their priorities for couples therapy? What are the major gridlocked issues that need to be addressed? What needs to change? What are some of the ways in which change can occur? The

Gottman therapist might suggest individual therapy concurrent with couples therapy, a psychiatric evaluation, group therapy, or a couple's intensive or marathon session as ways to address and improve both individual and relational difficulties. In addition, the Gottman therapist establishes an agreement on how the couple will do homework on their own (usually positive, friendship-oriented exercises) so the therapeutic work on conflict management has a greater chance of success. Once the treatment plan and agreements have been made, interventions can begin. A typical intervention session includes the couple raising a topic or issue, the therapist suggesting a Gottman intervention to help the couple explore and engage in dialogue about the issue with coaching and assistance from the therapist, perhaps some positive, connecting exercises or activities, and homework for the couple.

Gottman method couples therapy is meant to be structured, pragmatic, transparent, and most importantly, equip the couple with the skills and methods they can use on their own to have dialogues, manage conflictual issues, and build intimacy and shared meaning. Usually this takes 8–12 sessions of therapy after the assessment has been completed. However, when it is clear that building skills to address the three dimensions of a sound relationship—friendship, conflict management, and shared meaning—are not causing a substantial improvement in the relationship, the Gottman therapist may renegotiate the treatment plan for a longer period and begin addressing underlying barriers and dynamics that go beyond skills and techniques. While the Gottman therapist is integrating childhood and trauma histories, coping strategies, and other psychological concerns from the beginning, the longer-term treatment becomes more focused on working towards transformative change at a deeper psychological level with one or both partners.

References

Bustamante, R. M, Nelson, J. A., Henriksen, R. C., & Monakes, S. (2011). Intercultural couples: Coping with culture-related stressors. *The Family Journal: Therapy and Therapy for Couples and Families, 19*(2), 154–164.

Carstensen, L. L., Gottman, J. M., & Levenson, R. W. (1995). Emotional behavior in long term marriage. *Psychology and Aging, 10*(1), 140–149.

Driver, J., & Gottman, J. M. (2004). Daily marital interactions and positive affect during marital conflict among newlywed couples. *Family Process, 43*(3), 301–314.

Goldfried, M. R., & D'Zurilla, T. J. (1969). A behavioral-analytic model for assessing competence. In C. D. Spielberger (Ed.), *Current topics in clinical and community psychology* (pp. 151–196). Academic Press.

Gottman, J. (1979). *Marital interaction: Experimental investigations*. Academic Press.

Gottman, J., Coan, J., Swanson, C., & Carrère, S. (1998). Predicting marital happiness and stability from newlywed interactions. *Journal of Marriage and the Family, 60*, 5–22.

Gottman, J., Driver, J., & Tabares, A. (2002). Building the Sound Marital House: An empirically-derived couple therapy. In A. S. Gurman & N. S. Jacobson (Eds.), *Clinical handbook of couple therapy* (3rd ed., pp. 373–399). Guilford Press.

Gottman, J. M. (1994). *What predicts divorce: The relationship between marital processes and marital outcomes.* Lawrence Erlbaum Associates, Inc.

Gottman, J. M. (1995). *Why marriages succeed or fail and how you can make yours last.* Simon and Schuster.

Gottman, J. M. (1999). *The marriage clinic: A scientifically based marital therapy.* W.W. Norton & Company.

Gottman, J. M. (2011). *The Science of trust: Emotional attunement for couples.* W.W. Norton.

Gottman, J. M. (2014). *Principia Amoris: The New Science of Love.* Routledge.

Gottman, J. M., & Gottman, J. S. (2015). *10 principles for doing effective couples therapy.* W. W. Norton.

Gottman, J. M., & Gottman, J. S. (2016). What makes same sex relationships succeed or fail? Retrieved from www.gottman.com/about/research/same-sex-couples/ on January 31, 2016.

Gottman, J. M., & Gottman, J. S. (2018). *The science of couple and family therapy: Behind the scenes at the "love lab": completing general systems theory.* W. W. Norton & Company.

Gottman, J. M., Gottman, J. S., Cole, C., & Preciado, M. (2019). Gay, lesbian, and heterosexual couples about to begin couples therapy: An online relationship assessment of 40,681 couples. Journal of Marital and Family Therapy. doi: 10.1111/jmft.12395

Gottman, J. M., Levenson, R. W, Swanson, C., Swanson, K., Tyson, R., & Yoshimoto, D. (2003). Observing gay, lesbian and heterosexual couples' relationships: Mathematical modeling of conflict interaction. *Journal of Homosexuality, 45*(1). doi: 10.1300/J082v45n01_04

Gottman, J. M., & Navarra, R. J. (2011). Gottman method couples therapy: From theory to practice. In D. K. Carson & M. Kasado-Kehoe (Eds.), *Case studies in couples therapy: Research-based approaches* (pp. 331–344). Routledge.

Gottman, J. M., Notarius, C., Markman, H., Bank, S., Yoppi, B., & Rubin, M. E., (1976). Behavior exchange theory and marital decision making. *Journal of Personality and Social Psychology, 34*(1), 14–23.

Gottman, J. M., & Silver, N. (2015). *The seven principles for making marriages work: A practical guide from the nation's foremost relationship expert.* Harmony Press.

Hawks, M. W., Carrere, S., & Gottman, J.M. (2002). Marital sentiment override: Does it influence couples' perceptions? *Journal of Marriage and Family, 64*(1), 193–201.

Lebow, J., & Snyder, D. K. (2022). Couple therapy in the 2020s: Current status and emerging developments. *Family Process, 61*(4), 1359–1385.

Rajaei, A., Daneshour, M., & Robertson, J. (2019). The effectiveness of couples therapy based on the Gottman method among Iranian couples with conflicts: A quasi-experimental study. *Journal of Couple & Relationship Therapy, 18*(3), 223–240.

Rajendrakumar, J., Manjula, V., & Rajan, S. K. (2023). Process of emotion regulation in Indian couples during Gottman's dreams-within-confict intervention: A mixed-methods design study. *Contemporary Family Therapy, 46*(1), 1–27.

9 Imago Relationship Therapy

Wade Luquet

History of the Model

Imago Relationship Therapy (IRT) was developed in the early 1980s by Harville Hendrix and Helen LaKelly Hunt. Hendrix introduced the model in his 1988 best-selling popular book *Getting the Love You Want: A Guide for Couples.* Hendrix explained that IRT was developed in his and Hunt's relationship and personal history.

> The source of the impulse that gave it birth is our similar yet quite distinct childhoods: the death of my parents and the absence of Helen's father, motivators of our primal search for healing through reconnection. Our divorces are another source, the aftermath of which led us to reflect on what happened to our marriages, to inquire into the nature of committed partnerships, and to resolve to find a way not to repeat the past.
>
> (Hendrix et al., 2005, p. 13)

Since its inception, Imago Relationship Therapy has become a widely used couples therapy practiced globally. Several thousand therapists are certified in the model through Imago Relationships International, and associations of Imago therapists can be found around the world, including South Korea, Canada, South Africa, the Middle East, Australia, and Germany, to name a few (https://imagorelationships.org/). Hendrix and Hunt have written multiple best-selling books on relationships, and several books for professionals interested in the model are also available (Hendrix et al., 2005; Hendrix & Hunt, 2021; Luquet, 2007; Luquet & Hannah, 1998). In addition, multiple peer-reviewed journal articles attest to the efficacy of the model (Gehlert et al., 2017; Muro et al., 2016a; Schmidt et al., 2016).

Basic Tenets of Imago Relationship Therapy

Imago therapists work under certain understandings of the purpose of close intimate relationships. From these tenets of IRT, therapists educate, guide, and teach couples how to use skills to achieve a healing, growth-producing, and authentic relationship. The tenets of Imago Relationship Therapy include the following:

1 Romantic relationships are an unconscious process. We are attracted to partners who embody our early childhood caretakers' positive and negative characteristics.
2 Romantic love is fleeting and drug-induced. Its purpose is to bring two people together unconsciously to work on their relationship consciously.
3 The purpose of the relationship is to heal childhood wounds and resolve issues from the past. Our partners unconsciously provide a pathway to healing through issues brought up in the

DOI: 10.4324/9781003369097-9

power struggle when they mirror aspects of our early childhood caretakers. They provide an opportunity for growth and healing. Our partner's characteristics are our **Imago Match**.

4 When couples work together intentionally when power struggle issues emerge, they can bring unconscious issues forward and resolve them together through understanding and behavior change.

5 The three-part Couples Dialogue utilizing mirroring, validating, and empathizing between partners is the key skill for couples to master in the Imago process. Using calming and centering techniques, the listening partners are taught to tolerate the anxiety they are experiencing so they can listen fully to their partner's pain, desires, or wishes. When partners are fully heard, they feel a sense of calm and being seen. When the receiving partner learns to intentionally listen without reacting, they hear their partner more fully and empathy develops, and they develop a deeper understanding and connection.

6 As empathy develops, partners can respond to Behavior Change Requests by understanding the reason behind the request rather than feeling coerced to change. The couple's conflicts become an opportunity for healing and growth, and they recognize how each contributes to the conflict based on past needs. Couples learn how to use the dialogue and behavior change requests to meet the needs of their partner while at the same time stretching into parts once unavailable to them.

7 Couples replace judgment with curiosity about the other. As they become less fearful of each other, couples become genuinely curious about the other's thoughts, feelings, and experiences, or what philosopher Martin Buber calls "the otherness of the other" (Buber, 1948, p. 23).

8 Couples practice intentional appreciation of each other daily. They replace negative interactions with positive appreciations. This aligns with John Gottman's (2013) research that happy, stable couples have a caring behavior ratio of five positive behaviors to every one negative. The flip side to this is that for every one negative behavior the couple must counteract with five positive behaviors. Positivity creates a sense of safety; the brain can let its protective instincts down to allow for more intimacy and connection.

9 The couple commits to ongoing growth and connection using the skills learned in Imago Relationship Therapy. They support each other's growth and development and commit to using the skills learned to create a conscious and intentional partnership addressing unresolved issues and narratives and helping each other reach dreams and goals. Couples can create a relationship based on mutual respect, empathy, and love by addressing unresolved issues and practicing new skills.

Conceptualization of Problem Formation

Steve and Carissa's relationship began like that of most others in love's throes. They found themselves talking endlessly on the night they met and continued their conversation resulting in multiple nights together, eventually leading them to an exclusive relationship. Their attraction and developing love were mysterious but exciting. They are confused now that their passion has changed. For Imago Therapy, developing romantic love is not a mystery; rather, it is viewed as drug-induced and fueled by an unconscious process. Couples in love are consumed by a chemical swirl of dopamine, serotonin, phenylethylamine, norepinephrine, oxytocin, and vasopressin (Cacioppio, 2023). It feels good to be in love, and couples want to be in each other's presence to experience this rush of emotion and excitement. The question that IRT asks is, "Why that person?" Of all the people they met that night, what started the reaction between Steve and Carissa? And, like many couples, what made it go away? What changed?

Part of that answer is that staying in this drug-induced state would be impossible, if not exhausting. This type of romantic love is a temporary condition. Like many drugs, such as cocaine and other addictive substances, the body gets used to the high and requires a heavier dose to maintain the euphoria. However, you only get so much in romantic love before the feeling fades. In IRT, we call these chemicals "nature's anesthesia." Nature, in its wisdom, anesthetizes partners from each other's faults. For most, as they build their lives together, the drug fades, and the power struggle begins. Couples must learn to deal with the struggles and find a new way to love.

Steve and Carissa followed this pattern, and now they must deal with what they have become as a couple. IRT conceptualizes the problems that develop for couples as arising from unmet childhood needs and the resulting mechanism they learned to cope with as a child. These unmet needs form the basis for the unconscious selection of a partner who helps them replay their childhood issues and, it is hoped, have a different outcome that heals the past wounds.

The human brain learns patterns. Our relationships with early caregivers shape our brains, our expectations of love, and our relationships with others. When our caregivers could not meet our needs, we developed coping mechanisms to protect ourselves from further emotional distress. Learned behaviors such as withdrawing, clinging, pleasing others, or becoming controlling become relationship patterns, and we seek a partner who matches our needs. Our partners often have opposite coping strategies, such as pursuing, distancing, self-absorption, and aloofness. When the euphoria of love wears off, the couple discovers they have found someone with the traits they despise the most, and the power struggle sets in. Only when the couple becomes conscious of this and intentional in their relationship can the healing occur and a deeper real love emerge between them.

Initially, Carissa had no issues with Steve going out with his friends. Because he had to be a good child following his parents' divorce, he enjoyed the freedom Carissa gave him in the marriage. She had things to do, so it was not a problem. But things eased up for her and she found herself alone a lot. Being alone felt familiar to her because her mom continued to teach throughout her childhood. Though her mom was home at 3:30 pm, she often graded assignments and wrote lesson plans, leaving Carissa and her sister mostly alone. Her father was a proud and honorable man who spent long hours at work, knowing his wife was home with the kids and they were safe. Carissa would deal with this by spending hours in her room working on math problems which later benefited her in her present job, but also was used to escape feelings of loneliness. Now she seemed to be in the same situation with Steve gone long hours at work and spending a couple of nights a week with his friends.

Deep down, she hoped that having a baby might lessen some of her loneliness and keep Steve home a bit more. But the difficulties they were having getting pregnant added to the stress between them. Her recent explosion over the cat litter box was just a symptom of stress and isolation. Steve's inability to see the issue as important to Carissa made her feel lonelier and left Steve feeling confused.

IRT would see the coping mechanisms learned in childhood and used by both Steve and Carissa as creating the conflict and disconnection they are experiencing now. These behaviors, Carissa now wanting closeness and Steve wanting space to enjoy himself, trigger their early wounds and create fear and disappointment. They find themselves fighting more or withdrawing. When Carissa yells at Steve, he minimizes her reaction, making her angrier. When she escalates, he gets quiet and plays dead, hoping the anger will wash over her and peace will return. But even if it does, it is only momentary as their real issue remains unconscious and is continually triggered by learned behaviors. Their fight-and-flight response is a normal and predictable behavior for all animals when feeling threatened. Peace will only come to them when they feel safe and can uncover the unconscious patterns of the past and heal those early wounds by becoming intentional in their conversations, with each understanding their triggers and the wounds of their partners.

According to IRT, the relationship is an opportunity for growth and healing if partners can learn the skills of safe relationships. In this case, the therapist will help Steve and Carissa become aware of past experiences and coping mechanisms and teach them ways to communicate and meet each other's needs healthily. They will be taught how to create a more conscious, safe, and fulfilling relationship and bypass the patterns causing conflict and pain. It will take time for their brains to acclimate to patterns of safety rather than patterns of defense and reactivity. Time and experience can bring trust back into the relationship and restructure old patterns into newer and safer patterns that will allow Steve and Carissa to feel some of the playfulness and nurturing of their early relationship.

Conceptualizing Diversity

Since its inception in the 1980s, Imago Relationship Therapy has been used across the world. It is an especially popular model of couples therapy in South Korea, Russia, South Africa, and many Middle East countries. Multiple research papers have been written attesting to the efficacy of IRT for world-wide populations (Hosseini & Movahedi, 2016; Oh & Minichiello, 2013). Sheydanfar et al., (2021) compared the effectiveness of 10 90-minute sessions of Emotionally Focused Couples Therapy and Imago Relationship Therapy with 24 Iranian couples. Using the Enrich Couple Questionnaire (MSQ), the research found that both treatments were effective, with the Imago couples scoring higher in marital satisfaction. In a controlled study in Tehran City, Seidabadi et al. (2021) compared changes in 30 couples using the well-researched Solution-Focused Therapy with those using IRT and found them both equally effective. While certain adjustments may need to be made to accommodate cultural differences, IRT's basic skills and understanding of relationships are portable between diverse cultures.

IRT recognizes that diversity issues can have a significant impact on relationships. As with many therapies, IRT practitioners in the United States and their clients tend to be overwhelmingly white. However, a number of ethnically diverse practitioners have utilized IRT theory and skills with great success when combined with the individual practitioner's understanding of cultural strengths and differences. Weiser and Thompson (1998) write that Imago Therapy can play "a significant role in the emotional, spiritual, and psychological growth of the African American couple" (p. 101). To work effectively, "it is essential for the therapist also to recognize and appreciate African American history, the uniqueness of their struggle, and their contribution to the American Culture" (p. 101). Because of the long history of control by white institutions, African Americans often approach therapy with caution. Weiser and Thompson hypothesize that African Americans proceed through Imago Therapy in four stages: Suspicion, Creation of Safety, Empowerment, and a Reclamation of [the] Spirituality taken from them when their "ancient spiritual connectedness was lost through internal fears and doubts" (Weiser & Thompson, 1998, p. 103). IRT can powerfully impact diverse couples by emphasizing connection and trust.

Mixed-race couples like Steve and Carissa are becoming an increasingly common pairing (Parker & Barrasso, 2021). Carissa's parents did their best to shield her from overt racism in their small Florida town; however, some racism is built into the system, and there are many micro- and macro-aggressions Carissa may have been exposed to in her lifetime. It will be essential for Steve to understand some of the generational struggles Carissa and her family have endured for her to feel truly connected to him. It is not enough to be color-blind and assume that love conquers all. It will be important for him to be curious about her and her entire family. IRT and the dialogue process they will learn supports the notion of being curious and not judgmental.

Carissa's work ethic and her parents' work ethic, which often left her and her sister by themselves, may be related to the fact that African Americans face obstacles in the job market, including finding jobs and having their performance evaluated more intensely than their white counterparts (Weller, 2019). In a 2019 report for The Center for American Progress, Weller reports that African-Americans have less access to good-paying jobs, job stability, and wealth than whites. Perhaps

Carissa's parents worked long and hard hours, knowing that to keep their middle-class status, they would have to work longer and harder than their white colleagues. This is a message they passed on to Carissa, who worked hard to obtain her accounting degree, but at the cost of being romantically alone until she met Steve.

It may also be important for the therapist to lead the couple into a dialogue about the possibility that Steve's time with his friends is also a manifestation of the power and privilege as a white male that he might assume in the relationship. If Steve is unaware of this power dynamic, he must address it so the relationship can become equal and healthy. Therapists must understand how cultural traditions and beliefs affect couple relationships (Bain, 1998; Kleinberg & Zorn, 1998; Martin & Bielawski, 2011; Smith, 2023). Couple dynamics are often governed by long-standing societal rules that no longer work in a modern marriage and therapists must understand how these changing rules interact with cultural norms.

IRT views diversity as an opportunity for growth and learning in relationships. The dialogue process encourages couples to acknowledge and explore their differences. This will help them develop greater empathy and understanding of each other's experiences and perspectives. The therapist will help Steve and Carissa identify and understand how their cultural backgrounds and experiences have shaped their relationship expectations and behaviors. In the safety of the dialogue process, they will be encouraged to communicate openly and honestly about their differences and seek to understand and respect each other's perspectives.

The Role of the Therapist

The Imago therapist is a teacher and active facilitator of the Imago processes that couples will learn in order to work through the issues that brought them to therapy. The IRT therapist's role is to facilitate communication and understanding between the couple by creating a safe and non-judgmental environment where the couple can explore the root causes of their problems and listen to each other with deep empathy and understanding. It begins with learning the basic skill of IRT, the Couples Dialogue (Hendrix, 1988; Luquet, 2007).

The **Couples Dialogue** is a three-part communication process where couples learn to mirror, validate, and empathize with what their partner is saying to them. The steps of the Couples Dialogue are:

1 **Mirroring**: The receiving partner, the one who is listening, repeats back as closely as possible what they heard the sending partner, the one who is speaking, say. They would start the mirror with the statement, "If I heard you correctly…" or "If I am getting this right, you said…," ending the mirror with, "Did I get that?" If the sending partner says yes, the receiving partner asks, "Is there more about that?" and stays safe and curious for two or three rounds of mirroring. If the answer is no, the sending partner clarifies what was said until the receiving partner hears fully what is said as intended.
2 **Validation** requires the receiving partner to see what was said from the sending partner's point of view. They do not have to agree with what was said, but rather see that their partner sees things in that particular way. When they get it, the receiving partner would say to the sending partner, "That makes sense," or "What makes sense to me about that is… ." If the receiving partner still cannot see the sense of the sending partner's point of view, it is possible they need more information so it makes sense. The receiving partner is guided by the therapist to stay safe and curious and ask the sending partner to say more that would help them understand.
3 Empathy: When the receiving partner is able to make sense of what has been said, they can offer an **empathetic statement**. They would say something like, "I can imagine that might make you feel sad, disappointed, and frustrated." The couple can repeat the dialogue process several times

and switch the sender and receiver as needed to resolve an issue. The Couples Dialogue is the main skill taught in IRT and even if the couple learns and uses only this skill, the relationship can improve.

Though awkward at first, couples can quickly learn the process through the psychoeducational process taught by the Imago therapist. Couples are first taught about the brain processes present in their frustrations and fights. Like any mammal, our brains are programmed to keep us alive when we experience danger through the fight-or-flight response. When we sense danger, we will fight, run, freeze, hide, or submit to avoid the perceived threat and stay alive. Conflicts with partners are interpreted as dangerous and trigger our brains to react to protect us. The brain does not know that most couples' conflicts do not result in physical threats or death. We might recommend a different therapy or some protective measure if abuse is suspected.

The brain is an anticipation machine, and any threat is a threat (Seigel, 2018). The body is prepared to react and shuts down all logical and empathetic processes to survive. Having a small model of the brain or an illustration of the brain is helpful to teach couples about the structure and function of the triune brain. Couples can visually see the reptilian, mammalian, and cerebral cortex parts of the brain, and the therapist can explain how each section plays a part in their frustrations (see Luquet [2007] for more information). Giving couples an experience of this protective phenomenon adds a layer of learning through an experiential understanding. This can be done by asking the couple to discuss for three minutes a frustration, in the way they usually do at home. It may take a minute, but couples are usually able to find a common frustration and enter into a mini-argument that can be used both as an illustrative experience for the couple and an assessment feature for the therapist. Couples can now see that they use the defenses of fight, flight, playing dead, hiding, and submitting as protective mechanisms in their arguments. The therapist can also point out to them that because their brains are in a defensive posture, any attempt to fix the problem will be temporary at best.

When couples understand that the protective factors of the brain are at work in their frustrations, they can become curious about how to engage in dialogue differently. The first step is creating a safe platform for them to connect and be able to listen to each other fully. Couples are taught the value of breathing and centering themselves. They are guided through the process of creating a safe place in their mind where they can visualize themselves listening to their partner. They are urged to stay in that space while listening to their partner in the dialogue process they have been taught, and if they find themselves triggered, to call a "time out" and re-center themselves rather than react to the statement that triggered them. They should be reminded that they will have their turn, just not now.

Eye contact and eye softening are also emphasized as a means of self-regulation. Porges (2011) refers to self-regulation as a way of creating safety in the social encounter. Because we are social creatures with a brain anticipating danger, we look for social clues, including eyes, eyebrows, and posture. Looking someone in the eye for one minute decreases the need for protection and allows for a more authentic dialogue. Couples are encouraged to spend a minute looking into each other's eyes and softening their facial features to relax the protective systems they have been utilizing in their reactive dialogues.

During these dialogues, the therapist's role is different from what is usually taught in psychotherapists' graduate training. IRT therapists are trained to pay more attention to those who are listening than those who are talking. The sender is given instructions to use **"I" statements** and keep their statements manageable so the receiver can mirror back what was said to them accurately. Using "I" statements decreases blame to the receiver and lessens their reactivity to the statements, whereas "you" statements place blame on the receiving partner and would increase their reactivity. The therapist must also be alert to hidden "you" statements in the form of "I think that you... ."

This is not an "I" statement, and the receiving partner will react as if accused. The sender should be re-directed to make the statement one about how they feel or an action they may take as a result of the behavior: "I feel anxious and want to walk out of the room when we get into discussions about money."

Giving attention to the receiver is important because what is being said can trigger them and they can easily revert to a reactive fight/flight response. The therapist pays attention to the receiver's facial movements, posture, and breathing. When distress is observed in the form of a changing breathing pattern, a furrowed brow, or an eye roll, the therapist intervenes by softly saying, "Breathe" or "Stay in your safe place" to the receiver. Until the brain learns that the conversation will not cause them harm, the couple will need reminders to stay safe and work through the anxiety. Once it is learned, the couple should be able to do the dialogue independently.

Steve and Carissa are now four sessions into their therapy. They have learned the Couples Dialogue and how to use self-regulation techniques to create a safe space for the conversation. They are seeing some improvement in their conversation at home. They did arrive at the session with an issue they would like to discuss.

Therapist: Welcome back. This is our fourth session, and you have learned a few skills and a little about each other. How did the week go?
Steve: Not bad. We do have an issue we would like to discuss.
Therapist: OK, we will do that. First, if you would, tell me something fun you did this week together that you enjoyed.
Steve: We went to a movie. It was a romantic comedy. Usually, I'm not too fond of those, but this one was not bad. I actually liked it!
Carissa: And I appreciate that you did this with me. It was a fun night.
Steve: It was a fun night! I'm glad we were able to do it and be together.
Therapist: That's great! Would you all do something like that again?
Steve: I think so. I enjoyed it a lot.
Carissa: I'm glad to hear you say that.
Therapist: Great. These enjoyable times will keep you in the relationship, so let's encourage more of that. So, let's get you two talking about this issue that has come up.
Steve: Well, what happened was…
Therapist: Whoa! Just a second. You'll be talking to each other in the dialogue process.
Steve: Oh yeah. I forgot. Sorry.
Therapist: Well, you know what to do. Steve, are you going to be the sender on this one?
Steve: I am.
Therapist: (*softly*) OK, time for you both to go to your safe place… Feet on the floor… Take a breath… Picture that place you created to do this work… See it… Feel it… Hear it if it has a sound… Smell it if it has a smell… Sit in the space for a minute or so and when you are ready, open your eyes and look into each other's eyes for a minute.

The therapist waits while the couple begins their self-regulation to be able to hear each other. After about a minute of the couple looking into each other's eyes, the therapist picks up the conversation.

Therapist: Carissa, when you are ready, say to Steve, "I can hear you now." And remember, Steve, use "I" statements and avoid "you" statements.
Steve: OK, Carissa, I felt upset on Sunday when I finished building that bench for the patio that you wanted me to build, and when I showed it to you, I mean, you said thank you, but it was not enthusiastic by any means. And you found that one extra hole I drilled. It felt critical to me.

Carissa:	So on Sunday, when you showed me the bench I asked you to build, you did not feel that I thanked you enthusiastically, and I found fault with it with the extra hole. It felt critical to you. Did I get that?
Steve:	Yes.
Carissa:	Is there more?
Steve:	Yes, I was hoping for a big thank you and a hug and maybe holding off on criticism for a bit.
Carissa:	So you were hoping for a big thank you and a hug. And you hoped that I would hold off on criticism. Did I get that?
Steve:	You did. And your reaction was difficult for me since I worked hard on it.
Carissa:	So my reaction was difficult for you to hear since you worked so hard on the bench. Did I get that?
Steve:	Yes.
Therapist:	Carissa, can you validate that? Does that make sense to you, knowing Steve?
Carissa:	It does. What makes sense to me about that, Steve, is that you like to be recognized for your work and you worked very hard on this bench. I can see where you would have liked a little more from me.
Therapist:	And how would you guess that would make Steve feel?
Carissa:	I would imagine that would make you feel sad, unappreciated, and discouraged.
Steve:	It did, yes.
Therapist:	Steve, do you remember feeling like that as a kid?
Steve:	Yes, I do.
Therapist:	Can you tell Carissa about that? And Carissa, can you return to your safe place and ground yourself so you can fully hear Steve?
Steve:	When I was growing up, it seemed like I could never do things right for my dad. He always found fault in what I did, and I did not feel appreciated for what I did around the house.
Carissa:	So when you were growing up, when you did things around the house, you did not feel appreciated like you wanted, and your dad always found fault with what you did. Did I get that?

Steve and Carissa continued this dialogue for 15 minutes under the therapist's guidance. The therapist monitored Carissa's breathing and posture to ensure she remained relaxed and self-regulated. The therapist listened to how Steve phrased things to ensure that pointed words like "you" or "you always" or other phrases that feel like an attack are avoided. With the proper guidance, the couple could have a productive conversation that brought about an empathetic response from Carissa. She understood that Steve's lack of acknowledgment as a child for his accomplishments is what brings on his strong reactions. She is now able to act toward giving Steve what he needs. She may also discover that what Steve needs is what she most needs to grow into—she did not get much praise either, and good work was just expected without notice.

The Imago therapist plays an active and directive role in guiding the couple through improving their relationship by facilitating communication and understanding between the couple. They do this by creating a safe and non-judgmental environment, helping couples learn to self-regulate their protective structures so they can fully hear the other. Specifically, the therapist helps the couple identify the root cause of their problems, often related to unmet childhood needs. Not all unmet needs manifest themselves in the couple relationship, and some might resist the idea altogether. For those couples, learning the Couples Dialogue process might be sufficient along with the Behavior Change Request. But most couples will clearly see that their frustrations are triggered in the present relationship, but have their roots in the past. The therapist will teach the couple several communication skills to address those unmet needs in the problem-resolution stage.

In addition, the Imago therapist teaches the couple several methods to learn to empathize with each other, validate each other's feelings, and communicate their feelings in a non-threatening and non-blaming way. Overall, the Imago therapist serves as a guide, teacher, and coach, helping the couple to repair their relationship and build a deeper, more meaningful connection.

Conceptualization of Problem Resolution

Conflict is part of any relationship. Imago views conflict as a point of growth where couples can use the tools provided to them to understand the source of the conflict. One way of viewing this is to think of relationship problems as having an upstream source and a downstream presentation. Couples see therapists when their frustrations become overwhelming, and they need help. Unfortunately, they usually wait a long time before seeking help—on average, couples wait two to six years from when they know they need help until they start therapy (Doherty et al., 2021). And what might be a big frustration for one couple might be a mild annoyance for another. The energy behind the big, recurring frustrations usually manifests where the couple finds an early childhood wound that gets triggered and needs understanding, empathy, and a behavior change from the partner. The upstream source fuels the downstream presentation. While many couples therapy models deal with the problem presentation, IRT is just as interested in the source and has multiple tools for couples to use to understand what triggers their partner.

Early in therapy, Imago therapists have couples fill out **The Imago Work-up** (Hendrix, 2008; Hendrix & Hunt, 2021; Luquet, 2007;). Steve and Carissa were asked to think back on their childhoods and make a list of the following:

1 The positive traits of their early childhood caretakers, typically a mother and father, but can include others.
2 The negative traits of their early childhood caretakers, typically a mother and father, but can include others.
3 What is something they needed as a child but did not get, i.e.: to be told they were smart, to be hugged, to be able to make up their own minds, to be taken seriously.
4 A list of at least three childhood frustrations and what they did when they got frustrated, i.e.: screamed and yelled, got quiet, cried, used sarcasm.
5 A list of positive childhood memories and how they felt when participating in those events, i.e.: happy, strong, connected, seen.

(Luquet, 2007, p. 97)

These memories are then put into a formula of sentence stems (in italics below) that reveal the Imago. The **Imago** is an image that developed in our childhood of positive and negative traits of our early childhood caretakers that we unconsciously use to find our romantic partner. From this exercise, partners can see what made them the choice for their partners and how their interactions trigger strong reactions based on unmet childhood needs. Having this understanding starts the process of developing the empathy necessary for them to open themselves up emotionally to each other.

For Steve and Carissa, their Imago Work-Up came out as follows:

Steve for Carissa:

I'm trying to get a person who is: sad, angry, tired, unaware, controlling, deceitful
To always be: loving, smart, kind, driven, competitive, resourceful

So that I can get: to be told I was good enough
And feel: happy, worthy, proud, free, and independent.
I stop myself from getting this sometimes by: working harder, but giving up, leaving the house,
  giving up because there is no making them happy.

Carissa's Imago Work-Up for Steve:

I'm trying to get a person who is: busy, dominant, demanding, unavailable, and quiet
To always be: smart, strong, open, kind, a hard worker, and open-minded
So that I can get: to know that what I was doing was good enough
And feel: proud and connected.
I stop myself from getting this sometimes by: [being] scared of getting close to men, looking for
  ways to be praised, and learning to stay by myself and being sad.

The Imago Work-Up was eye-opening for Steve and Carissa. Not everything they wrote fit their
partner; some were qualities they took on themselves. But the work-up allowed them to see that
they had unconsciously chosen someone with traits similar to their parents and that many of their
current frustrations matched those of their childhood. Carissa wanted a closer relationship with her
father and her work to be noticed and praised by both parents. She worked hard in school and at
her job and still did not feel like she was being noticed the way she needed to be. Steve recognized
that he had given up on trying to make Carissa happy, which is what he did as a child. He was
now doing what he did then and escaping by being with his friends. Of course, this leaves her
alone and sad, and he is still not getting what he needs. And from this, they recognized how their
behaviors affected each other. Recognition of unconscious patterns is important to the success of
IRT. Couples who learn that their present frustrations have an unconscious link to their past tend to
have greater empathy toward the other (Muro et al., 2016b; Schmidt & Gehlert, 2017) and can see
how their present reactive behavior triggers their partner. Partners who understand this can become
intentional in their relationship and lessen negative interactions.
    Steve and Carissa participated in additional sessions that deepened their empathetic connection,
including the Parent/Child Dialogue and holding exercises (Hendrix & Hunt, 2021; Luquet, 2007).
    The **Parent/Child Dialogue** places the couple in an "as if" situation. The receiving partner
listens to the sending partner "as if" they were one of their parents. The sending partner talks to the
receiving partner "as if" they are their parent at the age they need to talk to them. The receiving
partner asks three questions and mirrors softly after each question.

1 I am your mother/father. What was it like to live with me?
2 I am your mother/father. What did you need from me that you did not get?
3 I am your partner now. What can I do for you to help heal those wounds?

For the **holding exercise**, the couple cradles each other and they talk about their childhood. The
sender is given the sentence stem to start the dialogue, "When I was a little girl/boy/person…" and
talks about what it was like for them as a child. The receiving partner mirrors back softly. From this
vulnerable, comfortable, and safe position, couples usually share deeper material than they have
in the past and bring a new understanding of how their childhood shapes their present. (For more
information on these two exercises and an illustration of the holding position, see Luquet, 2007).
    When Steve and Carissa saw the pain that their reactive behaviors were causing each other
related to their childhood experiences, they became interested in changing their behavior to lessen
the frustrations they were experiencing and causing.

When couples feel coerced into changing a behavior, the change is often temporary or done with resentment. When a couple opens up emotionally and understands the pain and frustration their behavior causes, they are more willing to take corrective action. IRT does this through a **Behavior Change Request,** a method of finding the hidden desire behind a frustration and putting together a positive, measurable, doable, and time-limited request for change that is actionable and less coercive to the receiving partner. The frustration, desire, and the request are often connected to a childhood wound and the request would be healing to one partner, and would require a stretching of behavior, or what we would consider growth, for the receiving partner. The Behavior Change Request process is described below for Steve and Carissa.

IRT views frustrations as a desire stated negatively. Human brains interpret negative comments as danger and go on the defense, becoming non-receptive to the desires of the other. If Carissa says to Steve, "You are gone all the time!" he has no choice but to defend himself, "No, I'm not!" This then sets her off, and the argument cycle begins. But under her statement is a desire or a wish, "I wish you were home with me more often" or "My desire is that we spend more time together." These statements do not need a defensive response, especially when the partner understands the wound beneath the statement. Steve now understands that Carissa felt lonely as a child because both of her parents worked so hard to help her go to college. She spent many hours in her room studying and felt lonely, with only her less academic sister to talk to about it. Steve knows this now, and Carissa's Behavior Change Request dialogue would go like this.

Therapist: Carissa, underneath that frustration you have with Steve going out with his friends, there may be something that you want. Maybe a wish or a desire.

Carissa: Yes, I think so.

Therapist: Can you give it words? It's hard to hear a frustration and much easier to hear a desire or wish. Steve, can you go to your safe place, breathe, and center yourself, and hear Carissa? Let her know when you are ready to hear her.

Steve: Yes, I can do that. (Takes a breath and says softly) I can hear you now.

Carissa: I was alone so much growing up. I thought it was normal, but now I know it is not. So when you are away with friends, I get really lonely and sad.

Steve: So if I am getting this right, when you were growing up, your parents left you and your sister alone so much that you thought it was normal, but now you know it is not normal. And now when I am away, you feel lonely and sad. Did I get that?

Carissa: Yes, you did.

Therapist: Great, Steve. Carissa, I sense you want something from Steve to help with that wound. Can you let him know what you need from him? Start it with, "My desire is…," and let him know what your wish is.

Carissa: My desire is that you and I can spend some uninterrupted time together talking and listening to each other's hopes and dreams. You know, laughing and supporting each other.

Therapist: Steve, can you mirror that?

Steve: Sure. What you would like is for us to spend some uninterrupted time together talking and listening to each other about our hopes and dreams. You want that time to be fun and supporting each other.

Carissa: That's right.

Therapist: Great! Now Carissa, let's get a little more specific so Steve knows exactly what you need to feel less lonely and feel supported as you just stated to him. We call this a Behavior Change Request. Certainly, he will not be able to spend all day, every day with you. Let's figure out what you need and put it into a specific, positive, and do-able request. Let's give him maybe two things he can do over the next two weeks. And I'll start you off. "Three times over the next two weeks, I would like you to…"

Carissa: Three times over the next two weeks, I would like you to spend one hour taking a walk in a park and listening to me talk about our future and my desire to start our family, using the dialogue we learned when needed.

Steve: OK, so three times over the next two weeks, you would like to go on a walk with me and talk about our future. And you would like us to listen to each other using the dialogue we learned in therapy when we need to so we can hear each other. Did I get that?

Carissa: You did.

Therapist: Good! Carissa, is there a second request that you can think of that would be healing to you?

Carissa: Yes. Twenty percent of the time when your friends call to go out, I would love if you could tell them that tonight I need to spend time with my wife and we find a movie on TV to watch together.

Steve: Oh wow! That's a tough one for me. You know how much I love going out with them. (*chuckles*) OK, so what would be healing to you is twenty percent of the time when the guys ask me to go out that I let them know that I need to spend time with my wife and we watch a movie on TV together. Did I get that?

Carissa: Yes, you did.

Therapist: Steve, is there any one of those that you could commit to?

Steve: I think I can do them both, but I want to try to commit to turning the guys down twenty percent of the time to spend time with Carissa.

Carissa: That would be nice.

Therapist: And say to Steve, "Thank you! That would help to heal my childhood wound of…"

Carissa: That would help heal my childhood wound of feeling alone and unimportant, and that other things are more important than me.

Therapist: And make me feel…

Carissa: It would make me feel important, worthy, and noticed, so thank you!

Steve: You're welcome.

Steve and Carissa learned to use this process to discuss their frustrations less reactively. They could reduce their negative interactions significantly, learn to respond to each other's needs, and feel less coerced by their partner because they understood why a change in behavior was requested. The request will be challenging for both of them. One of the things emphasized in IRT is that partners do not have what the other partner needs. Rather, what one partner needs is what the other partner most needs to grow into. Growth and change are seldom easy and involve stretching into new behaviors. With the addition of an empathetic connection between the couple, they can make these changes because they want to, not because they have to make the change.

Imago Relationship Therapy conceptualizes problem resolution as a process of addressing and healing underlying wounds that contribute to conflict and difficulties in relationships. IRT believes that most relationship problems are rooted in childhood experiences that shape how individuals relate to others in their adult lives. In IRT, problem resolution involves identifying and addressing the unconscious wounds and unfinished emotional business individuals bring into their relationships. Through structured communication and empathy building, IRT helps couples develop deeper understanding and compassion for each other's emotional experiences, as Steve and Carissa are beginning to do. This can facilitate healing and resolution of conflicts.

Overall, IRT views problem resolution as a collaborative process that requires both partners to take responsibility for their emotional wounds and work together to create a more fulfilling and harmonious relationship and to have the skills and knowledge to deal with frustrations as they arise.

Case Transcript

This chapter began with the basics of Imago Relationship Therapy, including its history, how it views problem formation, diversity, the role of the therapist, and problem resolution. It has explored how Steve and Carissa have learned and used some of the skills taught by Imago therapists to help couples understand their relationship's frustrations and ways to deal with them so they can make changes without feeling coerced. And learning the Imago model begins in the first session.

Steve and Carissa were not in a good way when they arrived for their first session. Carissa was angry at being left alone so much and worried about what kind of father Steve would be. Steve was confused because he thought he was doing well in the marriage. Both were uncertain about the future of the marriage. After some chit-chat, the therapist asked them an important diagnostic question, "Tell me the story of how you met." Gottman (2013) reports that how a couple remembers their story is predictive of divorce. What Gottman calls the "Story of Us" is important not so much for the actual story, but for the retelling done with detail and positivity. For those who remember details and tell the story positively, there is a greater than 90 percent chance the marriage will make it. For those who tell the story negatively and with few details, the chances of recovery for the relationship are less certain.

Fortunately, Steve and Carissa remember their meeting fondly. They recalled that night in the club, talking and flirting, and how time seemed to fly by that night. They could not wait to see each other again and continue the conversation. It was a glorious time, as they recalled, and they wished they could return to that feeling. The therapist let them know it might not return to that exact state because of the chemicals involved in the romantic love process. Still, they can find a different and possibly deeper love as they begin to understand what's behind their present frustrations and learn new skills.

The IRT therapist teaches the couple how their brains protect them from perceived harm when their fight-or-flight response emerges. Even if there is no real harm, the brain goes into a defensive posture lighting up the reptilian brain and the vagal nerve system (Porges, 2011). To illustrate this, the therapist will ask Steve and Carissa to show for three minutes what a typical frustration would look like at home. Here is a small part of that interaction:

Carissa: You are always with your friends. I'm tired of being alone all the time.
Steve: But you were OK with it before. And I need some time away with my friends. I need to unwind.
Carissa: I feel like that's all you do is unwind. And I am really concerned because we are trying to have a baby and I'm worried about what kind of father you will be.
Steve: I'm going to be a great father! I'm going to play with the baby and take them places. I'm really looking forward to all the things we are going to do.
Carissa: And how do you think I feel when you come home from being with your friends and we have to go right upstairs to have sex when I'm ovulating? A little romance would be good.
Steve: What do you mean?! I leave early to come home so we can have our baby! I would think you would see that as a sacrifice too.
Carissa: You just don't get it.

No doubt this conversation is going nowhere and adding to the pain they are both experiencing. They are not hearing or understanding each other, and some intervention will be needed to change the pattern.

The therapist leads them through skills to bypass the fight-or-flight response in their power struggles and calm their nervous system during their dialogue. Steve and Carissa will learn breathing and centering techniques and how to create a safe place in their minds to listen fully to their partner without reacting. They will learn to tolerate some of the anxiety to retrain the brain that they are not in danger of injury or death. From this place of calm and safety, they will learn to fully listen to each other in the Couples Dialogue process—a three-part communication skill that is the basis of Imago Therapy. If they leave learning only one thing in the therapy, it would be best to learn this process which is why it is introduced in the first session. In dialogue, they will be taught to take turns by fully hearing their partner before it is their turn to respond. In the dialogue that follows below, the therapist's thought process will be highlighted in italics.

Steve determined that the best place for him to hear Carissa would be for him to visualize himself in his childhood treehouse. He recalled retreating to this space when he was upset and was able to find comfort and calm himself down in this very private part of his yard. The therapist helps Steve to become fully immersed in his safe place.

Therapist: (*softly*) OK, Steve, what I want you to do is put both feet on the floor and take a deep breath. Uncross your arms. Close your eyes... Take another breath... And I want you to picture yourself in your treehouse... Can you see it?... See where you are sitting... Feel the floor... The treehouse might have a smell ... wood ... fresh rainfall. There might be familiar sounds ... birds chirping ... trees rustling... Get yourself fully there... And remember how this feels and remember how to get back to this place when your discussions make you the least bit anxious. This is your safe place... A place you created and know that you are perfectly safe in this space. Are you fully there Steve?

Steve: I am.

Therapist: Good. I'm going to ask you to open your eyes now and Carissa is going to talk to you. Try to keep yourself in the treehouse even when you want to respond or disagree with what Carissa is saying. Listen to her fully, and you will get your chance to respond when she feels fully heard.

Steve: OK.

Therapist: Carissa, could you tell Steve what you need to say in a sentence or two. Tell him what you need to say using "I" statements such as "I feel sad when..." or "I feel lonely when..." And when you are done, he will mirror what you said to you to ensure he got it. Can you do that?

Emphasizing short manageable sentences in "I" statements.

Carissa: Yes.

Therapist: Steve, when you are ready, say to Carissa, "I can hear you now."

Making sure Steve is ready to hear.

Steve: Yes, I can hear you now.

Carissa: Steve, I feel alone when you are out with your friends, and I am all alone in the house.

Therapist: Steve, can you mirror that back?

Teaching them the dialogue process for the first time.

Steve: If I am hearing you correctly, you feel really lonely when I am with my friends and you are home alone.

Therapist: Ask her, "Did I get that?"

Steve:	Did I get that?
Carissa:	Yes, you did.
Therapist:	Ask her, "Tell me more about that?"

This encourages Steve to be curious rather than judgmental.

Steve:	Tell me more about that?
Carissa:	I'm not in school anymore, so I don't have a lot to do at night. I don't have a lot of friends and I really want to spend time with you. I can't just spend my time watching TV alone. I need you home and spending time with me.
Steve:	Why don't you just…
Therapist:	Nope!! Steve, let's go back to your safe place. Now is not the time to fix anything. Now is a time for listening. Can you take a breath and go back to the treehouse?

Steve is becoming triggered and retreating to old ways of responding. This was a re-direct by the therapist to stay with the dialogue process.

Steve:	Sorry, yes, I can.
Therapist:	Do you need Carissa to repeat what she said.
Steve:	I think so.
Therapist:	(*to Steve*) Deep breath.
Carissa:	I'm really lonely at night. I don't have a lot to do since I am not in school and I don't like watching TV alone. Things have changed, Steve. I didn't mind you being with your friends before, but now we are thinking about a family and I'm home by myself with nothing to do. I'm really worried about us.
Therapist:	(*softly*) Steve, can you mirror that?
Steve:	So, you are saying you are lonely at night when I am with my friends. Things have changed and it was OK before, but now that you have less to do at night, you are lonely and don't really like to watch TV by yourself. And you are worried about how we are going to be in the future now that we are thinking about having children. Did I get that?
Carissa:	Yes, you did.
Therapist:	Steve, the second part of this process is validation. Validation is not agreeing. It's saying that if I were looking at the world through your eyes, I could see that you would feel that way. That makes sense to me. Can you see what Carissa said from her point of view? Does it make sense to you?

The therapist is teaching the couple how to engage in validation with one another.

Steve:	Yes, I can see that.
Therapist:	Can you tell her? That makes sense to me. Or what makes sense to me about that is… And let her know.
Steve:	What you are saying makes sense to me. What makes sense to me about that is that I know you were busy when we first got married and it was probably best that I was out so you could get your work done. But now you have less to do and I did not change my lifestyle. And I can see how that would worry you in the future when we have kids if I keep going out as I am doing now. I can see how that would be a worry to you.
Therapist:	Great. Steve, the third part of this is called empathy. Can you take a guess at how Carissa might be feeling about this? You don't have to be right. It's just an attempt

to connect on a feeling level with her. You would say something like, "I imagine that might make you feel…" And take a guess at what might be going on for her.

The therapist next teaches empathy to the couple.

Steve: I can imagine that it might make you feel lonely, sad, and worried.
Therapist: Ask her, "Did I get that?"
Steve: Did I get that?
Carissa: Yes, you did.

At this point, the therapist might ask Carissa to pick one of the feelings and talk more about it. The therapist will work to keep Steve in a safe place listening to Carissa in deeper ways than they are used to communicating. Their dialogue continues.

Therapist: Carissa, can you talk to Steve about one of those feelings he offered to you?

Working with the couple to go deeper into the issue.

Carissa: Yes, I want to talk about feeling lonely. I do feel lonely a lot. I put a smile on my face when you go out and tell you to have a good time, but really, I'm quite lonely by myself and I find myself thinking about work when I really should be relaxing.
Steve: So you are saying that you are quite lonely when I leave even though you put a smile on your face and tell me to have a good time. Deep down you feel all by yourself and think about work a lot. Did I get that?
Carissa: You did.
Steve: Is there more about that?
Carissa: Yes. You know, I used to be able to cover up my feelings about this. I was so used to feeling alone growing up, but with the possibility of a baby, I don't want to do this alone and don't want our baby to have one parent.
Steve: But you know…
Therapist: (Interrupts) No, not yet, Steve. Let's see where this goes for Carissa. Go back to your safe place… Take a breath… And see if you can mirror what she said.

Steve was noticeably triggered by the comment. He was directed back to the process and maintaining safety.

Steve: What I heard you say is that it is getting harder to cover up how you feel. You did that for so long, you are worried now that when the baby comes along you will be lonely and you don't want to be the only parent in their life. Did I get that?
Carissa   (*getting teary*) Yes, you did.
Therapist   (*softly*) Carissa, it sounds like this is bringing up something from your childhood.

The therapist is helping Carissa connect the present issue with a past issue to increase the understanding of the frustration.

Carissa: I think so.
Therapist: Can you give it words and tell Steve about it? Steve, listen with your heart on this one.
Carissa: When I was a kid, my parents worked a lot. They had to work a lot; there was no choice. We were not rich, but their jobs made us comfortable. My parents were proud

of what they accomplished and knew they needed to keep it up, or they could lose it. If one of them lost their job, it would be all over.

Steve: So when you were a kid, your parents worked a lot, and you were often by yourself. You said that they had no choice. They had to work to keep up the life they provided for you and your sister. They were not rich, but what they did made the family comfortable. They felt they needed to keep it up or they could lose it. Did I get that?

Carissa: You did.

Steve: Can you tell me more about that?

Carissa: Yes, and I think this is one of the things you don't understand, Steve, because you are white.

Therapist: Stay safe and hear this, Steve.

The therapist is letting Steve know that what Carissa is about to say is important to her, and might be triggering to him.

Carissa: We were a black family living in the South. My mom's education and my dad's hard work made us middle class, but many forces were working against us. We know we are constantly being watched for when we make a mistake.

Steve: So as a middle-class black family living in the South, you were constantly being watched at your jobs, and people were looking for you to make a mistake. Did I get that?

Carissa: Yes, my parents tried to protect us from this, but their message always was that you have to work twice as hard. Others are watching and you could lose it all. I knew why they were not there for me. They were working and trying to keep all the balls in the air. One slip and the balls all end up on the ground, and there is no guarantee of recovery.

Steve: So your parents tried to protect you from the prejudice in your town, but you could see that they had to work twice as hard as others or lose it all if they made a mistake. You said you knew why they were not there for you because they were working to keep all the balls in the air. They felt that if they made one slip, they could lose everything and there was no guarantee they could recover. Did I get that?

Carissa: Yes, and that message was impressed on me which is why I tend to work so hard. And I am tired. I want to be able to let down a little. I want to be able to make a mistake once in a while without worrying that my career is over.

Steve: And you picked up on that message and that's why you work so hard. And now you are tired. You want to be able to let down a little and know that your mistakes that anyone can make won't bring you down.

Therapist: Steve, does that make sense to you?

Steve: It really does and it explains a lot. What you are saying makes a lot of sense to me and I can see how tiring it must be for you, and your family, to keep up your high level of work. I can see how much you all work to stay where you are.

Therapist: And how would you guess what she might be feeling?

Steve: I can imagine you feel tired, lonely, and constantly anxious that you could lose it all. You are always on! You are always trying to be your best, and that's exhausting as well as lonely.

Carissa: It really is. Thank you for seeing that.

For a brief moment through dialogue, Steve was able to step into Carissa's world to see that she has been lonely for a long time. Some of the loneliness was due to him, and a lot was due to being left alone due to her parents' work ethic; an ethic necessary for them to maintain their status in their small Florida town. While Carissa may have been shielded from overt racism, her parents could not shield her from the systemic racism inherent in systems that distrust black workers and look for flaws to exploit. It is not fair or just, and the result for Carissa was a supported, but often lonely childhood. She learned to have a good work ethic which helped her become successful in her job, but she did not know how to relax and enjoy what she had accomplished. Later in her Behavior Change Request, Carissa would ask Steve for some of his time. And because he was able to see what this meant to her, he was more likely to be able to grant her request without feeling coerced or bitter. He now knows why she needs time and a chance to let down.

Of course, Steve will also have his turn for Carissa to listen to him in dialogue and his needs may be the opposite of hers. Steve had to be good as a child after his parents' divorce and had difficulty openly having fun during his teenage years. He has undoubtedly been making up for this with his frequent nights out with his friends. As Carissa listens to his story, she will begin to understand how his family impacted his carefreeness as a teen. He may request a more reasonable amount of time to spend with his friends. Opposite needs and desires are not unusual, but rather a place of growth in the relationship. As stated earlier, what one partner needs is what the other partner needs to grow into. Partners need to stretch into new behaviors to meet their partner's needs and for their own personal growth.

Steve and Carissa will leave the session with homework to practice dialogue three to five times for 20 minutes over the next week until the next session. They will be told that it will feel awkward and they may get it wrong, but they are just learning, and they will practice more in the next session. They will also be given instructions and information about **caring behaviors**, giving their partner what they need to feel cared for in the relationship. Gottman's (2013) research found that happy, stable couples express caring behaviors at a ratio of five positive behaviors for every one negative behavior. Steve and Carissa will be instructed to be polite and kind and do things the other likes to do until the next session.

In subsequent sessions, the therapist will add additional skills to increase empathy between the couple and teach them the Behavior Change Request process. Steve and Carissa will also develop a vision for their relationship so they can act toward the shared image of their future together. Now that the bloom of early romantic love is gone, they will need to develop a new way of thinking about themselves and will come up with visionary ideas such as: We go out once a week; We are good parents to our children; We save money for the future; We take one agreed upon vacation per year; and We talk about disagreements using Couples Dialogue.

They will also develop a list of caring behaviors that, when given by their partner, would make them feel loved and cared for in the relationship, keeping in mind that care for one person may not be considered care by the other. While Steve might like ice cream, Carissa might like a smoothie instead, and if he gives her ice cream, she might not feel as grateful as he would expect. A long list of caring behaviors will be developed by both Steve and Carissa—a back rub, making a cup of tea, asking if there is something I can do to help, taking a walk—and presenting them to each other will allow each of them to give a caring "gift" that can be appreciated by the other.

Conclusion

Steve and Carissa are an interesting, and typical, couple who sought couples' therapy to work on their relationship. They initially had a passionate connection driven by chemistry, but as time passed and the chemicals faded, they realized they needed help. Imago Relationship Therapy taught them the purpose of their relationships and gave them substantial skills to maintain and deepen their connection. Through Imago Therapy, they learned how to create a sense of safety within the relationship by grounding themselves and managing reactive tendencies. They also developed active listening skills through the Couples Dialogue, allowing them to understand and empathize with each other emotionally. Additionally, they acquired the ability to make reasonable behavior requests that would require personal growth for both of them. They have begun envisioning a future for their marriage and are committed to taking actions that will demonstrate care and love for each other.

Steve and Carissa were able to accomplish this with 12 weeks of therapy with the Imago therapist. A 2017 random-controlled study of 14 couples (Gehlert et al., 2017) supports the hypothesis that a 12-week dose of IRT can produce significant change as measured by the Marital Adjustment Test (Locke & Wallace, 1959). Though there was some loss of effect, the positive MAT scores remained significant at the 12-week follow-up. It is often recommended that couples commit to a minimum of 6 to 12 sessions, with some needing 16 weeks or longer depending on the severity of the problems and the clients' commitment to learning the Imago processes. Termination or a weaning off of regular sessions can take place after the couple learns the Imago processes discussed in this chapter and feels comfortable using them as needed on their own. It is also recommended that couples consider booster sessions with the therapist every few months to discuss any recent issues and to anchor the processes in the relationship.

Considering their willingness to learn and practice the Imago process regularly, it is highly likely that Steve and Carissa's marriage will have a positive prognosis.

References

Bain, H. (1998). Imago therapy with Hispanic couples. In W. Luquet & M. T. Hannah (Eds.), *Healing in the relational paradigm: The Imago relationship therapy casebook* (pp. 113–124). Brunner/Routledge.

Buber, M. (1948). *Between man and man* (Ronald Gregor Smith, Trans.). Macmillan.

Buber, M. (1996). *I and thou* (W. Kaufmann, Trans., 1st Touchstone ed.). Touchstone. (Original work published 1923)

Cacioppio, S. (2023). *Wired for love: A neuroscientist's journey through romance, loss, and the essence of human connection*. Flatiron Books.

Doherty, W. J., Harris, S. M., Hall, E. L., & Hubbard, A. K. (2021). How long do people wait before seeking couples therapy? A research note. *Journal of Marital and Family Therapy*, *47*, 882–890.

Gehlert, N., Schmidt, C., Gingerich, V., & Luquet, W. (2017). Randomized controlled trial of Imago Relationship Therapy: Exploring statistical and clinical significance. *The Journal of Couple and Relationship Therapy*, *16*(3), 188–209.

Gottman, J. M. (2013). *What makes love last: How to build trust and avoid betrayal*. Simon and Schuster.

Hendrix, H. (1988). *Getting the love you want: A guide for couples*. St. Martin's Griffin.Hendrix, H. (2008). *Getting the love you want: A guide for couples*. Macmillan.

Hendrix, H., & Hunt, H. (2021). *Doing Imago therapy in the space in-between*. W.W. Norton.Hendrix, H., Hunt, H. L., Hannah, M. T., & Luquet, W. (Eds.). (2005). *Imago Relationship Therapy: Perspectives on theory*. Jossey-Bass.

Hosseini, H. M., & Movahedi, A. (2016). Imago therapy: A strategy to improve couples lovemaking. *Mediterranean Journal of Social Sciences*, *7*(4 S1), 242.

Kleinberg, S., & Zorn, P. (1998). Multiple mirroring with lesbian and gay couples: From Peoria to P-Town. In W. Luquet & M. T. Hannah (Eds.), *Healing in the relational paradigm: The imago relationship therapy casebook* (pp. 135–199). Brunner-Mazel.

Locke, H. J., & Wallace, K. M. (1959). Short marital-adjustment and prediction tests: Their reliability and validity. *Marriage and Family Living*, *21*(2), 251–255.

Luquet, W. (2007). *Short term couples therapy: The Imago model in action*. Routledge.

Luquet, W., & Hannah, M. T. (1998). *Healing in the relational paradigm: The Imago relationship therapy casebook*. Brunner-Mazel.

Martin, T. L., & Bielawski, D. M. (2011). What is the African American's experience following imago education? *Journal of Humanistic Psychology*, *51*(2), 216–228. https://doi.org/10.1177/0022167809352379

Muro, L., Holliman, R., & Luquet, W. (2016a). The impact of the Safe Conversations Workshop with diverse, low income couples. *American Journal of Family Therapy*, *44*(3), 155–167.

Muro, L., Holliman, R., & Luquet, W. (2016b). Imago relationship therapy and accurate empathy development. *Journal of Couple and Relationship Therapy*, *15*(1), 1–16.

Oh, J., & Minichiello, V. (2013). Psychosocial development in South Korean couples and its effects on marital relationships. *Journal of Family Psychotherapy*, *24*(3), 228–245.

Parker, K., & Barrasso, A. (2021, February 25). In Vice President Kamala Harris, we can see how America has changed. Pew Research Center. Retrieved from www.pewresearch.org/short-reads/2021/02/25/in-vice-president-kamala-harris-we-can-see-how-america-has-changed/

Porges, S. (2011). *The polyvagal theory: Neurophysiological foundations of emotions, attachment, communication, and self-regulation*. Norton.

Schmidt, C., Luquet. W., & Gehlert, N. (2016). Evaluating the impact of the Imago couples workshop on relational adjustment and communication patterns. *Journal of Couple and Relationship Therapy*, *15*(3), 1–18.

Schmidt, C. D., & Gelhert, N. C. (2017). Couples therapy and empathy: An evaluation of the impact of Imago relationship therapy on partner empathy levels. *The Family Journal*, *25*(1), 23–30. https://doi.org/10.1177/1066480716678621

Seidabadi, S., Noranipour, R., & Shafiabady, A. (2021). The comparison of the effectiveness of solution-focused couple therapy and Imago relationship therapy (IMAGO) on the conflicts of the couples referring to counseling centers in Tehran city. *Journal of Counseling Research*, *19*(76), 4–23.

Seigel, D. (2018). *Aware: The science and practice of presence*. TarcherPerigee.

Sheydanfar, N., Navabinejad, S., & Farzad, V. (2021). Comparing the effectiveness of Emotionally Focused Couple Therapy (EFCT) and Imago Relation Therapy (IRT) in couples marital satisfaction. *Journal of Family Psychology*, *4*(2), 75–88.

Smith, P. (2023). *Black marriage, attachment and connecting in relationships: An observational mixed-methods study investigating the effects of the getting the love you want workshop on black couples' attachment, interactions, marital satisfaction and communication*. Unpublished Dissertation, Antioch University.

Weiser, H., & Thompson, C. (1998). Is Imago Therapy culturally relevant? Case studies with African-American families. In W. Luquet & M. T. Hannah (Eds.), *Healing in the relational paradigm: The Imago relationship therapy casebook* (pp. 113–123). Brunner-Mazel.

Weller, C. E. (2019, December 15). African-Americans face systemic obstacles to getting good jobs. Center for American Progress. Retrieved from www.americanprogress.org/article/african-americans-face-systematic-obstacles-getting-good-jobs/

10 Emotionally Focused Couple Therapy

Nicholas Lee, James L. Furrow, and Hannah S. Myung

History of the Model

Emotionally Focused Couple Therapy (EFT; Johnson, 2020) is an integrative approach in the treatment of couple distress. It is among a few couple treatment modalities with a robust line of empirical support for effectiveness in treating couple distress (Doss et al., 2022; Wiebe & Johnson, 2016). EFT was given its name to emphasize the pivotal role that emotions play in the organization of interactional patterns and experiences in intimate relationships (Johnson, 2020).

EFT was established in the 1980s when behavioral interventions for couple treatment were primarily used. The behavioral approach was known to be the most widely researched and recognized for its efficacious treatment in couple distress (Baucom et al., 1998). Behavioral interventions rooted in social learning theory and behavioral principles aimed to facilitate positive interactions through communication training, problem-solving, and behavioral exchanges, and contracts in which the therapist mainly took on a coaching role (Jacobson & Margolin, 1979). Relationships were conceptualized as transactional and "quid pro quo." The beginning formulation of EFT sought to address the lack of validated couple treatments with more focus on humanistic approaches rather than behavioral interventions.

In their initial outcome studies, Susan Johnson and Les Greenberg (1985a, 1985b) observed therapy sessions of distressed couples working to repair their relationships. Their work drew from humanistic-experiential views (Gendlin, 1974; Perls et al., 1951; Rogers, 1951) and systemic theories, including structural family therapy (Minuchin & Fishman, 1981), which supported a framework that guided their observations and understandings focused more on process rather than on the individual. Their humanistic-experiential emphasis gave attention to how partners process and construct their experiences and the systemic approach focused on each partner's responses in the context of interactions. The integration of the humanistic-experiential and systemic approaches allowed for a clearly delineated couple therapy model that engaged a couple's intrapersonal experiences *and* interpersonal patterns (Johnson, 2020).

Furthermore, Johnson included attachment theory (Bowlby, 1969) in her observations of couple dynamics and questioned the viewing of relationships as only rational bargains, arguing instead that relationships are better understood as affectional bonds (Johnson, 1986). Attachment theory eventually became a primary framework for conceptualizing patterns of relationship distress and also a map to relationship reparation (Johnson, 2020). From an attachment perspective, couple distress is understood in the context of insecure bonds and separation. As partners experience prolonged periods of distress, the sense of attachment security is threatened, and attachment-related fears are triggered.

Attachment-related affect plays a significant role in the organization of attachment responses. Negative attachment-related affect that is continually experienced results in predictable behaviors that are characterized by avoidant and anxious responses. Over time, partners become stuck in

DOI: 10.4324/9781003369097-10

insecure patterns of responding. Relationship repair becomes difficult as partners become more prone to rigid ways of relating to one another.

The attachment framework serves as a map for the couple therapist by focusing on the couple's attachment insecurities and highlighting attachment longings and needs for closeness and security. The attachment approach guides therapists in helping partners access, resynthesize, and restructure emotional bonds and interactions. In summary, Johnson and colleagues (1999) suggested four treatment assumptions characteristic of emotion and adult attachment in healthy couple relationships. First, intimacy is best understood as an attachment bond in romantic relationships. Second, common patterns of couple conflict often interrupt partners' abilities to form and sustain secure attachment. Third, engaging emotional experience is critical to transforming intrapersonal and interpersonal dynamics. Fourth, emotional responses must be addressed in therapy to change a couple's negative interactional patterns. Also, a couple's ability to express attachment needs and desires is adaptive and facilitates intimacy (Johnson, 2020).

Empirical Support and Process Research

Research using clinical trials and process-based studies are a hallmark of the EFT approach. EFT meets the highest criteria for evidence-based practice with extant research demonstrating absolute, relative, and contextual efficacy (Sexton et al., 2011). Johnson and colleagues (1999) conducted an initial meta-analysis of the primary randomized controlled trial (RCT) studies and reported an effect size of 1.31, which was more robust than commonly reported effects for couple therapy at that time (e.g., Dunn & Schwebel, 1995). Couples receiving EFT showed significant decreases in relationship distress with over half (70–73%) of the couples demonstrating treatment recovery. Recent meta-analyses and reviews have continued to support the notion that EFT is an efficacious treatment for couple distress (Beasley & Ager, 2019; Johnson & Wittenborn, 2012; Rathgeber et al., 2019; Wiebe & Johnson, 2016). A more recent and comprehensive (with inclusion of experimental and quasi-experimental designs) meta-analysis of EFT (as derived by Johnson, 2020) studies found an effect size of .93 for pretreatment to posttreatment improvements, and an effect size of .86 for pretreatment to follow-up (Spengler et al., 2022).

Findings from EFT process research show support for the model's theory of change, reveal therapy factors predictive of successful outcomes, and inform clinicians in treating couple distress. Theoretically derived key change events in EFT have been task analyzed and delineated, including withdrawer re-engagement (Lee et al., 2017b), blamer softening (Bradley & Furrow, 2004), and attachment injury resolution (Makinen & Johnson, 2006; Zuccarini et al., 2013). More recent process research also examined the emotional processes involved in these key change events (Myung et al., 2022). In Johnson and Greenberg's (1988) initial process-outcome study, couples who appeared to benefit from EFT had significantly higher levels of emotional experiencing and affiliative responses than couples who did not show improvement. Similarly, higher levels of emotional experiencing and increases in affiliative interactions were observed in more resolved couples receiving EFT in a study with couples facing chronic illness (Couture-Lalande et al., 2007) and couples with attachment injuries (Makinen & Johnson, 2006).

Researchers have also identified specific therapist interventions that correspond to successful treatment outcomes. Zuccarini et al. (2013) identified interventions associated with successful resolutions of attachment injuries. Similarly, EFT therapist interventions and process themes have been identified in successful blamer softening (Bradley & Furrow, 2004) and withdrawer re-engagement change events (Lee et al., 2017b). Furrow and colleagues (2012) found that the therapist's emotional presence and engagement predicted increased levels of clients' emotional experiencing necessary in the process of successful softening. Blamer softening is a significant change event in EFT that is predictive of increases in relationship satisfaction (Burgess Moser et al.,

2016; Dalgleish et al., 2015a) and has been identified in couples showing improvement (Burgess Moser et al., 2016; Johnson & Greenberg, 1988). The combination of outcome and process research studies have furthered the validation of the efficacy of the model and a deeper understanding of its process of change. Taking study findings on process factors for change, Brubacher and Wiebe (2019) further provided a concrete and detailed map for clinicians applying these active change ingredients in therapy.

Treatment Applications with Specific Populations and Concerns

EFT has empirical support for treating various clinical issues including depression (e.g., Wittenborn et al., 2019), posttraumatic stress disorder (Weissman et al., 2018), and low sexual desire (Macphee et al., 1995). EFT has been shown to be a supportive intervention for improving relationship functioning and experiencing empathic caregiving for the cancer population (McLean et al., 2013). Outcome research showing support for EFT in addressing attachment injuries (Makinen & Johnson, 2006) has demonstrated treatment effects remaining stable at a three-year follow-up (Halchuk et al., 2010). EFT has received support for reducing couple distress for partners raising children with autism (Lee et al., 2017a), as well as with chronically ill children (Walker et al., 1996) with improvements observed at a two-year follow-up (Cloutier et al., 2002). Improvements have also been shown to occur across the trajectory of multiple follow-up time points, indicating a growth pattern, in distressed couples (Wiebe & Johnson, 2016).

Throughout the years, EFT has expanded its applicability to different populations including same-sex couples (Josephson, 2003), older couples (Bradley & Palmer, 2003), remarried couples (Furrow & Palmer, 2007), families (Furrow et al., 2019; Johnson et al., 1998), and individuals (Johnson & Campbell, 2022). A practical understanding of attachment theory and EFT has been made accessible for the general population through Johnson's (2008) book, *Hold Me Tight*, which has been translated into 20 different languages and has been implemented in workshops, psychoeducational settings, and relationship enrichment programs. In *Love Sense* (Johnson, 2013), she provides the general public with a scientific understanding of emotional bonding and offers practical advice for partners in managing and strengthening secure attachment bonds. The focus of this chapter will be on exploring the application of EFT with couples.

Treatment Limitations

EFT is particularly appropriate for working with couples because of its application of attachment theory for understanding and intervening in adult intimate relationships. However, it is worth mentioning the contraindications for EFT when working with couples. The approach is not suitable for couples who clearly wish to separate, couples who are already separated and are ambivalent in working toward reconciliation, and couples where one or both partners are involved in an extramarital affair. Therapists should assess and help clarify the needs and goals for the couple and make appropriate recommendations as deemed necessary, which may include individual work for those who are separating. Also, the therapist should assess for areas that are threatening the couple's sense of safety in the relationship including ongoing abuse. The abused partner's experiences and expressions of vulnerability can be detrimental and place the partner at a higher risk for harm in an abusive context. Last, while recent research on EFT has expanded to include couples who hold minoritized identities, earlier research has predominantly included couples who come from culturally dominant identities. Continued research with non-white and non-heterosexual populations is needed to further generalize the effectiveness of EFT, as well as elaborate on mechanisms of change with these populations (Spengler et al., 2020, 2022).

The following sections examine the EFT approach to problem formulation and problem resolution using the case of the Hogarths. Examples are provided to demonstrate how an EFT therapist
might conceptualize this couple's distress, understand aspects of diversity, and intervene over the
course of treatment.

Conceptualization of Problem Development

In EFT, each partner's emotional experience provides a reliable guide from relational distress to a
more intimate relationship. The EFT therapist focuses on each partner's emotional responses that
drive partners further apart. These negative interactional patterns reinforce increasingly defended
positions and keep partners in a cycle defined by a dance of distance and distress (Johnson, 1998).
Emotions animate each partner's actions and reactions as the couple struggles to regain their
connection. Attachment theory provides the therapist with a map for the behaviors and motivations
that make a couple's negative pattern predictable, understandable, and ultimately changeable.

Negative Interactional Patterns

The EFT therapist focuses on emotion as both a source of distress and a resource for its resolution.
The reasons for a couple's conflict are secondary to powerful **negative emotional patterns** that
create self-absorbing negative affect states (Johnson, 2020). Couples who are caught in cycles of
escalating distress may have chronic disagreements, but it is each partner's inability to regulate
negative affect that puts their relationship at risk for dissolution. These insidious patterns develop
over time as couples navigate around issues of vulnerability, and fears mount as partners increasingly manage their needs on their own rather than as a couple. As conflict and crisis increase, these
patterns take prominence and cascade couples toward greater isolation and emotional disengagement (Gottman, 1998). The process of EFT engages partners through these rigid interactions and
transforms these cycles by accessing, expanding, and engaging the underlying attachment-related
emotions and needs that are the basis of a more secure emotional bond (Johnson, 2019).

Systemically, EFT conceptualizes couple distress as an interactional pattern composed of partners' **secondary emotional responses** (Johnson, 2020). These secondary responses are informed
by more vulnerable **primary emotions** of hurt, sadness, and fear that are reinforced by the painful
interactions of the couple. Together, each partner's responses to these negative experiences form
more rigid positions (e.g., pursuit, withdrawal). As partners seek to regain their emotional balance
in reaction to underlying concerns, the withdrawing partner quickly retreats in the face of the critical response of a more pursuing partner, which engages more pursuit from that partner and consequently greater withdrawal. Understanding the couple's positions and patterns begins with an
understanding of this critical recognition of primary and secondary emotion.

The Hogarths enter therapy following a period of time dealing with issues pertaining to infertility.
They have been trying to conceive a child for the past three years with no success, including several rounds of in-vitro fertilization. They acknowledge a growing sense of disconnection between
them and their interaction in session points to Carissa's growing frustration and Steve's dismissive
and callous tendencies. Steve takes the position of a withdrawer within the relationship, evidenced
by his history of leaving and spending time with his friends, participating in golf outings, and his
general dismissiveness toward Carissa's bids for his attention and time. Carissa takes the position
of pursuer within the relationship, evidenced in her frequent initiations for connection, communication, and intensifying her attempts at gaining Steve's attention through frequent criticisms
and complaints. Underlying Steve's dismissive and callous secondary emotional position in the
relationship is likely more vulnerable, primary emotions such as hurt, sadness, and feelings of
inadequacy as a partner. Similarly, underlying Carissa's secondary emotional experience of anger

is likely a sense of loneliness, hurt, and feeling rejected by Steve. Over time, Steve and Carissa have become entrenched in these positions such that it has placed great strain on their attachment bond with one another.

Attachment Bonds

Johnson (1986) recognized that what was at stake in couple distress was more than the social exchange of partner's personal interest, but rather an enduring emotional bond. Following attachment theory (Bowlby, 1969) and its application to romantic love (Hazan & Shaver, 1987), Johnson proposed that EFT offers much more than an explanation of couple conflict, but rather a theory of love (Johnson, 2013). Attachment theory not only provides the EFT therapist with a comprehensive approach to the couple's patterns of distress, but also the motivation underlying each partner's drive to connect and grow.

The primary motivation of couples seeking help in therapy is not simply the reduction of conflict but the need to renew and restore their intimacy as a couple. Research on couple conflict and its treatment has tended to focus on resolving conflict and negative relationship problems (Fincham et al., 2007), while couple therapies have lacked a systematic theory of intimacy (Roberts, 1992). Johnson (1986) initially proposed that relationships were built on emotional bonds and not simply a series of negotiated bargains between partners. Attachment theory (Bowlby, 1969) and its application to adult relationships (Hazan & Shaver, 1987) provide the EFT therapist with an overarching theory for the motivation and functions of romantic love where a couple's bond is best understood as an emotional tie that governs the relationship and one's experience in that relationship.

For the Hogarths, questioning the future of their relationship is a reflection of both the precipitating events that brought them to treatment, but also a deeper, more extensive experience of a lost connection in their relationship. Adults in more secure relationships are better able to express their needs and respond to those of their partners, especially when these needs are experienced in the context of vulnerability (Simpson et al., 1996). The results of a more secure style are evident in couples reporting a more intimate, satisfying, and trusting relationship (Collins & Read, 1990). For Bowlby (1988), the ability to maintain contact with one's attachment figure is essential to survival, and these relational needs are integral to well-being from the cradle to the grave.

Through EFT, couples can move to more effective dependence, which results in more coherent expressions of self and personal autonomy (Dalgleish et al., 2015b). Attachment theory provides the EFT therapist with a map for understanding a distressed partner's predictable responses. Using an attachment lens, the EFT therapist can focus on the relational insecurities, longings, and needs that organize a partner's actions and relationship experience (Johnson, 2019). At the heart of the relationship is an emotional tie that defines the importance of the other (e.g., attachment figure) and the relationship itself (i.e., attachment bond). The experience of insecurity and separation distress in a romantic relationship takes precedence in one's actions and experience (Johnson, 2020). Attachment theory enables the therapist to conjecture about the meaning and motivation at the heart of a partner's responses. Primary or core emotions are understood as attachment-related emotions informed by a human need for social bonds with one's partner which is of ultimate importance.

A partner's behaviors in a distressed relationship can be understood as attempts to manage the inability to effectively respond to a threatened attachment bond. The patterns of anxious pursuit and avoidant withdrawal become predictable responses for couples where partners are no longer emotionally responsive and accessible. As these patterns persist, efforts to respond and repair are met with increasing disengagement. Building on Bowlby's (1988) observations of parent and child relationships, Johnson (2020) recognized that patterns of separation distress in couples follow a similar predictable sequence, where a partner's angry protest over the experience of distress often gives way to anxious efforts to regain closeness and when these remain unsuccessful, partners withdraw into depression and despair.

The level of despair is painfully clear at this point in the Hogarths' relationship. Questions about the future of the relationship are a reflection of the enduring pain and distance that neither Steve nor Carissa have been able to address. The focal issue for the couple is the impact of infertility, yet the way the couple responds to this issue is indicative of a long-term pattern of demand and distance. Couples caught in these vicious cycles of insecurity increasingly rely on less effective means of coping or relationship survival (e.g., fight, flight, freeze). The loss of emotional connection with an attachment figure can trigger "**primal panic**" which is a primary emotional system associated with social loss and a primary source of psychic pain (Panksepp, 1998). The impact and routine experience of fear reduce the couple's ability to make their way back to the secure relationship they desire and need. Fear blocks the couple's efforts to express their basic needs for contact, care, and comfort, and as a result, couples rely on secondary strategies to manage the increasing insecurity in their relationship. The therapist's understanding of these blocks normalizes the struggle that the Hogarths face in connecting, especially after struggling with Carissa becoming pregnant. The level of distress is a source and a result of the ways each partner responds, often in automatic ways, to the threats experienced in the relationship.

Emotions play a central role in the organization and expression of attachment-related dynamics for couples. Each partner's response to distress in the moment is influenced by their attachment histories that impact the appraisal, interpretation of, and response to an emotionally threatening interaction (Johnson & Whiffen, 1999). Partners with more insecure attachment styles are more likely to experience negative views of self (e.g., fear of rejection) or negative views of others (e.g., fear of abandonment). In response, these insecure styles result in a range of reactive behaviors from anxious and clinging responses demanding reassurance to distancing avoidant responses (Pietromonaco & Barrett, 2000). Through the lens of attachment, the actions of pursuit and withdrawal can be further understood in terms of the specific interactions and patterns happening between the partners. The more anxious pursuing partner tends toward amplifying the anxiety of felt insecurity, while the more avoidant partner is more likely to deny or minimize this anxiety (Johnson & Whiffen, 1999). Partners' attachment strategies are evident in the secondary emotional responses that fuel the couple's negative interactional pattern and perpetuate the couple's felt insecurity.

Change in these patterns results from new experiences, new information, and new interactions. The process of EFT provides partners with new experiences of the couple's problematic pattern through accessing, processing, and engaging the attachment-related affect underlying the more reactive roles that dominate even their best moments of trying to connect.

The attachment strategies endure in the presence of experiences that confirm the felt insecurity (Mikulincer & Shaver, 2016). From an EFT perspective, emotion is seen as "an organizing force in working models rather than an outcome of them" (Johnson, 2009, p. 266) and these models are revised through emotional communication (Davila et al., 1999).

Therefore, change in a couple's relationship results from new experiences that disconfirm past fears and expectations and inform models of self and other (Johnson & Whiffen, 1999). Johnson (2009) suggested that EFT offers corrective emotional experience that provides partners with new experience of and new meaning to what has become a familiar and expected outcome (e.g., negative pattern) and these changes through experience and meaning promise new possibilities for the relationship. She states that "when both partners then send clear and more coherent emotional signals and so create a closer and more attuned interpersonal dance, they literally are able to shape a new and transformative emotional world for each other" (p. 279). For Steve and Carissa, the therapist focuses on the fundamental attachment dynamics of their emotional bond, and this will require forming a new connection organized by the shared engagement of attachment-related emotions and needs in an accessible and responsive way. They must change their dance.

The therapist will guide Steve into encountering his felt sense of inadequacy around being able to provide Carissa with the experience of being a mother. It is this sense of inadequacy and a negative view of self that drives Steve to either lash out in anger at Carissa's complaints or find distance from her through activities with his friends. Likewise, the therapist will guide Carissa into an experiential understanding of her pain, hurt, and rejection. Carissa's deep pain surrounding the infertility and Steve's responses to her drive Carissa's increasing anger, frustration, and criticisms. In EFT, anger and criticism are reframed within the context of attachment-related separation protest, whereas withdrawal is reframed as a form of self-protection versus being cold and uncaring.

Conceptualizing Diversity

EFT is humanistic and empathic at its core. As such, it sees the panoply of human connection and intimate relationships as valid, equal, and part of what it fundamentally means to be human. According to the EFT theoretical framework, our need for safe and secure attachment within the context of our romantic relationships is universal across cultures. However, there is also the recognition that culture plays a significant role in how emotion, which governs how we respond and make sense of our attachment relationships, varies based upon culture-specific emotional display rules. Johnson (2020) wrote that "we are wired for connection no matter who we are. The EFT therapist attempts to implement this stance in every session. It is of course true that EFT must be adapted to specific populations" (p. 201). While attachment-related processes, as well as the powerful role that emotion plays in shaping our relational worlds, are shared cross-culturally, the EFT therapist must consider the implications of how the differing worldviews and lived experiences of individuals from different cultures play out within the context of treatment.

In Stage 1 of EFT, the therapist focuses on building an alliance, assisting the couple in making sense of the issues that beset their relationship, and begins the process of explicating attachment-related emotions that have gone unacknowledged for each partner. Linhof and Allan (2019) suggested that EFT treatment, integrated with narrative and story-based interventions around dominant cultural narratives of power, oppression, and invalidation of the relationship, is well-suited for treatment with intercultural couples. Indeed, dominant cultural narratives about the self, one's relationship, and what is a "healthy and normal relationship" can have a profound influence on relationship well-being and the course of treatment. The **CARE framework** (i.e., Context, Attachment, Relationship, Emotion) provides the EFT therapist with a phenomenological approach to the impact of context on vulnerability and its expression in both the therapist and the couple relationship (Johnson & Campbell, 2022). This framework provides a cultural and contextual lens to explore the socio-cultural influences shaping each partner's experience of safety and security.

For Steve and Carissa, internalized experiences of oppression via microaggressions, racism, and broader cultural messages about their relationship are valid and must be openly addressed and brought into the therapeutic conversation. The EFT therapist needs to acknowledge how negative societal messages about interracial couples have shaped their unique and shared experiences. It is important to note here that discriminatory behaviors, attitudes, and messages sometimes do occur within the couple's own families of origin, as is the case with Steve's father, as well as their broader community. The EFT therapist might ask, "How do the two of you respond *together* when you experience discrimination about your relationship?" or "Carissa, are you able to go to Steve when you have experienced microaggressions from the family and ask for his support?" "Are there others you turn to for support in these times, and what is that like for you?"

In addition to examining the influence of negative societal messages about interracial couples on the relationship, the EFT therapist needs to explore how culture plays a role in the formation of the couple's unique relationship structure. For instance, Seshadri and Knudson-Martin (2013) suggested there are multiple ways in which partners integrate different cultural attitudes, values, and practices into their relationship. These can range from integrated, where partners celebrate, validate, and incorporate both cultures into their relationship structure, to unresolved structures, which occur when partners are unsure of how to successfully incorporate their cultural differences, leading to possible conflict and tension. Here again, the EFT therapist can explore with Steve and Carissa how they have managed to integrate their cultural differences within one another, especially as they navigate the challenges of attempting to start their own family.

In Stage 2 of EFT, the therapist focuses on restructuring the attachment bond between partners, first through the process of withdrawer re-engagement, which is then followed by blamer softening. The result of this stage is the beginning formation of more secure attachment responses and behaviors with one another. In this stage, more so than Stage 1, emotional expressions of attachment-related fears, needs, and wants become deeply poignant. It behooves the EFT therapist to be attuned to how the depth of emotional experiencing, how emotions are shared, and the degree of emotional vulnerability displayed can vary based upon culture-specific rules and practices. In Stage 3 of EFT, the couple begins to implement new solutions to old, more long-standing issues, as well as beginning to cement new patterns of interaction that continue to promote secure attachment (Johnson, 2020). For Steve and Carissa, bringing their cultural differences to the fore in how they work together to address long-standing problems provides a springboard for each to reflect on the inherent strengths in their relationship. The EFT therapist might ask, "How do you two see your cultural and racial differences as a strength in how you face these challenges?" or "When you two experience discrimination because of your relationship, how will the two of you stand together going forward? What will that look like?"

Since its inception in the late 1980s in Canada, EFT training and practice has been disseminated throughout the world. There are 30+ International Centers for Excellence in EFT (ICEEFT; www. iceeft.org), affiliated training centers and communities in North and Central America, Europe, the Middle East, Asia, Australia, and New Zealand. The Hold Me Tight relationship enhancement program based upon EFT has been translated into numerous languages including Chinese languages, Dutch, Farsi, German, Polish, and Spanish to name a few. As the dissemination of EFT has spread around the globe, culturally contextualized research has been conducted on various issues related to the training and professional practice of EFT. For instance, research has been conducted on cross-cultural training practices and experiences in Spanish-speaking countries (Rodríguez-González et al., 2020), in Hungary (Koren et al., 2021), in South Africa (Lesch et al., 2018), in Taiwan (Tseng et al., 2023) and among Chinese Canadian couples (Wong et al., 2017). Additionally, research has examined the application of EFT to intercultural couples (Linhof & Allan, 2019), rural men (Ceniza & Allan, 2021), polyamorous and same-sex couples (Edwards et al., 2023; Hardtke et al., 2010; Josephson, 2003), military/veteran couples (Ganz et al., 2022), and how EFT clinicians adapt their work with diverse couples (Allan et al., 2023).

The Role of the Therapist

According to Johnson (2020), the EFT therapist has three essential roles: (1) process consultant, (2) choreographer, and (3) collaborator. The EFT therapist is first and foremost a **process consultant** who guides the process of change for partners as they explore and engage in new experiences together. The therapist relies on interventions that invite accessing and processing of emotional experience as the partners' unfolding experience is explored from session to session. The engagement of moment-to-moment experience follows the moves of the EFT Tango (Johnson, 2020) and the power of the model to effect change through a series of corrective emotional encounters.

The EFT therapist **choreographs** new levels of engagement as partners move through de-escalating reactivity to taking new positions of vulnerability together. EFT sessions hold a therapeutic "safe haven" where a partner can be seen and understood in the distance and distress they experience as they seek to find a way out of entrenched cycles of negative affect (Johnson, 2020). As an attachment resource, the EFT therapist guides partners through the co-regulation of emotional experience, enabling shifts from reactive stances in their relationship drama toward the core underlying experiences that shape new interactions of more secure relating. The therapist maintains an active and attuned presence that invites a constructive dependence that promotes a more coherent and congruent expression of relationship needs and desires.

As a **collaborator**, the EFT therapist joins the partners with an open and curious stance, seeking to make sense of their experience and their goals in therapy. The therapist's empathic presence provides a critical resource for creating a level of emotional safety that begins with each partner's experience and provides acceptance and validation for their uncertainty and concerns. This collaboration relies on the therapist's own genuineness and authenticity as a bridge between the self-protective pattern that defines the couple's reactive cycle and a growing exploration of the inner world of each partner and their interaction with one another. This active and transparent presence is evident in the therapist's reliance on empathic attunement, validation, and empathic conjectures. Overall, the EFT therapist is ever-attentive to the alliance, recognizing that from this secure base, partners will find clarity in their goals for therapy.

Conceptualization of Problem Resolution

EFT helps partners access and expand their emotional experience, especially softer and more vulnerable emotions. Once shared, these emotions provide new patterns of engagement that are characterized by new levels of responsiveness and accessibility (Johnson, 2020). There are three primary change events—conflict de-escalation, withdrawer re-engagement, and blamer softening—that mark major shifts in the resolution of couple distress. The EFT process of change is composed of three stages and nine specific steps. In a recent development, Johnson (2019, 2020) proposed the EFT Tango as a macro intervention used by therapists in working the EFT process in session (see Figure 10.1). The Tango illustrates five essential foci that shape how a therapist guides partners through the EFT process.

The **EFT Tango** highlights the essential actions a therapist takes in ordering and engaging emotional experience in session. Presented as a sequence, a therapist may flexibly move between the different foci. In Move 1, the therapist focuses on a couple's here-and-now experience. Often these are moments of reactivity or emerging vulnerability. The therapist actively explores and engages this experience, giving attention to each partner's immediate responses. This shift draws attention to the interpersonal and intrapersonal cycles that drive insecurity and create opportunities for vulnerability. In Move 2, the focus shifts to one partner's experience and expands and processes a live emotional moment. In ordering this experience, the therapist helps a partner contact bodily felt experiences, perceptions, and action tendencies associated with this felt state. The experience is often deepened through the therapist's use of evocating interventions that focus on the granularity of a vulnerable moment of core emotion. This sets up the sharing of this experience with one's partner, and in Move 3, an encounter is choreographed and enacted. Move 4 follows the enactment with a focus on processing this new encounter with the partner who shared and the other who received this newly shared experience. The final move of the Tango involves summarizing the shared encounter and contrasting this new experience with the couple's or partner's typical experience.

The focus of the Tango shifts from processing partner experience in the context of the couple's reactive cycle in Stage 1. Through de-escalation of a couple's reactivity, a Stage 2 tango is more likely to explore intrapersonal themes associated with a partner's view of self or view of partner. The change process is illustrated below with descriptions of each step and how they might apply to the treatment of Steve and Carissa.

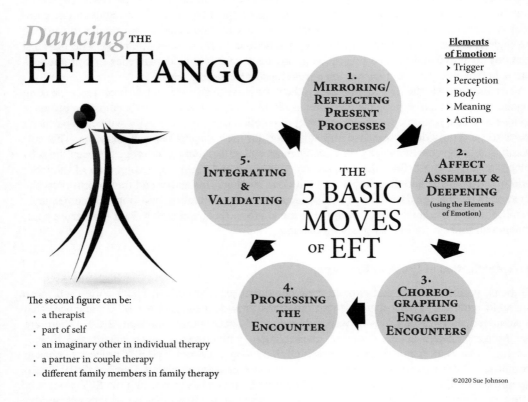

The second figure can be:
. a therapist
. part of self
. an imaginary other in individual therapy
. a partner in couple therapy
. different family members in family therapy

©2020 Sue Johnson

Figure 10.1 The five basic moves of EFT.

Stage 1: Cycle de-escalation

The focus of Stage 1 is a de-escalation of the couple's negative interaction cycle which is evident when partners share in identifying their pattern and make it their common problem. This shift results in lessened reactivity and greater relationship flexibility. Partners are less likely to use negative attributions and can exit rigid patterns of pursuit and withdraw. As Johnson (2020) notes, this initial shift is a "first-order" change as partners modify their actions to move away from their conflict cycle, but neither partner is able to move toward a new position of engagement in the relationship.

Step 1: Assessment. Creating an alliance and identifying the relational conflict issues between spouses from an attachment perspective.

Step 2: Identify the negative interactional cycle that maintains attachment insecurity and distress. In Steps 1 and 2, the EFT therapist establishes a working alliance with the couple and begins to track their relationship pattern. As an experiential therapy, EFT actively attunes to the experience of each partner, providing acceptance and validation of their unique perceptions and emotions. From an attachment perspective, the therapist's alliance with each partner provides a secure base to begin to explore their relationship, especially through the "here-and-now" focus of each therapy session. The therapist's responses validate clients' experiences from a genuine non-blaming stance and promote a shared working alliance. The alliance is established through eliciting and processing each partner's experience of the problem and through carefully tracking the unfolding negative interaction pattern.

In working with the Hogarths, the therapist would isolate a difficult moment that the couple recognized as typical of their presenting problem, such as Carissa's frustration with Steve's lack of responsiveness and availability. The therapist would begin to track and reflect both Steve and Carissa's experience as they re-live this past argument in the moment. In this process, the therapist would provide empathic reflections and validation of Carissa's frustration in "not getting through" and her anger at feeling dismissed by Steve. In turn, the therapist would work with Steve on his own hidden frustration at Carissa's unrelenting expectations. As the therapist walks through the rising tension, their focus shifts to Carissa's underlying hurt and fears about her importance in Steve's life and his fears about failing her and their future together.

Step 3: Accessing the primary/unacknowledged emotions underlying each partner's interactional positions and attachment needs.

In Step 3, core emotional experiences become the focus as each partner begins to access and expand the underlying emotions that drive their reactive response in their negative cycle. The therapist uses empathic conjectures and questions to elicit the salient emotions associated with attachment-related needs and fears. For example, the therapist may reflect and intensify Carissa's fears of being invisible and unwanted by Steve, normalizing the desperation of these feelings and connecting them with this sense of panic which often drives her critical responses and accusations.

These core emotions come alive in the present moment. Experiences are not simply labeled, but are explored as a means of bringing focus to the attachment-related dynamics underlying each partner's self-protective responses. So, as Carissa recounts her exasperation with Steve's minimizing, the therapist can track Steve's physical distancing in the conversation as he looks away in frustration. In noticing Steve's immediate response, the therapist uses **evocative questions** to bring his emerging experience to the foreground by acknowledging the importance of these responses. "It's hard to hear what she is saying, and the way her words come across? What's happening inside you now as you turn away?" The therapist tracks and reflects immediate responses as "action tendencies" associated with felt emotion that partners can be guided toward.

The vulnerability experienced in each partner's core emotion promotes a new awareness of what is at stake in a couple's conflict cycle. Steve's hurt is evidence of Carissa's importance to him, and his insufficient efforts to make things better between them seem to underscore his felt sense of disappointment, leading to his withdrawal in shame. Listening to the other's experience of the genuine hurt, sadness, and fear creates a new picture of the familiar postures of a distancing withdrawer and a demanding pursuer. The therapist uses an attachment lens to reframe the meaning and motivations associated with these felt emotions that have become real in session. Accessing and expanding these emotions helps to communicate the fears and longings both partners share for a different relationship and begin to change the underlying music in the relationship.

Step 4. Reframing the problem in terms of the negative cycle, the underlying emotions, and attachment needs.

In Step 4, the therapist summarizes the couple's interactional cycle in greater detail, including the predictable positions partners take, along with the experience of each partner's underlying emotional experience. The therapist reframes the patterns as a relationship problem that has come between both partners and explains that this obstacle is keeping them from what they want and need. Often the therapist reframes the cycle by summarizing the pattern as it has played out in this specific circumstance, enabling the therapist to emphasize what a partner does (i.e., reactive responses) and what is going on in those moments at a deeper level (i.e., core emotions).

In this case, the therapist shifts the focus from Steve's defensive withdrawal and Carissa's anxious pursuit to the ways these action tendencies take center stage in an escalating pattern of insecurity. Steve relies on a minimizing carefree approach to weather the intensity of Carissa's protests and leans away from the pain of her disappointment. Carissa's fear leads to an angry desperation when she feels Steve pulling away, and then she challenges his avoidance as a lack of regard or concern for their relationship. Together, their efforts to connect and respond in moments of uncertainty take them away from the vulnerability they feel as both become lost in the escalating negativity of their cycle.

Cycles are often framed as a block that comes between the partners, which has the effect of externalizing a predictable dynamic in their relationship and inviting partners to face this obstacle together. The negative attributions and polarizations associated with their conflict cycle lose their power as partners gain clarity about their experience and that of their partner. No longer alone in a fight for their needs, the couple can come together against the cycle that so easily entangles and defeats them. A possible challenge facing the Hogarths is differences in family experience and the ways in which racial identity, family support, and a history of infertility may influence their experience of safety and vulnerability as a couple.

Following the **CARE approach** (Johnson & Campbell, 2022) to assessment, the EFT therapist would identify the potential influence of race matters on the couples' experience as an interracial couple and potential threats to safety and vulnerability given Steve's father's uncertain acceptance and support of their relationship. The EFT therapist would assess infertility as a factor impacting the couple's negative interactional cycle and sexual intimacy (Brigance et al., 2021). For some couples, infertility and its treatment can have a differential impact on partners that results in a breach of trust. These couples may work through aspects of the injury and achieve de-escalation, but the risk and vulnerability required in Stage 2 (accessing their primary emotions) may interrupt a couple's progress until the "attachment injury" is fully addressed (Makinen & Johnson, 2006). In the case of the Hogarths, partner avoidance may mask deeper injuries in the trust of their relationship around vulnerabilities associated with race differences and medical treatment for infertility.

Stage 2: Restructuring Positions

Stage 2 in EFT focuses on each partner moving to a new level of emotional engagement. In **withdrawer re-engagement**, a previously withdrawn partner asserts their interest in the relationship with greater openness and accessibility to the other. This change event typically precedes the softening of the more demanding pursuing partner. The engaged withdrawer is more emotionally available and capable of responding to the needs and fears underlying a pursuer's anxious demands (Lee et al. 2017b). In **blamer softening**, the more critical partner is able to reach out to the other with their attachment-related fears and needs (Bradley & Furrow, 2004). The softening creates a shift from control to closeness that fosters new levels of shared vulnerability that result in a prototypical bonding event. This offers healing of past hurts and injuries, as well as a new definition of the relationship itself (Burgess Moser et al., 2016).

Step 5. Promoting identification with disowned needs and aspects of self and integrating these into relationship interactions.

The Stage 2 process follows the same three steps for withdrawer re-engagement and blamer softening. In Step 5, the therapist gives more attention to each individual, focusing on accessing, expanding, and deepening the underlying emotions associated with each partner's position (e.g., withdrawer, pursuer). As the focus shifts into deeper emotional experiences and the history of anxious or avoidant attachment strategies, the therapist facilitates new experience and meaning associated with views of self (e.g., "I am unlovable") and views of other (e.g., "You might leave me"). These **attachment schemas** are poignant expressions of implicit attachment fears and longings, which inform the actions and experiences couples encounter in separation distress (Johnson & Whiffen, 1999). The therapist actively processes these new experiences and meanings while fostering the engagement with and acceptance of this emerging experience by the other partner.

Steve's pattern of withdrawal has a long history. In reflecting on his difficulty in staying with the intensity of Carissa's anger and hurt, the therapist helps Steve contact his own sense of help-lessness and struggle to respond to Carissa's concerns. Staying with this experience, the therapist repeatedly heightens Steve's uncertainty and invites him to focus on the more vulnerable longings he feels in those moments. The therapist stays focused on these emerging feelings in session as the process unfolds, encouraging Steve to take ownership of his withdrawal and begin to share the fears that drive his self-protection. Through empathic conjectures and validation, the therapist helps Steve identify his attachment-related fears and longings to engage with Carissa differently in these moments. As this process unfolds, the therapist engages vulnerable experiences by inviting Steve to share directly with Carissa.

Step 6. Promoting acceptance of the partner's new construction of the relationship and new inter-actional behavior.
In Step 6, witnessing one partner's emerging primary emotion and vulnerability often draws the listening partner toward greater care and connection. The power of deeper expression of attachment affect is organizing and clarifying. Steve's sharing invites Carissa into a deeper level of understanding, which the therapist seeks to make explicit through evoking its impact, acknow-ledging the listening partner's acceptance, and then acting on this acceptance through sharing this with the other partner. In situations where the listening partner struggles to accept their partner's newfound vulnerability, the therapist validates their mistrust or uncertainty about these new emo-tional revelations. The therapist uses their alliance to validate the partner's mistrust, which itself can be reframed and organized around the listening partner's need and longing for a vulnerability in their partner that is trustworthy and real. In doing so, the therapist holds hope that a new trusting connection is possible when partners begin to share at this level, even if time is needed to develop trust and consistency.

Step 7. Facilitating the expression of specific needs and wants and creating emotional engagement. The key change events, withdrawer re-engagement and blamer softening, are completed in Step 7.
In Step 7, the process of restructuring positions culminates as partners move toward one another, enacting the expression of their attachment needs for security and care. As attachment-related fears and needs are crystallized in the context of that partner's experience, the therapist uses **enactments** to prompt the couple to share and respond to the essential needs that define their connection. **Engaged encounters** in EFT involve the therapist directing partners to turn toward each other and share from their experience. This enactment may involve intensifying an individual's emotional experience or fostering a deeper emotional connection as a couple (Furrow et al., 2022). As such, Step 7 enacts attachment security where partners successfully risk, receive, and respond to one another's attachment bids that each partner feared expressing in the context of their history of dis-tress (Johnson, 2020).

Steve typically hides his vulnerability from Carissa for fear she will reject him if she were to really see his need for her support and comfort. Bowlby (1988) argued that the experience of fear can block humans from making bids for attachment. Ironically these blocks obscure the attachment-related signals that coordinate proximity seeking in more secure relationships (Mikulincer & Shaver, 2016). As Steve shares his fears with Carissa, the therapist focuses Steve's attention on his unspoken attachment needs (i.e., what he most needs from Carissa in these moments). The therapist heightens his fear and invites an encounter focused on Steve's immediate need. For example, the therapist might say in this moment of fear, "Steve, as you look at Carissa right now, and you see she is here for you, what do you need most from her in this moment? Can you ask her right now?" The therapist's more directive stance provides a resource for Steve to risk a new level of engagement. Steve could respond to Carissa, "I need you to believe me. I need you to believe in me. I want us to work, but I need you to support me, to be on my side, and not just criticize and disrespect me. I need you to give me the benefit of the doubt and believe I do love you."

In the above examples, we illustrate the process of Steve's withdrawer re-engagement, which sets the stage for working toward Carissa's blamer softening. Softening events predict successful treatment outcomes in EFT (Burgess Moser et al., 2016). Blamer softening is perhaps the most challenging change event for the therapist (Johnson & Talitman, 1997). For Carissa, the process of reaching Steve with her attachment may prove challenging because of past difficulties specific to the couple's infertility (Brigance et al., 2021), or to Carissa's vulnerability from race- related trauma or discrimination (Nightingale et al., 2019; Young et al., 2023). Specifically, as an African American woman, Carissa may have felt her needs were secondary and been pressured to take a "strong woman" persona (Guillory, 2022; Young et al., 2023). As the therapist begins the Stage 2 process, the block in Carissa's ability to risk more vulnerable emotions with Steve may be justified by her experience of Steve's more capricious responses to a future pregnancy and residual injuries from their struggle to conceive (Brigance et al., 2021). Consequently, the therapist may shift to a focus on attachment injury resolution before proceeding with Stage 2 change events.

Stage 3: Consolidation

Step 8. Facilitating the emergence of new solutions to old relationship problems.

Step 9. Consolidating new positions and new cycles of attachment behavior.
The final stage of EFT focuses on consolidation of the progress of the couple to regain a secure connection in their relationship. Couples revisit persistent conflicts often rooted in differences in background, values, or preferences (e.g., money, parenting, family relationships) from new positions of accessibility, responsiveness, and emotional engagement (Johnson, 2008). Past issues may trigger their negative pattern, and in Step 8, the therapist helps the couple identify their previous work in moving away from the reactive cycle to new positions of security. The therapist returns the focus to the underlying themes and experiences previously worked through in Stage 2 and enables the couple to face these persistent concerns with the resources they have in their secure connection. Steve's interactions with his father about his relationship with Carissa is an area that Steve and Carissa must navigate. Though Steve's relationship with his father has improved in recent years, they both avoid conversations about Steve's marriage to Carissa given the father's prejudice. The EFT therapist would help the couple use their renewed security to face these tensions together and identify how Steve can more effectively confront these painful interactions, advocate for Carissa, and intervene against the father's microaggressions.

In Step 9 the couple has renewed confidence in what they have accomplished. Couples are able to reflect on changes they have made as the therapist heightens these differences and the narrative the couple now shares. The therapist focuses on the couple's successes and positive examples where they have been responsive and accessible to one another. **Attachment rituals** are discussed as an opportunity for the couple to take intentional steps to invest in the secure bond they have renewed (Furrow et al., 2022). For the couple, this may mean finding an activity that signals reassurance for Carissa and appreciation for Steve. This can be as simple as sharing written notes with one another or setting aside a specific time when the focus is on the needs and hopes they share.

Case Transcript

The session begins with a focus on their hopes for therapy, inviting a process for establishing a working alliance around their relationship goals.

Therapist: I'm wondering if we can begin with a hope or two that each of you has for our work together. I want to get a sense of how the two of you have thought about this time and how you feel about your relationship.

Here the therapist begins the alliance and assessment process indicative of the initial phase of EFT where the therapist joins the couple through engaging each partner's experience and their understanding of the relationship.

Carissa: Sure, I hope we can talk about priorities. Sometimes it feels lately like we are headed in two different directions and lately, I am not so sure we want the same things.

Steve: Yeah, we are in a tough spot lately. Maybe it's work or trying to have a child, but recently there's a lot of pressure to make things better and somehow with all these expectations, we're not able to make it better. It gets so intense, and nothing really gets resolved.

Carissa: What he means is I am too intense, expect too much, and I am the real problem here. (*Rolls her eyes*)

Steve: I didn't say that. That's not what I meant. Do we have to start like this?

Therapist: (*Interjecting with energy, matching growing intensity*) OK. Yes. I can see that, coming in, you both have concerns that can quickly take off into frustration and difficulty. Both of you have something to say here about how hard this is, and I want to understand what it's like for you even as we get started here. This is a hard place to be and right now I hear you both saying we need to find a way to talk about the things that matter in our relationship, and we are struggling to find a way to reach each other in these conversations. Am I getting it?

The therapist quickly joins the escalating tension in the session, attuning to the emerging frustration and matching the growing intensity with acceptance, empathic understanding, and a curiosity about how their fights go.

Carissa: Yes, it's hard to talk about this without a fight or Steve taking off.

Steve: It's hard to see the point of arguing if it's the same conversation over and over, and she's not really wanting to deal with the issue at hand. It's always something bigger.

Therapist: Right, so let's just start here, because you are both trying to be heard here and I appreciate how much this matters to both of you. Can you tell me more about what it's like when you try to talk about priorities and expectations? What happens between the two of you?

The therapist invites the couple to focus on a specific experience to track their interaction pattern: Tango Move 1.

Carissa: Well, the other day we got into it over the cat's litter box. I walked into the house and there was an awful smell and I asked Steve if he had taken care of it. It's his responsibility. And he dismissed it all.

Steve:	More like I gave my version of things, which you didn't like. Then you made it about me. "What's wrong with you?" (*Mockingly*)
Therapist:	So, Carissa, you asked Steve about the cat litter, and Steve, you gave your take on this, and that was challenged and then you reacted which left you, Carissa, feeling dismissed. Then what happened next?
Carissa:	I got angry. He was out with his friends while I was working late. He could have dealt with the cat litter when he got home. That would have been considerate but instead, he gives me excuses and makes this about my attitude.
Steve:	You were already upset when you walked in the door.
Therapist:	So, Carissa is angry, trying to engage you, then? (*Glances at Steve*)
Steve:	I backed off. Things were getting worse and nothing I said was going to make it better. I already failed in her eyes, and her anger is going to make her point regardless.
Therapist:	So, you back away, saying to yourself, "Things are getting worse. She's angry with me" and you see you have disappointed her in some way, and you move away.
Steve:	Sadly, I do that more and more these days. (*Looks away, then shakes his head*) I don't get her intensity, why she thinks I don't care, but I guess that doesn't matter because we just end up in the same place repeatedly.
Therapist:	So, that's hard. Disappointing. You look away. That's tough because you see what's happening here, she's angry, and you are pulling away trying to manage the moment. And Carissa, you see him pulling away and that's hard for you too?
Carissa:	Yes, I get we are different. We grew up differently and when it comes to emotions and feelings, I can come on strong, but I can't get his attention. And then he disappears for hours, and I am really on my own with all of this.
Therapist:	Right, so you both handle emotions differently at times and his response to your anger is to pull away leaving you alone and is that where this gets harder for you, unbearable at times?
Carissa:	Uh huh. (*Tears*) It didn't used to be like this but the infertility, job demands, and family issues are too much, and it just seems the distance between us is growing. He wants to be with his friends more than me. I feel like I am the only one seeing this, or the only one who cares.
Therapist:	Hmm, yes, this is a lonely place. A painful place? You feel like Steve is pulling away and going away from you. All the while, Steve, you are stepping back from the anger and her disappointment and the distance seems to grow between you. And then you find yourself alone not knowing if you matter to the other person. It makes sense that both of you have at times stayed away from these conversations because they land in such hard places. How do you come back together after one of these fights?

Tracking the cycle, the therapist also reflects the emerging underlying emotions of each partner and holds more poignant moments with understanding and care.

Steve:	It can take a couple of days. I think Carissa usually checks in with me and then we find our way back to talking and connecting…
Carissa:	(*Interrupting*) And we never get back to the issue. So, we never resolve the problems we have, and it wasn't always this way.
Therapist:	Right, you can remember times when the distance was less, and you felt more connected. More like a team. More together? (*Both nod in agreement*)

This moment provides an opportunity to explore a positive interaction with the couple where a positive cycle of responsiveness and availability can be explored. In this case, Carissa jumps back to the negative cycle, and the therapist will follow up on this positive pattern in a future assessment session.

Carissa:	Yeah, it's been a while though and Steve seems more interested in spending time with his friends than me. I try to talk to him, but he doesn't want to talk. He gets quiet or goes away.
Steve:	That's because nothing I do is good enough and you have no problem pointing out the problem is me!
Carissa:	(*Exasperated*) I'm just trying to talk with you. We don't talk anymore!
Steve:	(*Sarcastically*) Why would I want to talk with you when you just pick at me?
Carissa:	(*Looking to the therapist*) I try to talk to him, but he doesn't want to talk. He gets so defensive and childish.
Steve:	That's because you attack me and there's no room to even have a conversation.
Carissa:	(*Furious*) I'm just trying to talk with you, but you're not there. You don't care!!!
Therapist:	(*Interrupting*) So this is what it's like, what happens at home? You both get stuck in this terrible loop where you (*to Carissa*) try to come to Steve, sometimes with simple things, and he explains or gives an excuse dismissing your concern. It's like Steve says to you, "This isn't a problem, What's the big deal?" All this comes off as indifferent and uncaring. Then you try again to get through, then things escalate like right now?

The therapist introduces the notion of the negative pattern of interaction—called **the cycle**—*as the primary problem in the relationship. This is indicative of Step 4 in the EFT treatment process. The therapist is drawing attention to this cycle in the present moment, highlighting each partner's position.*

Carissa:	Exactly…
Therapist:	And Steve, you feel the edge and intensity in her response, and it sends this message that this is not about the cat litter, this is about you, another example of you failing her, doing it wrong, again.
Steve:	Yes, there's an attitude there, like she is going to push her point till it either makes me angry and I blow, or I go away. It's ridiculous. Almost treating me like a kid.
Therapist:	I see … so the two of you get caught in this pattern where you are both left feeling quite disconnected and at odds. Carissa, you end up feeling discounted and dismissed and, Steve, you end up feeling criticized and belittled … am I getting that right?

Here again, the therapist continues to elaborate on the conflict pattern, each partner's position in it, and their emotional experience that drives the interaction.

Carissa:	All our arguments end in the same place. It doesn't matter what we fight about. He ends up defending himself and going away and then I end up alone in the bedroom, by myself, it's sad.
Therapist:	And over time this terrible pattern has eroded so much of the good faith you shared— what drew you together—being strong for each other at the beginning. (*Both Carissa and Steve nod*) Now it's working against you. Can we take a deeper look here? See what's happening. I know it's tense right now, I feel that, but that's just what happens with this pattern, so let's understand it together. Can we do this together?

The therapist replays the cycle frame, acknowledging the tension in the room and offers themself as a resource seeking buy-in for going deeper into the conflict pattern.

Therapist: Carissa, can you talk more about that sadness that can show up— you, all alone in the bedroom? Can you help me understand that sadness?

The therapist is using an evocative question to further explore Carissa's sense of sadness. Within EFT theory, sadness is conceptualized as a primary emotion that carries an adaptive action tendency. Moreover, Carissa's sadness often goes unacknowledged by Steve. By drawing attention to her sadness and processing it experientially, the therapist can then shape a new interaction between Carissa and Steve that addresses her attachment-related sadness.

Carissa: I don't know … It's hard to describe. It's just this strong feeling of dread I have after our fights. I feel sick. Then I retreat upstairs to the bedroom and sit there, sad. It's pathetic.

Therapist: (*Tentatively*) You retreat in pain? Alone. In dread. Heartsick over all this. This all hurts a lot … yes?

The therapist gently reflects Carissa's primary emotional experience, inviting her to explore it more.

Carissa: It hurts when he pushes me away, dismisses me, doesn't engage. But I am not going to show it—it's not the way I was raised. You don't let others see that side of you. That's just not OK. Especially when he doesn't get it.

Therapist: Can you help me? It's not OK? Sadness is not OK?

Carissa: No, showing it. You don't let others see this. You must be strong, power through, don't make it about you. So, it just feels pathetic to find myself crying myself to sleep at times.

Therapist: Oh right. You know how to be strong in the face of pain and hurt and it also makes a lot of sense to me that when the person you count on and truly want to be close with pushes you away, like you don't matter, like you're too much drama, it hits hard. As I say this, I see what looks like pain in your face. It's like talking about it is touching that hurt right now? Would it be OK just to make some space for a bit of the hurt you carry, alone?

The therapist validates and acknowledges the attachment salience of her sadness (wanting to be close yet pushed away) and then draws attention to how her primary emotion is emerging within the here-and-now moment. Move 2 of the EFT Tango.

Carissa: (*Avoids eye contact*) Well, I am used to being disregarded at work or questioned or not seen for what I bring. Then there are times on the street when we are together, you see that look. The disapproval or question as if you don't measure up. They talk to Steve, and I am invisible. You know silly crap like that. I am not going to cry over that, that's just what I know.

Therapist: Right, I see your strength. Survival strength. Makes sense that you keep your strength even as you are carrying on. I also see that this pain or disrespect and disregard is something you know in the outside world and the last place you expect it is with Steve. He's been a safe place for you and now that seems to be broken somehow. Not as safe. Not so sure.

Carissa: Yes. It's been hard for us. First, my father-in-law and his prejudiced attitudes, then the infertility process, how do you feel safe, much less wanted, or chosen? It's like there's pain between us and when we try to get close, anger is all we have. Makes me wonder at times, where I am in his world, did we make some horrible mistake? (*Her voice softens into sad tones*)

Therapist:　Of course, there has been pain at every corner lately and it's landed in the most vulnerable of places. Thank you for opening the door into this lonely pain. It makes so much sense that when you are alone, wondering whether you matter to Steve, struggling to find strength to go on, your body weeps, tired from all this hurt.

The therapist empathically reflects and validates her pain and sadness using the emotional handle of "weeping alone." Following the CARE model, the therapist attunes to her window of vulnerability and honors her strategies for holding safety, vulnerability, and dignity. Carissa sits silently for a moment, then the therapist continues.

Therapist:　Thank you for taking that step with me. I feel honored that you would share what feels like a really hard and hurtful place. I'm just wondering if you are ever able to talk with Steve about this private place, this hurt and pain you carry on your own? I get that you sometimes tell him about what concerns you, but I'm wondering if he knows about this part? The part of you that hurts alone…

The therapist invites Carissa to experientially imagine and reflect upon sharing her sadness with Steve. Attention is drawn to how the conflict pattern inhibits the expression of her primary emotional sadness. The therapist is setting the stage for an enactment where Carissa can express a measure of her sadness with Steve. The therapist is moving toward an engaged encounter; Move 3 of the EFT Tango.

Carissa:　I don't know. That's not what I do… I mean… It's hard to be open like that, especially from this place.

Therapist:　Yes, it takes a lot to trust that he would be open, especially given how hard things have been lately. And it would also make sense in a world where your value is questioned and you can be dismissed, being strong and carrying the pain is better than sharing it. Am I getting it?

Carissa:　Yes.

Therapist:　OK, let me check with Steve to see where he's at. I see his eyes have been on you the whole time you have been sharing. (*Carissa nods*) Steve, when you hear Carissa talk about being strong and carrying this pain from her outside world, the disregard, the hurt of discrimination, and the legacy of pain that bears, the way that when you are caught in these struggles, you go away or dismiss her concerns, and that hurt hits on the inside in a way that is unbearable at times. So, Steve, what is it like for you right now as you hear Carissa talk about this pain she carries around on the inside? Did you hear the pain in her voice? What happens inside for you as you hear her pain right now?

The therapist draws Steve's attention to his wife's sadness, that stems from the layers of pain from being disregarded, and the ways in which this pain plays on a larger stage. The therapist then uses an evocative question, inviting Steve to share his reaction to her hurt. According to attachment theory, primary emotional cues have the potential to pull a comforting response from partners. The therapist wants to capitalize on this and assist Steve in being emotionally accessible and responsive to Carissa. The therapist is processing Steve's response to the pain Carissa shared with the therapist to make clear Steve's availability.

Steve: Yes, I am used to the anger, and she's one of the strongest people I know, but it's the quiet here and soft feeling that seem so different. I don't think I have seen how the ways I respond could land her in this place, that she could hurt like this. I am used to seeing her anger but not this pain.

Therapist: You know, Steve, I get that. You are used to seeing Carissa as frustrated with you, or upset at your choices, so I can understand why this might be different to hear. What is it like for you right now as she touches on this pain that she feels … how when she can't find you it hurts so much?

Steve: It makes me sad, honestly, I hurt too. I have seen this pain before with the way my dad can be with her. It's so hard to see that she feels that pain with me.

Therapist: It's hard to see. Can you say more about that? What's coming up for you?

The therapist uses an evocative question targeted toward Steve's sense of sadness about his wife feeling hurt. Here Steve is having a different reaction toward his wife, one that is characterized by vulnerability instead of avoidance or anger.

Steve: I know we get stuck on a lot of things and the pregnancy issues have made this all so much more intense, and I just want to get away from it. But this feels different. I know I don't always understand what it's like in her world, being a woman of color, but I don't want to be the cause of that kind of pain. I go away from the drama and intensity, but I don't want to leave her alone hurting like this. (*Choking back emotion*)

Therapist: Steve, can you share this with Carissa right now? Can you share how you are seeing this pain right now and how it impacts you? Can you turn toward her right now and share what this is like for you?

The therapist choreographs an enactment focusing on Steve's felt response to her pain. The focus is on having him turn toward her rather than away.

Steve: I'm sorry Ceecee (*Steve's nickname for Carissa*). I didn't see how this was impacting you. I know I can shut down and wall myself off or tune you out when we fight, but I didn't realize how this impacts you. It's hard to see how I have hurt you.

Therapist: Thank you, Steve, I appreciate you sharing from your heart how Carissa's pain sits with you. Carissa, what's it like to hear Steve see your hurt right now?

Carissa: I know he's sincere and that's good. We don't talk about this. We usually just fight and go our separate ways. But this is more than us being different, more than racism, it's about whether I can count on him when it matters. Do I matter to him? (*Angry tones present*)

Therapist: Right, there's a bigger context here and he is seeing that more clearly, but what you also need him to see is how it hurts to question if you count in his world, if you matter. Carissa, can you help him understand what it's like when he goes away?

Now that the therapist has checked in with Steve and gauged his level of in-session responsiveness, an enactment is established whereby Carissa directly expresses her pain and hurt with Steve. This engaged encounter is the completion of Move 3 of the EFT Tango.

Carissa: I think so… (*to Steve*) It's painful when you shut me out. I know I can be harsh or difficult when I am hurting, but it's so hard for me when I feel like I can't get to you. I need you to try and hang in there with me and not be so quick to close me out.

Steve: I'll try my best. It's hard for me too… I don't see this soft side of you. I am used to you being unhappy with me about random things and I just assume you are mad at me about the infertility issues we can't seem to resolve.

Therapist: Thank you, Steve. I appreciate your honesty and openness in sharing how you have been making sense of the hardness of your conversations, especially around the infertility issue. I can see how these play into this pattern that can leave you both losing each other, and I see you both taking steps to begin to do something different.

In an initial session, the therapist may briefly process an engaged encounter, creating space for partners to share their experience. This is Move 4 of the EFT Tango.

Carissa: Thanks … it's hard…

Steve: Yeah … It's definitely not easy.

Therapist: That's right … in time, I think the two of you can team up against this cycle. Steve, we've heard a bit from Carissa about what seems to be happening for her under the surface during times of conflict. I'm wondering if you could also help me understand a bit more about how these difficult conversations can lead you to push away or leave the intensity and difficulty.

The therapist begins to explicate Steve's primary emotional experience much as was just done with Carissa. This is Move 1 of the EFT Tango.

Steve: I'm not sure what to say…

Therapist: Take your time and let's try to find what makes sense of your side of this pattern. What's it like when Carissa gets angry or frustrated, like just a minute ago when she asked you to be patient and not go away so quickly?

Steve: It's like a "gut check" feeling—like when something bad might happen.

Therapist: You have a gut check—like "Oh no, something bad going to happen here."

Steve: Yeah … It comes up when things go negative. It doesn't matter if it's about my going out with friends or not meeting her expectations. It could be anything really. Then I freeze.

Therapist: So this gut feeling happens quickly, then you shut down? I wonder if this is what Carissa is describing when she says she loses you emotionally?

Steve: Probably. The only thing I want to do at that moment is stop the argument. Sometimes I get defensive and push back; other times I just walk away.

Therapist: Steve, what is going on inside in that moment just before you walk away?

The therapist uses an evocative question to assist Steve in elaborating more fully about his emotional experience during a conflict with Carissa. Note how the therapist did not ask Steve, "What are you thinking at that moment?" Instead, the therapist draws attention to Steve's internal emotional experience. The therapist shifts to Move 2 of the EFT Tango.

Steve: I don't know… I'm pretty angry at that point. Frustrated … like what's the point? I am already a disappointment.

Therapist: Yes, it would be very frustrating to get tangled up in this argument and then want it to end … only to feel you're disappointing the person who really matters to you.

Steve: Yeah…

Therapist: Yes, I get there's a part of you that gets angry and frustrated, but I'm wondering if there is another part of you? A part that feels a bit poked at perhaps. A part that also feels hurt in these moments.

*Here the therapist uses a "**parts-language**" intervention to (a) highlight Steve's secondary emotional experience (his anger) and (b) conjecture about his possible primary emotional experience. At times, clients may struggle to identify their primary, attachment-related emotions. When this happens, the therapist can utilize what is called an "**empathic conjecture**" to assist clients in gaining a better sense of their primary emotional experience.*

Steve: It's hard being criticized for most things you do. It wears on me.
Therapist: Yes, this all can be quite draining. Hard for you when the message seems to be that you are falling short. It makes sense you might move away from these difficult conversations, especially when you don't feel like you have anything that will make things better.

The therapist reflects and validates Steve's secondary emotional response of going away from disappointment and the underlying desire to improve the situation.

Steve: Exactly, after so many of these fights you learn that it's not about finding a solution, it's about the fight. Honestly, it all is so defeating, and I want a break or at least not make things worse by the anger that can happen between us.
Therapist: Defeat. That's a strong word. Is that where the hurt is for you?
Steve: I hate that feeling that there's nothing I can do to make this better. In fact, without knowing it, I am making things worse for both of us, and I don't know how to deal with it when my efforts are criticized.
Therapist: Yes, I hear you. Defeating. Losing at something that really matters.
Steve: Yeah … makes me sad when I think about it. We've always had something special and now that's hard to find between us.
Therapist: As I hear it, you saw the loss and the longing for that connection, that feeling of being special together, feeling important to each other, desired. Am I getting it?
Steve.   It's sad, you know, this distance between us.
Therapist: What happens inside when you talk about sadness?
Steve: It hurts.
Therapist: Steve, I'm wondering if it's actually quite painful for you when Carissa comes to share her concerns? This quickly becomes a conversation about you failing and being a disappointment. And what you are longing for is a way to get back to the specialness you once shared.

The therapist utilizes another empathic conjecture to help Steve elaborate further on his emotional experience. The therapist "guesses" that Steve might be feeling some hurt and/or pain stemming from his wife's complaints about him. A good empathic conjecture is tentative and allows the client to "try on" the emotional experience to see if it fits.

Steve: Yes. That's it.
Therapist: What's it like for you to feel like Carissa is disappointed in you?
Steve: It's awful. It's a terrible sickening feeling.
Therapist: Steve, are you feeling that now?
Steve: Yeah … it's heart breaking. Not sure how we got here but it sucks.

Therapist: Those are powerful words, Steve. This breaks your heart. This matters, how she sees you matters.

Steve: Yes, she does! But I don't think she believes me.

Therapist: Right, that's what this cycle does, leave you both doubting each other in those things that really count. But right now, do you think you could let Carissa in on this part of you that's brokenhearted at hurt at the thought of disappointing her, losing the specialness you have together.

The therapist invites Steve to experientially imagine sharing his pain and vulnerability with Carissa. The therapist coordinates an enactment whereby Steve directly expresses a primary emotional experience (feeling like a disappointment) with Carissa. This is Move 3 of the EFT Tango.

Steve: I'll try. It's (*to Carissa*) really hard for me to talk about this. I feel like I constantly disappoint you; that I'm letting you down. So rather than have another argument about it I try to shut it down.

Carissa: I didn't know you felt that way.

Steve: I don't want to be a disappointment to you. That's why I feel like I must defend myself all the time. It's like I'm trying to prove to you I'm not that guy.

Therapist: Carissa, what's it like for you as Steve begins to open up about this place he goes to that says, "I feel like such a disappointment"?

The therapist processes Steve's engaged encounter. This is Move 4 of the EFT Tango.

Carissa: I don't like it. I don't want him to feel that way. I just want to talk and try to make us better. I didn't realize I had that kind of impact on him.

Therapist: I appreciate you both being able to go to a deeper place with each other because you are both beginning to see each other differently. The pattern takes over in times of uncertainty, and before you know it, the efforts you make to try to reconnect are erased by anger and distance. Carissa, you desperately want to address the issues within your relationship. So, you go to Steve and try to talk with him about what is concerning you. Only Steve, you don't hear it as concerns. You experience Carissa as criticizing you, which leads you to a place of feeling disappointment. Rather than sharing that with her, you become angry and shut her out or go away. And Carissa, when Steve shuts you out, you are left feeling lonely and hurt. Am I getting this right? (*Both Steve and Carissa nod*) I wonder if we can make addressing this cycle a primary goal of our subsequent sessions. You both did something different today; you had a different type of interaction. I want to support the two of you in teaming up against this cycle so you can hear one another's concerns and find ways back to being the team you once were.

The therapist summarizes the entirety of the conflict pattern, highlighting (a) each partner's behavior, (b) the behavior's relative impact on the other, (c) the primary emotional experience underlying the conflict pattern, and (d) how the negative cycle of interaction is a common enemy the couple can team up to fight against. This is Move 5 of the EFT Tango.

References

Allan, R., Edwards, C., & Lee, N. A. (2023). Cultural adaptations of emotionally focused therapy. *Journal of Couple & Relationship Therapy, 22*(1), 43–63. doi: 10.1080/15332691.2022.2052391

Baucom, D. H., Shoham, V., Mueser, K. T., Daiuto, A. D., & Stickle, T. R. (1998). Empirically supported couple and family interventions for marital distress and adult mental health problems. *Journal of Consulting and Clinical Psychology, 66*(1), 53–88. doi:10.1037/0022-006X.66.1.53

Beasley, C. C., & Ager, R. (2019). Emotionally focused couples therapy: A systematic review of its effect-iveness over the past 19 years. *Journal of Evidence-Based Social Work, 16*(2), 144–159. doi: 10.1080/23761407.2018.1563013

Bowlby, J. (1969). *Attachment and loss: Vol. 1. Attachment*. Basic Books.

Bowlby, J. (1988). *A secure base: Parent-child attachment and healthy human development*. Basic Books.

Bradley, B., & Furrow, J. L. (2004). Toward a mini-theory of the blamer softening event: Tracking the moment-by-moment process. *Journal of Marital and Family Therapy, 30*(2), 233–246. doi:10.1111/j.1752-0606.2004.tb01236.x

Bradley, J. M., & Palmer, G. (2003). Attachment in later life: Implications for intervention with older adults. In S. M. Johnson & V. E. Whiffen (Eds.), *Attachment processes in couple and family therapy* (pp. 281–299). Guildford Press.

Brigance, C. A., Brown, E. C., & Cottone, R. R. (2021). Therapeutic intervention for couples experiencing infertility: An emotionally focused couples therapy approach. *The Family Journal, 29*, 72–79. doi:10.1177/1066480720720973420

Brubacher, L. L., & Wiebe, S. A. (2019). Process-research to practice in emotionally focused couple therapy: A map for reflective practice. *Journal of Family Psychotherapy, 30*(4), 292–313. doi:10/1080/08975353.2019.1679608

Burgess Moser, M., Johnson, S. M., Dalgleish, T. L., Lafontaine, M., Wiebe, S. A., & Tasca, G. A. (2016). Changes in relationship-specific attachment in emotionally focused couple therapy. *Journal of Marital and Family Therapy, 42*(2), 640–654. doi: 10.1111/jmft.12139

Ceniza, M., & Allan, R. (2021). Conceptual and application considerations of emotionally focused therapy with white heterosexual working-class rural males. *The Family Journal, 29*(2), 200–207. doi: 10.1177/1066480720966525

Cloutier, P. F., Manion, I. G., Walker, J. G., & Johnson, S. M. (2002). Emotionally focused interventions for couples with chronically ill children: A 2-year follow-up. *Journal of Marital and Family Therapy, 28*(4), 391–398. doi:10.1111/j.1752-0606.2002.tb00364.x

Collins, N. L., & Read, S. J. (1990). Adult attachment, working models, and relationship quality in dating couples. *Journal of Personality and Social Psychology, 58*(4), 644–663. doi.org/10.1037/0022-3514.58.4.644

Couture-Lalande, M. E., Greenman, P. S., Naaman, S., & Johnson, S. M. (2007). Emotionally focused therapy (EFT) for couples with a female partner who suffers from breast cancer: An exploratory study. *Psycho-Oncologie, 1*(4), 257–264. doi: 10.1007/s11839-007-0048-7

Dalgleish, T. L., Johnson, S. M., Burgess Moser, M., Lafontaine, M. F., Wiebe, S. A., & Tasca, G. A. (2015a). Predicting change in marital satisfaction throughout emotionally focused couple therapy. *Journal of Marital and Family Therapy, 41*(3), 276–291. doi:10.1111/jmft.12077

Dalgleish, T. L., Johnson, S. M., Burgess Moser, M., Wiebe, S. A., & Tasca, G. A. (2015b). Predicting key change events in emotionally focused couple therapy. *Journal of Marital and Family Therapy, 41*(3), 260–275. doi:10.1111/jmft.12101

Davila, J., Karney, B., & Bradbury, T. N. (1999). Attachment change processes in the early years of marriage. *Journal of Personality and Social Psychology, 76*(5), 783–802. doi.org/10.1037/0022-3514.76.5.783

Doss, B. D., McKenzie, K. R., Wiebe, S. A., & Johnson, S. M. (2022). A review of the research during 2010–2019 on evidence-based treatments for couple distress. *Journal of Marital and Family Therapy, 48*(1), 283–306. doi.org/10.111/jmft.12552

Dunn, R. L., & Schwebel, A. I. (1995). Meta-analytic review of marital therapy outcome research. *Journal of Family Psychology, 9*(1), 58–68. doi.org/10.1037/0893-3200.9.1.58

Edwards, C., Allan, R., Marzo, N., Wynfield, T., & Hicks, R. (2023). The use of emotionally focused therapy with polyamorous relationships. *Family Process, 62*(4), 1362–1376. doi:10.1111/famp.12934

Fincham, F. D., Stanley, S. M., & Beach, S. R. H. (2007). Transformative processes in marriage: An analysis of emerging trends. *Journal of Marriage and Family, 69*(2), 275–292. doi:10.1111/j.1741-3737.2007.00362.x

Furrow, J. L., Edwards, S. A., Choi, Y., & Bradley, B. (2012). Therapist presence in emotionally focused couple therapy blamer softening events: Promoting change through emotional experience. *Journal of Marital and Family Therapy, 38*(1), 39–49. doi:10.1111/j.1752-0606.2012.00293.x

Furrow, J. L., Johnson, S. M., Bradley, B. A., Brubacher, L., Campbell, L. T., Kalos-Lilly, V., Palmer, G., Rheem, K., & Woolley, S. (2022). *Becoming an emotionally focused therapist: The workbook* (2nd ed.). Routledge.

Furrow, J. L., & Palmer, G. (2007). EFFT and blended families: Building bonds from the inside out. *Journal of Systemic Therapies, 26*(4), 44–58. doi:10.1521/jsyt.2007.26.4.44

Furrow, J. L., Palmer, G., Johnson, S. M., Faller, G., & Palmer-Olsen, L. (2019). *Emotionally focused family therapy: Restoring connection and promoting resilience.* Routledge.

Ganz, M. B., Rasmussen, H. F., McDougall, T. V., Corner, G. W., Black, T. T., & De Los Santos, H. F. (2022). Emotionally focused couple therapy within VA healthcare: Reductions in relationship distress, PTSD, and depressive symptoms as a function of attachment-based couple treatment. *Couple and Family Psychology: Research and Practice, 11*(1), 15–32. doi:10.1037/cfp0000210

Gendlin, E. T. (1974). Client-centered and experiential psychotherapy. In D. A. Wexler & L. N. Rice (Eds.), *Innovations in client-centered therapy* (pp. 211–246). Wiley.

Gottman, J. M. (1998). Psychology and the study of the marital processes. *Annual Review of Psychology, 49*(1), 169–197. doi:10.1146/annurev.psych.49.1.169

Guillory, P. T. (2022). *Emotionally focused therapy with African American couples: Love heals.* Routledge.

Halchuk, R. E., Makinen, J. A., & Johnson, S. M. (2010). Resolving attachment injuries in couples using emotionally focused therapy: A three-year follow-up. *Journal of Couple & Relationship Therapy, 9*(1), 31–47. doi:10.1080/15332690903473069

Hardtke, K. K., Armstrong, M. S., & Johnson, S. M. (2010). Emotionally focused couple therapy: A full-treatment model well-suited to the specific needs of lesbian couples. *Journal of Couple & Relationship Therapy, 9*(4), 312–326. doi: 10.1080/15332691.2010.515532

Hazan, C., & Shaver, P. (1987) Romantic Love conceptualized as an attachment process. *Journal of Personality and Social Psychology, 52*(3), 511–524. doi.org/10.1037/0022- 3514.52.3.511

Jacobson, N. S., & Margolin, G. (1979). *Marital therapy: Strategies based on social learning and behavior exchange principles.* Brunner & Mazel.

Johnson, S. M. (1986). Bonds or bargains: Relationship paradigms and their significance for marital therapy. *Journal of Marital and Family Therapy, 12*(3), 259–267. doi:10.1111/j.1752-0606.1986.tb00652.x

Johnson, S. M. (1998). Listening to the music: Emotion as a natural part of systems theory. *The Journal of Systemic Therapies, 17*(2), 1–17.

Johnson, S. M. (2008). *Hold me tight: Seven conversations for a lifetime of love.* Little, Brown & Company.

Johnson, S. M. (2009). Extravagant emotion: Understanding and transforming love relationships in emotionally focused therapy. In D. Fosha, D. J. Siegel & M. F. Solomon (Eds.), *The healing power of emotion: Affective neuroscience, development and clinical practice* (pp. 257–279). W.W. Norton & Company, Inc.

Johnson, S. M. (2013). *Love sense: The revolutionary new science of romantic relationships.* Little, Brown and Company.

Johnson, S. M. (2019). *Attachment theory in practice: Emotionally focused therapy with individuals, couples, and families.* Guilford.

Johnson, S. M. (2020). *The practice of emotionally focused couple therapy: Creating connection* (3rd ed.). Routledge.Johnson, S. M., & Campbell, T. L. (2022). *A primer for emotionally focused individual therapy (EFIT): Cultivating fitness and growth in every client.* Routledge.

Johnson, S. M., & Greenberg, L. S. (1985a). Differential effects of experiential and problem- solving interventions in resolving marital conflict. *Journal of Consulting and Clinical Psychology, 53*(2), 175–184. doi:10.1037/0022-006X.53.2.175

Johnson, S. M., & Greenberg, L. S. (1985b). Emotionally focused couples therapy: An outcome study. *Journal of Marital and Family Therapy, 11*(3), 313–317. doi:10.1111/j.1752-0606.1985.tb00624.x

Johnson, S. M., & Greenberg, L. S. (1988). Relating process to outcome in marital therapy. *Journal of Marital and Family Therapy, 14*(2), 175–183. doi:10.1111/j.1752-0606.1988.tb00733.x

Johnson, S. M., Hunsley, J., Greenberg, L., & Schindler, D. (1999). Emotionally focused couples therapy: Status and challenges. *Clinical Psychology: Science & Practice, 6*(1), 67–79. doi:10.1093/clipsy.6.1.67

Johnson, S. M., Maddeaux, C., & Blouin, J. (1998). Emotionally focused family therapy for bulimia: Changing attachment patterns. *Psychotherapy: Theory, Research and Practice, 35*(2), 238–247. doi.org/10.1037/h0087728

Johnson, S. M., & Talitman, E. (1997). Predictors of success in emotionally focused marital therapy. *Journal of Marital and Family Therapy, 23*(2), 135–152. doi:10.1111/j.1752-0606.1997.tb00239.x

Johnson, S. M., & Whiffen, V. (1999). Made to measure: Adapting Emotionally Focused Couple Therapy to partners' attachment styles. *Clinical Psychology: Science & Practice, 6*(4), 366–381. doi:10.1093/clipsy.6.4.366

Johnson, S. M. & Wittenborn, A. K. (2012). New research findings on emotionally focused therapy: Introduction to the special section. *Journal of Marital and Family Therapy, 38*(s1), 18–22. doi.org/10.1111/j.1752-0606.2012.00292.x

Josephson, G. J. (2003). Using an attachment-based intervention with same-sex couples. In S. M. Johnson & V. E. Whiffen (Eds.), *Attachment processes in couple and family therapy* (pp. 300–317). Guilford.

Koren, R., Wooley, S. R., Danis, I., & Török, S. (2021). Measuring the effectiveness of emotionally focused therapy externship training in Hungary done through translation. *Journal of Marital and Family Therapy, 47*(1), 166–182. doi: 10.1111/jmft.12443

Lee, N. A., Furrow, J. L., & Bradley, B. A. (2017a). Emotionally focused couple therapy for parents raising a child with an autism spectrum disorder: A pilot study. *Journal of Marital and Family Therapy, 43*(4), 662–673. doi:10.1111/jmft.12225

Lee, N. A., Spengler, P. M., Mitchell, A. M., Spengler, E. S., & Spiker, D. A. (2017b). Facilitating withdrawer re-engagement in emotionally focused couple therapy: A modified task analysis. *Couple and Family Psychology: Research and Practice, 6*(3), 205–225. doi.org/10.1037/cfp0000084

Lesch, E., de Bruin, K., & Anderson, C. (2018). A pilot implementation of emotionally focused couple therapy group psychoeducation program in a South African setting. *Journal of Couple & Relationship Therapy, 17*(4), 313–337. doi: 10.1080/15332691.2017.1417940

Linhof, A. Y., & Allan, R. (2019). A narrative expansion of emotionally focused therapy with intercultural couples. *The Family Journal, 27*(1), 44–49. doi: 10.1177/1066480718809426

Macphee, D. C., Johnson, S. M., & Van Der Veer, M. C. (1995). Low sexual desire in women: The effects of marital therapy. *Journal of Sex & Marital Therapy, 21*(3), 159–182. doi:10.1080/00926239508404396

Makinen, J. A., & Johnson, S. M. (2006). Resolving attachment injuries in couples using emotionally focused therapy: Steps toward forgiveness and reconciliation. *Journal of Consulting and Clinical Psychology, 74*(6), 1055–1064. doi.org/10.1037/0022- 006X.74.6.1055

McLean, L. M., Walton, T., Rodin, G., Esplen, M. J., & Jones, J. M. (2013). A couple-based intervention for patients and caregivers facing end-stage cancer: Outcomes of a randomized controlled trial. *Psycho-Oncology, 22*(1), 28–38. doi: 10.1002/pon.2046

Mikulincer, M., & Shaver, P. R. (2016). *Attachment in adulthood: Structure, dynamics, and change.* (2nd ed.). Guilford.

Minuchin, S. M., & Fishman, H. C. (1981). *Family therapy techniques.* Harvard University Press.

Myung, H. S., Furrow, J. L., & Lee, N. A. (2022). Understanding the emotional landscape in the withdrawer re-engagement and blamer softening EFCT change events. *Journal of Marital and Family Therapy, 48*(3), 758–776. doi:10.1111/jmft.12583

Nightingale, M., Awosan, C. I., & Stravianopoulos, K. (2019). Emotionally focused therapy: A culturally sensitive approach for African American hetrosexual couples. *Journal of Family Psychotherapy, 30*(3), 221–244. doi: 10.1080/08975353.2019.1666497Panksepp, J. (1998). *Affective neuroscience: The foundations of human and animal emotions.* Oxford University Press.

Perls, F., Hefferline, R., & Goodman, P. (1951). *Gestalt therapy.* Julian Press.

Pietromonaco, P. R., & Barrett, L. F. (2000). Attachment theory as an organizing framework across diverse areas of psychology. *Review of General Psychology, 4*(2), 107–110. doi.org/10.1037/1089-2680.4.2.107

Rathgeber, M., Bürkner, P. C., Schiller, E. M., & Holling, H. (2019). The efficacy of emotionally focused couples therapy and behavioral couples therapy: A meta-analysis. *Journal of Marital and Family Therapy, 45*(3), 447–463. doi:10.1111/jmft.12336

Roberts, T. W. (1992). Sexual attraction and romantic love: Forgotten variables in marital therapy. *Journal of Marital and Family Therapy, 18*(4), 357–364. doi:10.1111/j.1752-0606.1992.tb00949.x

Rodríguez-González, M., Schweer-Collins, M., Greenman, P. S., Lafontaine, M. F., Fatás, M. D., & Sandberg, J. G. (2020). Short-term and long-term effects of training in EFT: A multinational study in Spanish-speaking countries. *Journal of Marital and Family Therapy, 46*(2), 304–320. doi: 10.1111/jmft.12416

Rogers, C. R. (1951). *Client-centered therapy.* Houghton-Mifflin.

Seshadri, G., & Knudson-Martin, C. (2013). How couples manage interracial and intercultural differences: Implications for clinical practice. *Journal of Marital and Family Therapy, 39*(1), 43–58. doi: 10.1111/j.1752-0606.2011.0026.x

Sexton, T. L., Gordon, K. C., Gurman, A., Lebow, J., Holtzworth-Munroe, A., & Johnson, S. M. (2011). Guidelines for classifying evidence based treatment in couple and family therapy. *Family Process, 50*(3), 377–392. doi:10.1111/j.1545-5300.2011.01363.x

Simpson, J. A., Rholes, W. S., & Phillips, D. (1996). Conflict in close relationships: An attachment perspective. *Journal of Personality and Social Psychology, 71*(5), 899–914. doi.org/10.1037/0022-3514.71.5.899

Spengler, E. S., DeVore, E. N., Spengler, P. M., & Lee, N. A. (2020). What does "couple" mean in couple therapy outcome research? A systematic review of the implicit and explicit, inclusion and exclusion of gender and sexual minority individuals and identities. *Journal of Marital and Family Therapy, 46*(2), 240–255. doi: 10.1111/jmft.12415

Spengler, P. M., Lee, N. A., Wiebe, S. A., & Wittenborn, A. K. (2022). A comprehensive meta-analysis on the efficacy of emotionally focused couple therapy. *Couple and Family Psychology: Research and Practice.* Advanced online publication.Tseng, C. F., Wittenborn, A. K., Morgan, P. C., & Liu, T. (2023). Exploring the effectiveness of emotionally focused therapy for depressive symptoms and relationship distress among couples in Taiwan: A single-arm pragmatic trial. *Journal of Marital and Family Therapy.* Advanced online publication. doi: 10.1111/jmft.12681

Walker, J. G., Johnson, S., Manion, I., & Cloutier, P. (1996). Emotionally focused marital intervention for couples with chronically ill children. *Journal of Consulting and Clinical Psychology, 64*(5), 1029–1036. doi.org/10.1037/0022-006X.64.5.1029

Weissman, N., Batten, S. V., Rheem, K. D., Wiebe, S. A., Pasillas, R. M., & Potts, W. (2018). The effectiveness of emotionally focused couples therapy with veterans with PTSD: A pilot study. *Journal of Couple & Relationship Therapy, 17*(1), 25–41. doi: 10.1080/15332691.2017.1285261

Wiebe, S. A., & Johnson, S. M. (2016). A review of the research in emotionally focused therapy for couples. *Family Process, 55*(3), 390–407. doi: 10.1111/famp.12229

Wittenborn, A. K., Liu, T., Ridenour, T. A., Lachmar, E. M., Mitchell, E. A., & Seedall, R. B. (2019). Randomized controlled trial of emotionally focused couple therapy compared to treatment as usual for depression: Outcomes and mechanisms of change. *Journal of Marital and Family Therapy, 45*(3), 395–409. doi: 10.1111/jmft.12350

Wong, T. Y., Greenman, P. S., & Beaudoin, V. (2017). "Hold Me Tight": The generalizability of an attachment-based group intervention to Chinese Canadian couples. *Journal of Couple & Relationship Therapy, 17*(1), 42–60. doi: 10.1080/15332691.2017.1302376

Young, J. Tadros, E., & Gregorash, A. (2023). Cultural consideration for using emotionally focused therapy with African American couples. *International Journal of Systemic Therapy, 34*(2), 63–82. doi: 10.1080/2692398X.2022.2159299

Zuccarini, D., Johnson, S. M., Dalgleish, T. L., & Makinen, J. A. (2013). Forgiveness and reconciliation in emotionally focused therapy for couples: The client change process and therapist interventions. *Journal of Marital and Family Therapy, 39*(2), 148–162. doi:10.1111/j.1752-0606.2012.00287.x

11 Solution-Focused Couple Therapy

Michael D. Reiter

History of the Model

Solution-focused brief therapy (SFBT) was developed by Steve de Shazer, Insoo Kim Berg, and colleagues at the Brief Family Therapy Center in Milwaukee, Wisconsin (de Shazer et al., 1986). de Shazer and Berg were introduced through John Weakland, one of the developers of the Brief Therapy model of the Mental Research Institute (MRI). After getting married, they relocated to Milwaukee and began seeing clients. They developed the Brief Family Therapy Center in 1978, originally located in their home and then in a main business location as well as branch offices. The model was developed in a team format, where one therapist worked with the clients in the room while one or more therapists watched the session from behind a one-way mirror (de Shazer et al., 1986).

Since they worked as a team, they developed a first session format that included introducing the set-up of the clinic, exploring the presenting complaint, exploring the exceptions to the complaint, developing the goals for therapy, beginning the solution-building process, utilizing a consultation break where the therapist and team members behind the one-way mirror discussed the case and developed an end-of-session message, and the therapist delivered the message (de Shazer et al., 1986). In future iterations of the model, SFBT therapists moved away from spending a lot of time exploring the presenting complaint, moving more quickly into goal negotiations. Some individual practitioners would take a thinking break (rather than a consultation break) to contemplate what had been talked about, construct an end-of-session message, and deliver feedback to the client (Berg & Szabó, 2005).

The SFBT model has roots in the brief hypnotherapeutic work of Milton Erickson and the Brief Therapy model of the Mental Research Institute (MRI) (see Fisch et al., 1982; Watzlawick et al., 1974). There are also components of Buddhist thought and Wittgensteinian philosophy (de Shazer et al., 2007). Borrowing from the clinical and conceptual ideas of Milton Erickson, SFBT holds that the key to brief therapy is **utilization**—utilizing whatever the client brings with them to therapy to help them move forward (de Shazer et al., 1986).

SFBT is a brief therapy model not because therapists limit the number of sessions (as the MRI model limited the number of sessions with a client to 10), but because their way of solving problems naturally tends to happen briefly (de Shazer et al., 1986). On average, clients will come to approximately 6 to 10 sessions. Based on ideas initially developed at the MRI, SFBT has espoused the following three basic rules (Berg, 1994):

1 If it ain't broke, don't fix it.
2 If it doesn't work, don't do it again; do something different.
3 Once you know what works, do more of it.

DOI: 10.4324/9781003369097-11

These rules shift the therapist's expertise from assessing the client and introducing new skills, since the client is viewed (in other models) as deficient in some regard, to utilizing the client's existing strengths and resources.

SFBT has philosophical underpinnings based on postmodernism and social constructionism.

Since meaning is created in conversation, therapy becomes a **language game** (Berg & de Shazer, 1993). Over the course of its development, SFBT has shifted from the strategic roots of the MRI brief therapy model to an understanding that change happens when people have conversations. Solution-focused therapy is predicated on what has been called **poststructuralism** (de Shazer, 1991; de Shazer & Berg, 1992) which holds that language is reality. Berg and de Shazer (1993) explained, "What we talk about and how we talk about it makes a difference, and it is these differences that can be used to make a difference (to the client)" (p. 7).

There has been a good amount of research to determine the efficacy of SFBT. Overall, the model is quite useful for clients. Gingerich and Eisengart (2000) reviewed 15 empirical studies on SFBT effectiveness and found they all supported the use of the model. Bond et al. (2013) evaluated the literature from 1990 to 2010 and reviewed 38 studies focusing on SFBT effectiveness. These researchers concluded that SFBT was effective overall, especially as an early intervention for non-severe problems. Today, SFBT has become one of the most popular and utilized therapeutic models around the world (de Shazer et al., 2007).

Conceptualization of Problem Formation

SFBT is considered a postmodern therapy that is predicated on social constructionism. In essence, therapy is a language game where the therapist and client co-construct meaning (de Shazer, 1994). Therapists do not mine the conversation to determine the Truth. Rather, they help create a "truth" that is true and useful for the client, a story of resources and competencies. There is not a Truth as to the Hogarths' relationship. It is never just a "good relationship" or a "bad relationship" or a "couple on the brink." What the relationship is becomes dependent upon the language game that is used at that moment (de Shazer, 1991). Each time they individually or collectively think and talk about their relationship, they come up with new understandings of it. In a hermeneutic fashion, each conversation about their relationship becomes a text that takes on new meaning. Currently, the way they are talking about their conversation leads to a meaning of a relationship in trouble. When they think about their marriage and communicate with the other, it is usually from a position that there is something wrong in the marriage and that, as a unit, they are in trouble.

Solution-focused therapists do not spend a lot of time exploring the past—especially in terms of problem etiology. Part of this is because the solution is not necessarily related to the problem (Nelson, 2011). Perhaps more than any other approach, much of the time spent in an SFBT session is focused on the future (Hoyt & Berg, 1998). Some SFBT therapists take pride in never talking about the problem as that, to them, only fosters problem talk. **Problem talk** is the conversation about what is going wrong and what the client does not want (Berg & de Shazer, 1993). All SFBT therapists want to shift problem talk to **solution talk**—talk about what has or can work. For those therapists who refuse to engage in problem talk, there is a concern that they become a **solution-forced therapist** (Nylund & Corsiglia, 2019). An alternative is using craft to acknowledge the client's problem focus and respectfully introduce solution talk into the conversation (Reiter & Chenail, 2016). Most likely, both Steve and Carissa have been using the time between setting up the session (and for years before that as well) and when they come in for the first session to think about all of the things that their partner does that concern, annoy, hurt, and scare them. If given a platform to talk about these concerns, they would likely spend many hours providing many examples of the other person's undesirable actions. This is common in many clients who come to therapy. However, this process is quite problematic as the more that the other person's deficits come into each partner's foreground, the more the other's beneficial behaviors move into the back-ground. This occurs in their view of the relationship as well. The more they view it problematically, the less they view it favorably. They will then likely take an **either/or position**: either our relation-ship is good or we are in trouble. The either/or position prevents them from holding a **both/and position** that will offer more possibilities: We can both have troubles in our relationship, and it can be a good relationship.

As per the rules of SFBT, if something doesn't work, a client should not do it again. Rather, they should do something different. However, sometimes clients are unaware of what they are doing that isn't working. People tend to try more of the same solution (Watzlawick et al., 1974). That is, the way that people attempt to solve a problem doesn't fix it. Conversely, it is the failed solution attempt that intensifies the problem and becomes a problem in itself. As de Shazer et al. (1986) explained,

> Clearly, people come to therapy wanting to change their situation, but whatever they have attempted to do to change has not worked. They have been getting in their own way, per-haps have accidentally made their own situation worse, and have developed unfortunate habit patterns.
>
> (de Shazer et al., 1986, p. 209)

Steve and Carissa have consistently gotten in their own way and have developed patterns that maintain their concerns. We will talk in the next section about how they do this.

Basic Assumptions of SFBT

SFBT makes a distinction between **difficulties** and **complaints**. "Difficulties are the one damn thing after another of everyday life, which clients frequently call 'problems'" (de Shazer et al., 1986, p. 210). The Hogarths are having several difficulties including not feeling as connected to each other as they have been in the past (and how they want to be in the present), obstacles in Carissa becoming pregnant, and each having different beliefs about how they should spend their time. These difficulties did not only happen once but have been present for a while. If something happened only once it would not be a difficulty. For instance, one day Steve had kept his phone by the side of the bed and during the night had received some text messages that pinged when received by the phone. The pinging of the text messages woke Carissa in the middle of the night. In the morning, she talked with him about this, and he first apologized and then told her he would keep his phone in the other room. This then was just a situation and did not occur again to become a difficulty.

Every individual, couple, and family have difficulties. This is just a normal aspect of life. What brings people to therapy is that the difficulties become bigger than they are. That is, difficulties morph into complaints.

> Complaints consist of a difficulty and a recurring, ineffective attempt to overcome that diffi-culty, and/or a difficulty plus the perception on the part of the client that the situation is static and nothing is changing; that is, one damn thing after another becomes the same damn thing over and over.
>
> (de Shazer et al., 1986, p. 210)

Complaints are maintained by clients thinking that what they are doing around the difficulty is the only thing they can do; that what they are doing is the only logical thing they could have done. Steve and Carissa are like every single couple in the world; they have difficulties. The question as to whether things get better or worse for them is how they attempt to handle the difficulty. For them, these cycles of avoiding talking about their difficulties and then having serious arguments where they attack the other person have led them to come to therapy with complaints. Their ineffective attempts to overcome the difficulty include seeing the other person as being "the problem" and pushing to get the other person to change in the way that they want. The more that they use these ineffective solution attempts—these ways that are maintaining the difficulty as a complaint—the more they become stuck in thinking that the way out of this is more-of-the-same behavior. They are increasingly perceiving that the other is to blame. They are arguing more. They are verbally attacking each other more when they argue. In essence, their way of trying to deal with their difficulty is making things continually worse.

This more-of-the-same process is quite problematic in that people are connecting to ways of being that are not useful to them rather than to aspects of self that are helpful. SFBT holds that couples will decide to come to therapy when the way they view their situation does not allow them to have access to ways of thinking and being that they find satisfactory (Hoyt & Berg, 1998). That is, they are viewing their situation in a way that disconnects them from their already existing skills, strengths, and competencies. There is little likelihood that Steve and/or Carissa go into an interaction thinking about how happy they are and how much they want to support one another. They are not tapping into their listening skills, caring, or past moments of enjoying one another. Rather, they are entering their engagements with one another with an expectation of defensiveness, aloofness, moodiness, and argumentativeness. These ways of being have become their primary tools of engagement rather than the ways of being they had with one another when they were beginning their relationship and were happy with one another. The more that they continue to have interactions in this manner, the more they consider their marriage to be on the brink of divorce.

Client Relationship Types

SFBT therapists attempt to understand how the client makes sense of the current situation. Not all people view things in the same way, including their relationship to the problem(s). Thus, therapists attempt to make sense of the client's view of the problem and how that will impact the relationship they have with the therapist. There are three **client–therapist relationship types** (Berg, 1994). The first is the **visitor** relationship, which happens when the client is coming to therapy because they are being forced. This may be because of a court order or a spouse, partner, or family member who is pushing them to come to therapy. Visitors tend to not acknowledge that there is a problem and are reluctant to participate in the therapeutic process.

The second relationship type is the **complainant**. This person recognizes that there is a problem but believes that its solution rests upon someone else changing. The spouse or family member who pushed the visitor to come to therapy is likely the complainant. When coming to therapy, they are readily available to give information to the therapist so that the therapist can work their magic and change the identified patient. The complainant usually views themself as the victim of the person engaging in the problem. With the Hogarths, both Steve and Carissa are complainants. At the current time, they each think that the primary problem in their relationship is the other person. Steve thinks Carissa has become too negative, moody, and argumentative over the last couple of years. In his view, Carissa has lost the desire and/or ability to just relax and have fun. Carissa thinks Steve is not passionate about her anymore and that he is focusing more on things outside of their house and relationship than inside. For each, there is clearly a problem in the marriage, but each believes that the other person is at fault and in need of change.

The third relationship type is the **customer**. Here, the client recognizes that there is a problem and that their involvement is critical for the problem to be solved. While other people may be involved in the creation of the problem, the customer understands that they can make changes to how they are thinking, feeling, and behaving that will likely make things better for themselves and perhaps for other people. In therapy, the therapist will attempt to have conversations with the couple to see in what ways they may be customers for change. That is, the therapeutic discourse will focus on what each of them wants individually, as well as jointly, and how they can each enact differences to their current patterns so that their lives are closer to how they hope they will be. The more the therapist can hold space in the conversation for Steve and Carissa to experience their own change as being useful to achieve their goals, the greater likelihood they will each have hope, expectancy, and motivation to make those changes. Further, viewing themselves as a catalyst for change will help shift their lens of seeing the other as problematic to potentially viewing the relationship in a more hopeful and positively expectant manner.

Conceptualizing Diversity

Solution-focused brief therapy was developed in the 1970s and 1980s in the Midwest of the United States. However, over its 40-year history, it has grown and been implemented around the world. SFBT has been successfully utilized with a wide diversity of clientele including Latinos (Suitt et al., 2016), African Americans (Gilstrap, 2021), Native Americans (Meyer & Cottone, 2013), Asians (Hogan et al., 2017), Chinese (Kim et al., 2015; Yeung, 1999), Muslim Americans (Chaudhry & Li, 2011), elderly people (Dahl et al., 2000), and military couples (Tews-Kozlowski, 2011). While developed in the West, SFBT also has roots in the East as Buddhist philosophy helped underpin it, and Insoo Kim Berg, one of the primary developers, was born and raised in South Korea.

Berg acknowledged that there are differences in couples therapy between Eastern- and Western-born therapists and clients (Berg et al., 1999). One of the primary differences is a focus on the possibility of divorce. For many Eastern cultures, as well as different religious groups, divorce is likely not a possibility. However, in the United States, many clients and therapists have values that include individuality and openness to relationship dissolution. For the SFBT therapist working with the Hogarths, they need to keep in mind that Steve and Carissa were born and raised in the United States, primarily learning about marriage in the 21st century. Given that approximately 50 percent of U.S. marriages end in divorce, this may be a legitimate possibility for the couple.

SFBT is sensitive to culture and different lifestyles, especially through its focus on behaviors rather than feelings, the future rather than the past, and highlighting solutions rather than problems (Corcoran, 2000). African Americans and Mexican Americans may find compatibility with the model in that it is time-limited and highlights contextual factors.

These aspects of diversity are not the therapist's initial focus. Hoyt (2008) explained, "The approach tends to be apolitical, however, and sociocultural topics such as ethnicity, class, race, and gender roles are not usually discussed explicitly unless clients make them the focus of conversation" (p. 261). Thus, the Hogarths' therapist will not force these topics onto them, but will be sensitive to them should they arise and be willing to engage them in conversation as to how their social location plays a role in how they view their difficulties and in their past solution attempts.

Solution-focused therapists tend not to focus on generalities, of what a group of people are like, but rather on the uniqueness of the individual (couple, family) and their hopes for change (Berg et al., 1999). SFBT demonstrates respect, especially to ethnic minority clients, for their unique worldviews (Corcoran, 2000). Berg explained, "The culturally-sensitive couple therapist's challenge is to work with the client's agenda" (Berg et al., 1999, p. 46). de Shazer described this as holding a constructivist position where the client, from their unique culture, is doing the best thing to do based on their context and situation (interviewed by Hoyt, 2001). The SFBT therapist accepts the client's position and thus can quickly develop an alliance with the variety of clients they meet. Steve and Carissa are operating from their individual cultural position as well as the third culture they have developed throughout their relationship. Based on how each person views what it means to be a man, woman, husband, wife, White, Black, married, and an interracial couple, their ways of trying to deal with one another make sense for them. There is a good reason for their actions, and the therapist will need to build upon the worldview and values that the couple brings into the session.

Client values are quite important in solution-focused work. Berg stated that "couple therapy training and the predisposing values that clinicians tend to hold make cultural and sub-cultural issues very challenging" (Berg et al., 1999, p. 47). However, by attempting to learn from clients rather than just learning about them, SFBT therapists honor cultural diversity (Hoyt, 2008). When therapists impose their own values, viewpoints, and direction on clients, there is a possibility of cultural insensitivity. SFBT therapists tend to do just the opposite. As Hoyt and Berg (1998) explained, "By working within the goals, ideas, values, and world views that clients present, solution-focused therapy is sensitive to the cultures that clients bring to the consulting room" (p. 224). Whatever comes of therapy—the solutions that are collaboratively developed—must fit for the client.

While SFBT therapists believe that they are being culturally sensitive by not imposing values and expectations on clients and holding the client's expertise, worldviews, and agenda as primary, there have been some critiques of the model along the lines of diversity, power, and gender differences. Dermer et al. (1998) provided a feminist critique of solution-focused therapy, believing that it tended to overlook gender and power differences. These authors argue that SFBT "fails to appreciate the pressure to accept complementary roles due to unequal power distributions perpetuated through societal expectations" (p. 242). While the feminist perspective views therapy as a political endeavor, SFBT tends to view therapy as nonpolitical. However, given the field's awareness and movement toward social justice, issues of equality, equity, and intersectionality have become more common throughout therapeutic sessions.

Steve is a White cisgendered heterosexual male while Carissa is a Black cisgendered heterosexual female. Steve was born and raised in a metropolitan area and grew up in a middle-class family. Carissa was born and raised in a very rural area in a family that had economic difficulties. They are an interracial couple who are living in the South of the United States and are likely to periodically experience familial and societal discontent about their relationship. In the United States, there is not a single certain way for an interracial couple to be. The Hogarths' therapist will not expect a certain level of intimacy, gender role division, or even a desire for having or not having a child. Each individual and each couple is different. The therapist's job will be to bring forth the expertise of this couple, and what being a couple means to them.

The therapist will need to be sensitive to how Steve and Carissa make sense of their relationship. While their understanding of what it means to be a male, female, White, Black, heterosexual, couple, or potential parent is partially developed based on past interactions with social systems (e.g., parents, peers, dominant social discourses, etc.), these meanings are not fixed and static. They can change as the clients come into better contact with their own perceptions and belief systems. The SFBT therapist will not go into the session trying to change Steve and Carissa's meanings, but rather will attempt to see how their perceptions of what is have been useful for them and get them to bring these ways of thinking, feeling, and behaving to the forefront so that they are even more useful for the couple.

The Role of the Therapist

The role of the SFBT therapist is likely different from most other approaches in that they may be viewed as a consultant. Instead of directing the client as to where they should go, the therapist leads from one step behind (Cantwell & Holmes, 1994). That is, the therapist learns from the client where they want to go and helps the client to take steps in the direction the client wants rather than where the therapist wants. The therapist won't force anything on Steve and Carissa. The goals of therapy will be based upon what they want rather than on what the therapist wants. The therapist's role is to help them to get where they want to go. If they want to stay together or they want to get divorced, the therapist will utilize their own skills to help the clients to utilize their skills to move forward.

While the SFBT therapist acknowledges that there is an inherent hierarchical relationship in the therapeutic endeavor, they attempt to make this an egalitarian rather than an authoritarian relationship (de Shazer et al., 2007). Rather than trying to make interpretations of what the client is thinking or why they are doing whatever they are doing, the SFBT therapist accepts the client where they are at. This is a shift from the therapist as expert to the client as expert (Berg, 1994). de Shazer explained that in developing SFBT, they used to have a motto, "If the therapist's goals and the client's goals are different, the therapist is wrong" (Hoyt, 2001, p. 163). Unless Steve and Carissa have a goal that is harmful to self or others (e.g., stealing, hurting, or attacking others), the therapist will support it. This will be the case even if the couple's goal does not fit within the therapist's values, such as their deciding they want to explore swinging when the therapist doesn't believe in partner swapping. It is the therapist's responsibility to work ethically within the client's value system.

One of the most significant therapeutic SFBT positions is that of curiosity (Thomas & Nelson, 2007). This curiosity is focused on the client's experiences and meanings. Going along with the client as expert, rather than the therapist as expert, the SFBT therapist's curiosity attempts to bring forth clients' inherent knowledge of their own experience. This is so significant that Thomas and Nelson (2007) stated that if "the therapist is more focused on his or her own views than on the clients', it is not SFBT" (p. 5). The therapist is not coming in with a prescribed framework for how Steve and Carissa's marriage and perceptions should be. The therapist doesn't know the couple or how they think. This is what will occur in session, that their positions are brought to the forefront to see how they think, feel, and behave have been useful for them in the past, and how these aspects can be used to help them get to where they want to go.

SFBT therapists also operate from a place of respect. Therapists take a solution-focused stance which includes being positive and collegial (de Shazer et al., 2007). This may be most clearly seen in the goal-negotiation process where it is the client's goals that are the main focus rather than the therapist's. Some of the behavioral components of respect include setting a friendly tone, being casual and relaxed, having a hopeful mentality, and using positive words (Berg, 1994). The SFBT therapist will never be Steve and Carissa's friend, but they should not be an automaton. Given that the primary tool of the therapist is their use of self, they should come across as being present, genuine, and authentic.

Another important therapist position is that of being tentative (Thomas & Nelson, 2007). While there are similarities to the not-knowing position of Anderson and Goolishian (1992), being tentative helps remind the SFBT therapist that what they think is only a hypothesis and not the truth. This is a temporary understanding of what is happening to the client. More information, gained from a curiosity about the client's understanding, is needed to help the therapist better understand the client's position. There may be times when the therapist has an idea of what Steve or Carissa is saying and will check in with them to ensure that their own perception is what the couple is trying to get across. This will happen through words such as "It seems…," "Perhaps…," or "Is that right?"

The SFBT therapist takes a non-normative and non-pathologizing position (Hoyt, 2008; Thomas & Nelson, 2007). They believe that what the client is doing is logical and makes the most sense for the client at that point in time. This doesn't mean that the behavior is useful for the client, but it is not endemic to an internal fault of the client. Rather, when the client's context changes their behavior will change as well. Therefore, SFBT therapists have presupposition as a primary tool in their therapeutic pouch. **Presupposition** occurs when the therapist believes that something has occurred or will. The therapist working with the Hogarths will presuppose that they have had times where they got along in ways that they wanted to and that they will have times when they are getting along "well." Given that language is extremely important in this model, very few SFBT therapists have "if" as part of their lexicon. This is because "if" demonstrates that there is a possibility that what is being talked about may not happen. For instance, asking the couple, "Steve and Carissa, *if* you were getting along better, what would that look like?" This question introduces the possibility that they will not get along. Rather, the SFBT therapist would ask, "Steve and Carissa, *when* you are getting along better, what will that look like?" Here, the therapist has presupposed that they can, and will, engage in their desired behavior.

SFBT therapists believe that change is constant and inevitable (de Shazer et al., 1986). Given this, only a small change is needed. The therapist doesn't have to work with the client until the problem is completely resolved. Rather, they are there to help orient the client in the direction the client wants to go and then to get out of the client's way so they can build the momentum of their positive change. Further, change in one part of the system leads to system-wide change. Whether Steve comes to therapy alone, Carissa comes on her own, or they come as a couple, the therapist only has to assist in one person changing. That person's change will interrupt the patterns that have not been working—and even make the situation worse—and will likely shift to patterns that have previously been successful and can be successful in the future.

Conceptualization of Problem Resolution

SFBT therapists conduct a purposeful interview, one that helps clients to reconnect to previous ways of thinking and being that were useful to them (Lipchik & de Shazer, 1986). The basic view of the model was put forth in de Shazer et al.'s (1986) original article about the model:

> In short, our view holds that clients already know what to do to solve the complaints they bring to therapy; they just do not know that they know. Our job, as brief therapists, is to help them construct for themselves a new use for knowledge they already have.
>
> (Shazer et al., 1986, p. 220)

By building on the client's preexisting beliefs, skills, and strengths, SFBT therapists promote an expectancy of competency that helps build the client's hope for continued change (Reiter, 2010). If Steve and Carissa went to a therapist who explored all the problematic areas of their marriage, they might develop an expectancy of deficit and disorder within themselves, each other, and their relationship as a whole. SFBT, in contrast, will explore past aspects of their relationship that have brought benefit to them and highlight and expand these existing knowledges and behaviors.

Since the SFBT model is predicated on helping clients recognize their past successes, therapists point out what clients have done in their lives that have been useful for them. These statements are known as **compliments** (de Shazer, 1982). These compliments may be some of the first interventions with clients, demonstrating the therapist's respect and affirmation of the client's strengths and competencies (Berg, 1994). Since Steve and Carissa are coming in to discuss how they have been arguing and are not in sync with one another, the therapist may compliment them for being able to, in session, have five minutes of respectful conversation with one another. The therapist can also compliment past behaviors, such as when the couple was able to have a date night.

Questions as Interventions

Over the development of the solution-focused model, the implementation of asking a variety of questions has shifted from an information-gathering process to intervention in itself. Asking questions that help bring forth, into the therapeutic conversation, clients' desires and their past accomplishments in having attained those goals and desires has become the primary mode of thera-peutic change.

Given the SFBT therapist's assumption that change is constant and inevitable, there has likely been change between the time that the clients made the appointment and their attendance at the first session. When therapists can bring this difference to the forefront, they send a message early in the first session that the clients' situation is not hopeless. Rather, they have already made a positive change, regardless of how big it is, and have done so on their own. The way to bring this information into the conversation is through the **Presession change question** (Weiner-Davis et al., 1987). The therapist working with the Hogarths can begin the session asking about what has been better since they made the initial phone call. This will start the session on a positive note, with an expectation that the couple is not hopeless. Rather, asking this question implies that the couple has engaged in positive behaviors, something that can be built upon. Further, these positive changes occurred outside of therapy, which can be considered extratherapeutic factors, which account for the highest percentage of positive change for clients (Lambert, 1992). SFBT attempts to channel these preexisting extratherapeutic factors and get clients to intentionally engage them. Coming into this first session, Steve and Carissa are probably quite disenchanted with their relationship, thinking that not much is going well for them. The more they view the relationship as problematic, the less hope and expectancy they will have for change. However, if during the beginning of the session, the therapist explores what has been better since the session appointment was made, they realize that their marriage is not as problematic as they thought. Further, the behaviors that were relationship-supporting occurred before therapy started. Thus, it wasn't the therapist that made that change, but the clients themselves. This demonstrates that they already have the ability and know-how to make their lives better.

The third rule of solution-focused therapy holds that clients should do more of what is working. **Exceptions** are those times when the problem could have happened but didn't (de Shazer et al., 1986). Problems are not always present or always arising at the same level of concern. Steve and Carissa get along at certain times and argue at others. Even if they are mad at each other all week, there are moments they are more upset with each other. This also means that there are times when they are less upset; even if there aren't times when they are happy with each other. SFBT therapists explore these exceptions as they help to shift clients from an either/or to a both/and perspective. Steve and/or Carissa may believe that they must always love each other and be happy with one another for their relationship to be a good one. This can be problematic, since any time they are feeling unhappy with the other person, they will view their relationship quite negatively. The SFBT therapist will likely help them to see that they can both have arguments with one another and have a good relationship. Further, a lot of the sessions will be focused on how they have had aspects of a good relationship in the past and then have discussions of how the couple can intentionally engage in those behaviors again.

Many times, clients come to therapy with an abstract explanation of their concerns or hopes. For instance, Carissa might describe being unhappy or wanting a connection. Steve may say he is frustrated and wants a regular marriage. The SFBT therapist's job is to help clients articulate their desires more concretely. **Scaling questions** are designed to do this. The discussion about the scale is a means of co-constructing where the therapist and client jointly agree upon the terms of the client's meaning. Berg and de Shazer (1993) explained, "Our scales are used to 'measure' the client's own perception, to motivate and encourage, and to elucidate the goals and anything else that is important to the client" (p. 10).

Solution-focused scales are usually developed where 1 is what the client doesn't want and 10 is the goal. This is useful as most sports operate from a position where the person/team with the most points wins. Further, people usually try to attain more rather than less. Thus, moving up on the scale—gaining more points—is a known process and is a movement toward what people want more of in their lives. The first time the client provides an answer to the **scaling question**, the therapist and client have a baseline of where the client currently is. Any movement up the scale demonstrates that the client is making progress.

Scaling questions can also be used to bring forth goals. The therapist can ask the client what they would see when they are at some point higher on the scale. If Steve said he was at a 5 on motivation to make the marriage work, the therapist can ask, "What would be different when you are at a 6?" The amount of difference up the scale is not really important. However, talking about moving up the scale helps to promote hope and the expectancy of change. It is probably better to use very small incremental jumps up the scale. If starting at 5 with Steve, there would only be five "differences" to be noticed before getting to a 10 (i.e., 6, 7, 8, 9, & 10). However, if the therapist asked what he would notice when he was at a 5.1, there would be 50 differences. Regardless of the point on the scale being talked about, the therapist should follow up the client's answer with, "What else will you notice different when you are at that number?"

Perhaps the most famous solution-focused question is the **miracle question**. This question gets the client to imagine a future in which the problem is no longer present (de Shazer, 1988). The therapist asks the client to use their imagination and suppose that while they were sleeping a miracle happened—that the concerns that brought them to therapy were gone. They then explore what will be the first behavioral signs that let them know the miracle happened. The outcome of this question is the development of client-desired goals. While this question has been a mainstay of solution-focused practice, what is more important than the question itself is the therapist's follow-up to build the miracle picture. Perhaps the most important question to ask here is, "What else?" If Steve and Carissa's answer to the miracle question is that they will go on a date, there is now only one sign that their miracle happened (that they are moving toward their desired relationship). However, if asked what else they would notice, there will be a greater chance that any one of the pieces of their miracle picture will likely happen. They may go on a date, cook together, spend time with one or the other's family, or watch *The Bachelor* together. Any of these actions is a sign to them that they are headed in the right direction.

Starting with the second session, the SFBT therapist focuses on what is happening in the client's life that they want to continue to be happening (de Shazer, 1991). The primary way of doing so is asking the **What's better question**. This occurs very straightforwardly at the beginning of the second and subsequent sessions: "What is better since the last time we met?" Once the client provides an answer, the SFBT therapist would then amplify their answer, exploring how the client was able to create that positive change. If the client answers that things did not get better, or even got worse, the therapist would try to be more specific and find times during the past week when things were not as bad as other times. With couples, especially those who may have different views of whether things are better, the therapist can ask the one who perceived things as better about those moments, and ask the partner who didn't see positive change what they did to ensure that things did not get even worse than they are (Jordan, 2016).

As just explained, there may be times when clients do not believe that things have gotten better. They may even perceive that things have gotten worse. When this occurs, SFBT therapists will ask the client a **coping question**; what they did to ensure that things did not get even worse than they are (Berg, 1994). This question is used to meet the client where they are presently instead of trying to cheer the client up or reassure them. This is likely not going to work as the therapist is not meeting the client where they are. Coping questions validate the client's current concerns and then help the client to become aware of their strengths and resources that they might not have been aware of previously.

SFBT therapists also ask **relationship questions**, which ask a client about other people's perceptions of them (Hoyt & Berg, 1998). Since problems and solutions occur in interaction, bringing in other people's voices—what they would see differently for the client—helps to add further possibilities and pathways to solution. Anyone in the client's relational field can be included in a relationship question, such as parents, friends, co-workers, extended family, etc. To add a playful aspect to this question, the therapist can include the client's pets. For instance, the therapist could ask Steve and Carissa, "When the two of you are getting along in the way that you want, how will your cat, Alberta, know? What will she see as different between you two?" Their answers to this fun but serious question then become other aspects of the couple's goals.

Outside-of-Session Interventions

Early in SFBT's history, interventions were thought to occur outside of the session, based upon the therapist's homework intervention. Many of these interventions were grounded on the clinical work of Milton Erickson and/or those from the MRI school. Eventually, SFBT therapists viewed interventions happening in the room through the questions presented in the previous section. Many of the early interventions outside the session were viewed as being useful for a wide variety of clients since they were general enough to be used with a wide variety of clients and situations. These interventions were originally called skeleton keys (de Shazer, 1985) and then later, **formula tasks**. A common thread through all these formula tasks is the utilization of expectation (Reiter, 2007). These are all tools that the SFBT therapist has in their pouch. Based on the situation, some may be more useful for the clients than others. When working with Steve and Carissa, the therapist may not use any of these formula tasks. However, they may suggest one or more of them depending on the flow of the conversation.

The most famous solution-focused formula task occurs at the end of the first session and is aptly named the **first session formula task**. It asks clients to shift their lens when they are out of session from aspects of their life that they don't want to aspects that they do. With couples, they are usually asked to individually notice what is happening in their relationship that they want to go on happening or have more of. The next session can be spent talking about what they noticed. By not having them talk about it during the week, each member of the couple has a heightened sense of anticipation to find out what their partner liked that happened that week. Out of all the formula tasks, this one can be used with every client regardless of the presenting complaint. The intention here is to shift foreground and background for clients, from first looking for problems and not really seeing solutions to seeing solutions first and having problems fade into the background. Steve and Carissa are primarily seeing what they do not want the other person doing. For Steve, this is Carissa being moody and argumentative. For Carissa, it is Steve being aloof and not passionate with her. The more they focus on what they don't want the other person to be doing, the less they are seeing what they appreciate that the other is doing. Further, the more they are looking for what is not working in their relationship, the less they are looking for what is working. The first session formula task asks clients to put on a different lens so that they can see aspects of their lives that have been useful for them.

Originally developed in 1978, the **do something different task** highlights the second rule of solution-focused therapy: if it doesn't work, don't do it again; do something different. This formula task is used when one person of a couple is complaining about the behavior of the other person and thinks that they have tried everything to get the other person to change (de Shazer, 1985). The therapist encourages each member of the couple, when they experience the problem happening, to do something different, regardless of how strange, odd, weird, or illogical it is. Given that Steve and Carissa keep complaining about the other person and do not see the other changing, this formula task might be a possibility since it could get them out of their pattern that is maintaining the complaint.

In 1974, de Shazer developed the **structured fight task** that is used with couples who are complaining about their arguments that never seem to come to any resolution (de Shazer, 1985).

The therapist instructs them that, the next time they are about to begin an argument, they are to stop and engage in the following steps. First, they are to flip a coin to decide who goes first. Second, whoever wins the coin toss gets to bitch for 10 minutes without the partner interrupting them. Third, the other person gets to bitch for 10 uninterrupted minutes. Last, they are to have 10 minutes of silence, and if they think they need it to start another round with a new coin flip. The arguments between Steve and Carissa seem to be increasing without any resolution. The structured fight task would seem to be potentially useful for them so that they can have their arguments, but in a different way than previously, which would hopefully spark some type of change in how they interact with one another.

Over the course of the model's history, there has been a move away from some of the early formula tasks, although the first session formula task has maintained a significant role for practitioners. SFBT therapists tend to view the out-of-session homework activities as coming from the client (de Shazer et al., 2007). These homework assignments, sometimes called **experiments**, are viewed to be more effective if they come from the client. What all homework/experiments have in common is that they are future-focused and based on the client's strengths. de Shazer et al. (2007) explained, "These experiments are based on something the client is already doing (exceptions), thinking, feeling, etc. that is heading them in the direction of their goal" (p. 11). Thus, if an experiment is used with the Hogarths, it will likely highlight their ways of being that have previously been useful for them.

As discussed earlier, SFBT therapists attempt to understand their connection to the client and the problem, recognizing that not all clients come to therapy with the same position. Some clients are visitors, some complainants, and others are customers. Just about all therapists, from any orientation, prefer to work with customers; people who think there is a problem, and that problem resolution will come from them doing something different. Given this, SFBT therapists attempt to **utilize the client's position**. For the visitor, the therapist may just thank them for coming to the session. They are not likely to assign homework or an experiment as the likelihood that the client will do it is small, given their decreased motivation for difference. The therapist might ask them to just pay attention to what is occurring in their lives as perhaps they will see something that they want to be changed. When working with a complainant-relationship-type client, the therapist is likely to ask them to notice what happens in an interaction, as they are likely to see that it is not only the other person but their reaction that perpetuates the problem. They would then be more likely to change. With the customer-relationship type, the therapist will encourage them to do something—a behavior—as the client sees that there is a problem and that their change of behavior will likely lead to a solution.

Goal Negotiations

SFBT therapists believe it is important for the client to know when they have achieved their goals. Given this, they have conversations to help transform client goals so that they are more effective (de Shazer, 1991). These characteristics of **good goals** include them being small, measurable, realistic, salient, inclusive of the client's hard work, and the presence of behavior rather than its absence.

Good goals need to be **small**. This is especially important since clients do not come to therapy at the first sign of the problem. Rather, they attempt to solve it, and unfortunately their way of trying to solve it creates more of a problem. This leads to increased frustration around the problem. If it took a long time to work with the therapist, clients would likely not stay around in therapy. Thus, SFBT therapists help clients to winnow down large goals into small goals. This helps to increase the client's sense of hope, expectancy, and motivation (Lambert, 1992) as the small goal should be achievable for the next therapy session. Steve and Carissa have been experiencing frustration in their marriage for several years now. They may be coming to therapy as a last resort. If positive change takes a year or even many months, they may not be able to maintain their motivation to come to therapy. However, by developing multiple goals, with at least one being small enough that it can be achieved by the next session, they will more likely realize that their relationship is not hopeless. The attainment of the small goal could be seen as the first step in their growth as a couple.

Goals should also be **measurable**. They should be concrete enough so that anyone will know exactly when they happen. Therapists can ask, "How will you know when you've achieved the goal?" or "What will you be doing?" or "If I was a fly on the wall, what behaviors would I see from you?" If a goal was too abstract, such as "being happy" or "getting along," we wouldn't know when that happened. But if the goal is to "spend 15 minutes together in an outside activity," we will know when that happens.

Good goals should also be **realistic**. There is no point in helping people to develop a goal they will never achieve. That would just be cruel. Thus, SFBT therapists help clients to focus on goals that they will be able to obtain within the course of therapy. If Steve and/or Carissa said their goal was "to always be happy with one another," we would be setting them up for failure if we agreed with that goal. Here, the therapist would need to introduce the concept of both/and to shift the goal from either "we are happy" or "we should divorce" to "we can be both happy and have times of frustration."

SFBT therapists will also support goals that are **salient** to the client. This means that the client cares about achieving the goal. They will not be motivated to work toward a goal that is not theirs and that they do not believe in. SFBT therapists are extremely curious as to what the client wants to do differently and help them to get there. Thus, the goals for therapy always come from the client. Suppose Steve wanted out of the marriage. He would likely not work hard to make the marriage work. He would probably continue to spend a lot of time away from home and not show Carissa much care and concern. Carissa would not work hard at the relationship if Steve said he wanted an open marriage. However, the more that the goals are their goals, that they both want, the more motivation they will have to take active steps toward them.

Clients have a tendency to enter therapy believing that a person they are in a relationship with needs to change for things to get better. This demonstrates that they are currently in the complainant-relationship type. To help move them into a customer-relationship position, SFBT therapists help them to develop goals that are **inclusive of the client's hard work**. If the client states that another person would need to change, the therapist accepts that and expands the client's desires. This can be accomplished by saying, "Okay. So suppose they change like that, how will you then be different?" This question gets the client to begin to view themselves in a different way where they can begin to enact these behaviors, regardless of whether the other person changes. Working with Steve and Carissa, this will be an important conversational tool as the therapist wants to increase each party's personal agency. If Carissa complained that she wanted Steve around more, the therapist would follow up with, "Suppose he is around more. What will you two be doing then?" Or when Steve states that Carissa is argumentative, the therapist would say, "Okay. Suppose she isn't argumentative. How will you respond to her?" These questions help demonstrate the interactional nature of their relationship. Regardless of whether the other person makes a change, each person can be the way they want. Their change may lead to positive change in the relationship as a change in one part of the system leads to system-wide change.

Last, goals should be the **presence rather than absence** of behavior. This characteristic is extremely important since most people come to therapy stating that there is a behavior they don't want in their lives. For instance, Steve and Carissa might say they "don't want to be miserable anymore," "don't want to be in a loveless marriage," or "don't want to continue arguing so much." This absence of behavior is problematic since they might know where they don't want to go, but are not clear about where they want to go. The therapist needs to help develop a goal that is the start of something. When a client says, "I don't want X," the therapist's response would be, "How would you rather it be?" The answer to this question would become the client's goal.

Last, the partners in a couple may not have the same goals. One may want more closeness while the other wants more distance. The solution-focused tool when this happens is **bridging** (Hoyt & Berg, 1998). This happens when the therapist helps to bring forth the interactional aspect of the pieces of the clients' miracle pictures. Thus, what eventually develops in the therapeutic conversation is a shared vision of how the partners want their lives to be. The Hogarth's therapist will need to be attuned to what the overlap between each person's goals are. They will need to think, "Why does Steve want Carissa not to be so argumentative?" and "Why does Carissa want Steve to be around more and do things with her?" The bridge between their two desires is that they want a better marriage. Bridging helps to shift parties from being oppositional with one another to working together for a common cause. People are more likely to work together, and work harder, when they are focused on the same goal attainment.

Termination

As with most therapeutic models, solution-focused sessions are usually spaced one week apart. However, once clients begin reporting that things are better, the therapist may introduce the idea of spacing out sessions (de Shazer et al., 1986). The length is usually worked out collaboratively between the therapist and client, but what frequently happens is that they shift to every other week and then every three weeks with continued positive movement from the client. This spacing out of sessions tends to happen quickly as every session, including the first session, focuses on what has been better in the client's life.

SFBT therapists terminate therapy when the client believes that they do not need to come to therapy anymore. This may be because the problem is no longer present or not at a level that is concerning for the client anymore. Therapists might ask clients whether things are "better enough" that they do not need to schedule another session (de Shazer et al., 1986). It is not for the therapist to tell the Hogarths that they need to keep coming because the therapist thinks they need to work on one or another "issue" that the therapist believes is negatively impacting them. Rather, the therapist respects Steve and Carissa's decisions as to what their goals are and whether they have achieved them. If the couple explained that they were in a good place, but the therapist thought there were additional changes they could make, the therapist would accept Steve and Carissa's position. Given that positive changes gain momentum, there is a high likelihood that the couple will continue to move toward their goals even when they stop coming to therapy as they are focusing on what is working in their relationship.

There may be some concerns that SFBT does not address the underlying cause of the problem. Further, the client may have "problems" that they are not saying are concerns, but others, perhaps even including the therapist, might think these are potential issues for therapy. Therapy is considered successful when clients no longer experience the concerns that brought them in, not just when certain aspects of their life improve. This is because the SFBT therapist tries to meet the client where they are and does not take an expert position of what "should be."

Case Transcript

Therapist: Welcome. I am glad that you both came today. One thing I've found is that, for some people, they notice that between the time they have called to make the appointment and coming in, there has been some type of positive change, even if quite small. What has either of you noticed that is better since you first called for the session?

The therapist begins the session with the presession change question, attempting to initiate a conversation that is predicated on preexisting positive change. This is also an important start to a couple's session as they are likely to be primed to complain about one another rather than focusing on aspects of their relationship that are already working.

Carissa:	I don't think I've really seen anything.
Steve:	Me either.
Therapist:	Okay. Sometimes there might be positive change and other times we might not notice. Let me ask you both, then, what are your best hopes for this session? What will let you know, at the end of this session, that it was useful for you both to come?

The therapist has accepted that the couple may not have noticed something better, and does not push too much since this is the first session. Instead of asking them what brings them in, as many other therapists might, this opening attempts to bring their goals into the conversation from the very first moments of the session. It is also another conversation thread that moves away from potential complaints of one another to what they may find useful.

Steve:	Hopefully we'll be able to finally get along.
Therapist:	Okay. How will you know you are getting along?

The therapist attempts to make Steve's goal measurable.

Steve:	We'll be able to talk without arguing.
Therapist:	All right. So, there won't be arguing. How will you talk with one another instead?

Here, the therapist shifts the goal from the absence of something to the presence of something.

Steve:	It will be respectful.
Therapist:	Carissa, what about for you? What are your best hopes for today's session?

While the goal of respectful conversation is too abstract and not measurable, yet, the therapist wants to ensure that both parties are heard to increase both members' participation in the session. The more possibilities of goals the better, as movement to one or more goals is a sign that the couple is moving in the right direction.

Carissa:	Well, I'm hoping that Steve would understand that he is not a bachelor anymore and would put as much, well really, more focus on me than he does on his friends, his job, or his sports.
Therapist:	Okay. So, suppose he does put that focus on you today. What would you then do?

This question attempts to shift Carissa from a complainant position to more of a customer. By highlighting that the goal is interactional rather than intrapersonal, the therapist is subtly opening up space for Carissa to see that she has a role in their interactional process.

Carissa:	I'd be happier.
Therapist:	And when you are happier, what would you do with Steve that you might not previously do?
Carissa:	We'd probably smile with one another and laugh.

Therapist: Okay. So, both of you would like to get along better where there is more respect in the relationship, more smiling, and more laughter.

The therapist begins to bridge their desires so that they can see they are partners on this journey rather than adversaries.

Carissa/Steve: Yes!

Therapist: All right. I am going to ask you a very strange question. Hopefully, you have good imaginations. And the strange question is this. After we finish the session, you will go home and finish whatever you do for the rest of today. And eventually, you will go to sleep. During the night a miracle happens. And the miracle is that all the concerns that you came here today with are (*Snapping fingers*) gone, because of this miracle. However, you were sleeping so you don't know that this miracle happened. What will be the first sign for you tomorrow morning when you wake up to let you know that something is different?

The therapist asks the miracle question to build on goal development that has already begun in the session.

Steve: She would be nice to me when we woke up.

Therapist: What would she do that would demonstrate her being nice?

Steve: She'd smile at me.

Therapist: What would come next?

Steve: We'd have a pleasant conversation.

Therapist: And then what?

Steve: Maybe we'd kiss and who knows.

Therapist: So, that would let you know there was a miracle?

The therapist is tracking potential sequences to demonstrate the interpersonal nature of the miracle.

Steve: Yes. Lately, that would be a miracle if that happened.

Therapist: Carissa, what would be the first sign for you that a miracle happened?

The therapist shifts to Carissa to expand the miracle picture and highlight that both people would be seeing differences. Further, phrasing it as the "first sign" implies that there are many more signs that would let them know they are experiencing their relationship in the way that they want.

Carissa: He'd be attentive to me.

Therapist: What will he be doing to show you he's attentive?

Carissa: He'd make me breakfast. Ask me what I wanted to do that day. We'd spend time together and have fun.

Therapist: Okay. So, suppose he does all of that. What will you do in response?

The therapist accepts the client's ideas and adds the interpersonal aspect to them, opening space for the client to talk about her own behaviors that will be useful for the relationship.

Carissa: I'd be nice to him. We'd talk. We'd spend quality time together.

Therapist: It seems both of you are wanting to spend time together in a positive way. Is that right?

The therapist continues to bridge Steve and Carissa's desires.

Steve/Carissa: Yes.

Therapist: The day after this miracle happened, how would your friends know that something is different?

The therapist expands the miracle question by asking a relational question. The more different viewpoints and possibilities for ways the couple could have a good relationship the better.

Steve: They'd want to be around us. Some of them have let me know that they are concerned that when we've been around them, we've been sniping at one another, and it makes them uncomfortable.

Carissa: I didn't know that. Why didn't you tell me?

Steve: I didn't want something else to escalate between us.

Carissa: So, you allowed them to continue to think we've got problems?

Therapist: Let me interrupt you there for a second. You were saying that your friends would want to be around you. What would the two of you be doing that they'd want to be around you?

The therapist interrupts the beginning of an interaction that is focused on problem talk and shifts it to a focus on the behaviors of the couple that are measurable.

Steve: We wouldn't be arguing.

Therapist: How would you be instead?

The therapist attempts to shift the conversation from the absence of a behavior to the presence of a behavior.

Steve: We'd be fun. And nice to each other. We'd be smiling at one another.

Therapist: Carissa, what do you think your friends would see between the two of you so that they'd know the miracle happened?

Carissa: I didn't know they had a problem being around us.

Therapist: That was a bit shocking for you, hearing that. And it seems you are quite disappointed that they would have that perception and that Steve didn't tell you about it.

Carissa: That's right.

Therapist: And them not quite wanting to be around you two is from before the miracle happened. However, we are talking about after the miracle. What would they see that was different in the two of you?

The therapist is focusing on the focus of the conversation, acknowledging the client's focus on problems, and then opening space for solutions (Reiter & Chenail, 2016).

Carissa: I guess they would see us holding hands. Talking. Lots of smiling.

Therapist: Today, I've heard a lot that when things are going well with the two of you there would be a lot of smiling at one another. Is that right?

Steve: Yes.

Therapist: What have been the times in your couplehood where you were that way? Where smiling was present and a significant part of your relationship?

Here, the therapist asks an exception question, which will demonstrate to the couple that some of the pieces of their miracle have already been a part of their lives. This will likely increase their hope and expectancy that they can smile at each other again since they have previously been able to engage in this behavior.

Steve:	When we go out and do activities. Like Top Golf. Or Dave and Busters.
Therapist:	Carissa. When do you recall the two of you smiling with one another?

The therapist presupposes that there have been times that the couple has smiled at one another. This is done through the use of "when" rather than "if" or "have."

Carissa:	Sometimes when we cook together.
Therapist:	You two cook together? Wow. I know a lot of couples where the kitchen becomes a battlefield, where they are not able to be in there at the same time. How are you two able to do that?

Using vocal intensity, the therapist compliments the couple on engaging in a behavior that leads to a piece of their miracle picture. Further, the therapist increases the intensity of this compliment by pointing out that the couple can engage in positive behavior that many other couples have difficulties with. This should increase their sense of competence and connection with one another.

Carissa:	I don't know. We just seem to be able to do it.
Therapist:	(*Said with a smile*) So, in the kitchen, the two of you have the recipe for getting along!
Steve/Carissa:	(*Both smile and laugh*)
Therapist:	Let me ask you another strange question. I have a lot of them. On a scale of 1 to 10 where 1 is the lowest you have been and 10 is where you know this relationship is going to work, where are you at on that scale in terms of being motivated to make it work?

The therapist asks a scaling question, assessing where each individual is to obtain a baseline. This will allow the therapist and clients to track their progress throughout this and future sessions. The therapist makes sure to define the parameters of the scale, so everyone knows which end of the scale signifies where the client doesn't want to be and which end is movement toward the goal. Further, an aspect of what the clients want—motivation to be together—is being scaled, rather than something they don't want (e.g., arguing or unhappiness). This helps people to think about what they will do rather than what they won't do.

Steve:	I am at a 7.
Carissa:	I'm at a 6.
Therapist.	Wow. A 7 and a 6. Many couples come in to see me when they are at a 2 or a 3. Some are even at a 1 or a 0. There were clearly some issues that the two of you were dealing with. How were you able to make sure that things didn't get worse?

These statements provide another compliment to the couple. While one person's number is not necessarily equivalent to someone else's, this juxtaposition of Steve and Carissa's scale answer to that of other couples demonstrates that they have strengths in their relationship that they might not have realized. The therapist then asks a type of coping question, acknowledging that their relationship hasn't been where they have wanted it, but also demonstrating that they have been doing things, likely outside of their awareness, to prevent their relationship from being even worse. The therapist also subtly uses tenses (e.g., "were") to presuppose that whatever relationship difficulties they had were in the past, whereas the future will be different.

Carissa: We might be frustrated with each other periodically, but I don't think we hate each other.
Steve: I don't hate her. I love her.
Therapist: You do?
Steve: Of course. She's my wife!
Therapist: How much do you think she knows you love her?
Steve: I hope a lot. I know I probably don't tell her as often as I should.
Therapist: This sounds like something that is extremely important for the two of you. Can you take a moment and talk about this with one another?

The therapist is introducing a solution-focused enactment (Seedall, 2009). While enactments are not a mainstay of solution-focused work and are usually associated with other models, such as structural family therapy, they can be used as part of the solution-building process. When clients can engage in their desired behaviors in session, they gain a greater sense that they can continue those behaviors outside of the therapy room.

Steve: I love you. You know that, right?
Carissa: Sometimes I wonder.
Steve: Why?
Therapist: Let me interrupt for a second. When you talk with one another, talk about what you've seen in the other that lets you know they care about you and that they love you.

The therapist interrupted the enactment because they saw that there was a likelihood that the conversation would shift from solution talk to problem talk. Their encouragement was to focus on the presence rather than the absence of behavior.

Steve: How have you seen me show you love?
Carissa: Well, when you're out you might text me to ask if I want you to pick up something for me, like dinner from a restaurant I like. And you know I love you, right?
Steve: I know it's there. I know you are also disappointed a lot.
Therapist: And when she is not disappointed? What do you see then?
Steve: She can sometimes be a snuggler. And she's not snuggling with just anybody. Just me.
Therapist: Wow. Those are nice ways that you can see each other's love. Let me take a second and go back to those scales. Steve, you said that you were at a 7. What will be different in your relationship when you are at a 7.1?

The therapist is using the initial scale to build further potential pathways to solutions. The couple is coming to therapy because they are experiencing a lot of frustration and concern. If the therapist asked what he would notice when he is at an 8, that might be too far beyond his realistic expectation of how quickly the relationship might improve. The small difference, from a 7 to a 7.1, is inconsequential. What is important is that there is talk in the conversation about positive movement.

Steve: We'd probably have a good conversation. Not that it was that long. Perhaps only five minutes. But it was a conversation where we connected.
Therapist: Okay. So, you'd have a conversation, even if it was brief, where you felt connected with one another.

Steve: Yup.

Therapist: And Carissa, what would you notice different in your relationship when you are at a 6.1?

The therapist has accepted that their answers on the motivation scale are different. This doesn't necessarily mean that Steve is more motivated than Carissa. Since the scale is subjective, Carissa's 6 might equal Steve's 7. They don't have to have the same number. What is important is that they both see that they can each move up the scale.

Carissa: That we went out on a date with one another. We used to go out a lot, but we haven't in a long while.

Therapist: So, when you're at a 6.1, you two would have gone on a date together?

The therapist ignores the second part of Carissa's statement as it will likely lead to problem talk. Rather, the therapist acknowledges the client's original answer which will better contribute to the solution-building process.

Carissa: Yes.

Therapist: Okay. We are coming close to the end of our session. I would like to take a moment to go out of the room and think about everything that has been talked about today and then come back and let you know what I have thought about.

SFBT was developed through a team format where a consultation break was a standard component of the therapeutic session. It provided the therapist and the team space to consider what had occurred during the session, provide a summary, and think about what homework/experiment might be suggested. Even though this case is being seen by a solo practitioner, SFBT therapists can take a consultation break for themselves. This also increases the sense of expectation of the clients for when the therapist returns and what the therapist might say.

Therapist: (*Returning to the room*) I want to commend you both for coming here today. Other couples might have waited longer to come to therapy, or not come at all, leading to very serious issues in their relationship. Somehow, you both knew how important it was for you to come. You both value this marriage. And you were motivated enough to make it work that you scheduled and came today. That is very commendable. It seems things were pretty good at the beginning of your relationship and marriage, and you've been finding that you've been moving away from where you want to be. Today seems one of the first steps to getting back to what you want; spending time together, having fun, holding hands, kissing, smiling, being nice to one another, having good and respectful conversations, being attentive to one another, going out on dates, and where you really feel the other person's love. That is pretty amazing that you have had all of these experiences previously in your relationship. I wonder what your relationship will be like when you are both doing more of these types of things with and for one another.

In this summary, the therapist has highlighted all the small goals the couple has talked about wanting to show that they are moving toward their desired relationship. Included in this explanation is a mutualization and bridging of their goals. These goals fit the criteria of good goals in that they are (1) small, (2) measurable, (3) realistic, (4) salient, (5) inclusive of each person's hard work, and (6) include the presence of a behavior. The therapist compliments the clients again, demonstrating that they already have significant motivation to make their marriage work. They are not starting from nothing, but rather have a lot of competencies already existing in their relationship. What they need to do is more of these useful behaviors. While the couple may not have talked about every concern that brought them to therapy, SFBT sessions do not need to address every single complaint since the solution is not necessarily related to the problem. The more Steve and Carissa engage in the various desired behaviors that they brought into the conversation, the more focus they will have on how their relationship is going in a positive direction.

Therapist: I have a little experiment for each of you to do this week, which I think might be useful for you. Between now and the next time we meet, pay attention to everything happening in your life, the very very small things, and the very very big things, and everything in between that you want to continue to be happening or have happen more. Please don't talk about these things with one another. Perhaps you can keep a list in a journal or on your phone, or if your brain works better than mine, you can track all of these things you notice in your memory. And then next time we meet we will talk about them.

The therapist ends the session by introducing the first session formula task. The therapist perceived that Steve and Carissa both came into the session as complainants, thinking that the other person is the reason their marriage is having problems. However, over the course of the session, there were forays into each of them developing into customers for change. This end-of-session recommendation works well with those who may be complainants and/or customers. They are asked to notice their own behaviors as well as those of their partner. Many couples spend the time between sessions focusing on everything their partner is doing that they do not like so they can bring it up in session to get the therapist to change their partner. They don't realize that when they wear these problem-focused lenses and expect discord in their relationship, their behavior is changed, leading to some of the problems they are waiting to see. The first session formula task asks people to wear their solution-focused lenses and expect positive behaviors and interactions from and with their partner. When using this lens, there is a much greater chance that the wearer will interact with the other person in a more positive manner, which will increase the other's positive response which will increase the first person's positive response, etc. Rather than engaging in more-of-the-same problem behaviors that maintain client complaints, this task encourages more-of-the-same behavior of ways of being that have been useful for them—the exceptions to the problem.

Carissa: Okay. I can do that.
Steve: I can as well. Thank you.
Therapist: When would you like to come back?
Steve: Can we come next week, same time?
Therapist: Sure. I will see you then and look forward to hearing everything you've been noticing this week that you found useful.

The therapist ends the session with a reiteration of the homework assignment, seeing their relationship through a new lens.

References

Anderson, H., & Goolishian, H. (1992). The client is the expert: A not-knowing approach to therapy. In S. McNamee & K. J. Gergen (Eds.), *Therapy as social construction* (pp. 25–39). Sage.
Berg, I. K. (1994). *Family based services*. Norton.

Berg, I. K., & de Shazer, S. (1993). Making numbers talk: Language in therapy. In S. Friedman (Ed.), *The new language of change* (pp. 5–24). Guilford.

Berg, I. K., Sperry, L., & Carlson, J. (1999). Intimacy and culture: A solution-focused perspective. In J. Carlson & L. Sperry (Eds.), *The intimate couple* (pp. 41–54). Brunner/Mazel.

Berg, I. K., & Szabó, P. (2005). *Brief coaching for lasting solutions*. Norton.

Bond, C., Woods, K., Humphrey, N., Symes, W., & Green, L. (2013). Practitioner review: The effectiveness of solution focused brief therapy with children and families: A systematic and critical evaluation of the literature from 1990–2010. *Journal of Child Psychology and Psychiatry, 54*(7), 707–723.

Cantwell, P. W., & Holmes, S. (1994). Social construction: A paradigm shift for systemic therapy and training. *Australian and New Zealand Journal of Family Therapy, 15*(1), 17–26. DOI: 10.1002/j.1467-8438.1994. tb00978.x

Chaudhry, S., & Li, C. (2011). Is solution-focused brief therapy culturally appropriate for Muslim American counselees? *Journal of Contemporary Psychotherapy, 41*, 109–113. DOI: 10.1007/s10879-010-9153-1

Corcoran, J. (2000). Solution-focused family therapy with ethnic minority clients. *Crisis Intervention, 6*(1), 5–12. DOI: 10.1080/10645130008951292

Dahl, R., Bathel, D., & Carreon, C. (2000). The use of solution-focused therapy with an elderly population. *Journal of Systemic Therapies, 19*(4), 45–55. DOI: 101521jsyt200019445

Dermer, S. B., Hemesath, C. W., & Russell, C. S. (1998). A feminist critique of solution-focused therapy. *The American Journal of Family Therapy, 26*(3), 239–250.

de Shazer, S. (1982). *Patterns of brief family therapy*. Guilford.

de Shazer, S. (1985). *Keys to solution in brief therapy*. Norton.

de Shazer, S. (1988). *Clues: Investigating solutions in brief therapy*. Norton.

de Shazer, S. (1991). *Putting difference to work*. Norton.

de Shazer, S. (1994). *Words were originally magic*. Norton.

de Shazer, S., & Berg, I. K. (1992). Doing therapy: A post-structural re-vision. *Journal of Marital and Family Therapy, 18*, 71–81.

de Shazer, S., Berg, I. K., Lipchik, E., Nunnally, E., Molnar, A., Gingerich, W. C., & Weiner-Davis, M. (1986). Brief therapy: Focused solution development. *Family Process, 25*, 207–221.

de Shazer, S., Dolan, Y., Korman, H., Trepper, T., McCollum, E., & Berg, I. K. (2007). *More than miracles: The state of the art of solution-focused brief therapy*. Routledge.

Fisch, R., Weakland, J. H., & Segal, L. (1982). *The tactics of change: Doing therapy briefly*. Jossey-Bass.

Gilstrap, D. (2021). Solutions-oriented intervention models for African American mental health. In M. O. Adekson (Ed.), African Americans and mental health (pp. 105–114). Springer.

Gingerich, W. J., & Eisengart, S. (2000). Solution-focused brief therapy: A review of the outcome research. *Family Process, 39*(4), 477–498. DOI: 10.1111/j.1545-5300.2000.39408.x

Hogan, D., Hogan, D., Tuomola, J., & Yeo, A. K. L. (Eds.). (2017). *Solution focused practice in Asia*. Routledge.

Hoyt, M. F. (2001). *Interviews with brief therapy experts*. Brunner/Mazel.

Hoyt, M. F. (2008). Solution-focused couple therapy. In A. S. Gurman (Ed.), *Clinical handbook of couple therapy* (4th ed., pp. 259–295). Guilford.

Hoyt, M. F., & Berg, I. K. (1998). Solution-focused couple therapy: Helping clients construct self-fulfilling realities. In F. M. Dattilio (Ed.), *Case studies in couple and family therapy* (pp. 203–232). Guilford.

Jordan, S. S. (2016). What's better? Focusing on positives. In G. R. Weeks, S. T. Fife & C. M. Peterson (Eds.), *Techniques for the couple therapist* (pp. 165–168). Routledge.

Kim, J. S., Franklin, C., Zhang, Y., Liu, X., Qu, Y., & Chen, H. (2015). Solution-focused brief therapy in China: A meta-analysis. *Journal of Ethnic & Cultural Diversity in Social Work, 24*(3), 187–201. DOI: 10.1080/15313204.2014.991983

Lambert, M. J. (1992). Psychotherapy outcome research: Implications for integrative and eclectical therapists. In J. C. Norcross & M. R. Goldfried (Eds.), *Handbook of psychotherapy integration* (pp. 94–129). Basic Books.

Lipchik, E., & de Shazer, S. (1986). The purposeful interview. *Journal of Strategic and Systemic Therapies, 5*, 88–89.

Meyer, D. D., & Cottone, R. R. (2013). Solution-focused therapy as a culturally acknowledging approach with American Indians. *Journal of Multicultural Counseling and Development, 41*(1), 47–55.

Nelson, T. S. (2011). Solution-focused brief couple therapy. In D. K. Carson & M. Casado-Kehoe (Eds.), *Case studies in couples therapy: Theory-based approaches* (pp. 275–287). Routledge.

Nylund, D., & Corsiglia, V. (2019). Becoming solution-focused forced in brief therapy: Remembering something important we already knew. *Journal of Systemic Therapies, 38*(2), 81–87. DOI: 10.1521/jsyt.2019.38.2.81

Reiter, M. D. (2007). Utilizing expectation in solution-focused formula tasks. *Journal of Family Psychotherapy, 18*, 27–37.

Reiter, M. D. (2010). The use of hope and expectancy in solution-focused therapy. *Journal of Family Psychotherapy, 21*, 132–148.

Reiter, M. D., & Chenail, R. J. (2016). Defining the focus in solution-focused brief therapy. *International Journal of Solution-Focused Practices, 4*(1), 1–9.

Seedall, R. B. (2009). Enhancing change process in solution-focused brief therapy by utilizing couple enactments. *The American Journal of Family Therapy, 37*, 99–113. DOI: 10.1080/01926180802132356

Suitt, K. G., Franklin, C., & Kim, J. (2016). Solution-focused brief therapy with Latinos: A systematic review. *Journal of Ethnic & Cultural Diversity in Social Work, 25*(1), 50–67. DOI: 10.1080/15313204.2015.1131651

Tews-Kozlowski, R. (2011). Solution-focused therapy with military couples. In B. A. Moore (Ed.), *Handbook of counseling military couples* (pp. 53–87). Taylor & Francis.

Thomas, F. N., & Nelson, T. S. (2007). Assumptions and practices within the solution-focused brief therapy tradition. In T. S. Nelson & F. N. Thomas (Eds.), *Handbook of solution-focused brief therapy: Clinical applications* (pp. 3–24). Haworth.

Watzlawick, P., Weakland, J., & Fisch, R. (1974). *Change: Principles of problem formation and resolution.* W. W. Norton.

Weiner-Davis, M., de Shazer, S., & Gingerich, W. (1987). Using pre-treatment change to construct a therapeutic solution: An exploratory study. *Journal of Marital and Family Therapy, 13*(4), 359–363.

Yeung, F. K. C. (1999). The adaptation of solution-focused therapy in Chinese culture: A linguistic perspective. *Transcultural Psychiatry, 36*(4), 477–489.

12 Narrative Couple Therapy

Jill Freedman and Gene Combs

History of the Model

In 1981, at the Second Australian Family Therapy Conference in Adelaide, Australia, Michael White dropped in on David Epston's workshop. He was intrigued by the presentation and found David's ideas resonant with his own (White & Epston, 1990). They got together after the workshop, and we could think of this meeting as the birthplace of narrative therapy.

From 1982 through the early 1990s David, who lived in Auckland, New Zealand, traveled about twice a year to Adelaide to join Michael in seeing families, couples, and individuals (White, 2016). They would watch each other's work, reflect on it, and talk about what each was doing differently than in previous meetings. They also enjoyed a lively correspondence which included reading recommendations, most of which were from anthropology and sociology, not directly related to family therapy. They found this wider perspective very useful in developing their thinking about their work in therapy.

In those years, David and Michael were not interested in creating a finished, complete model. They resisted naming their work, saying that naming it would reduce their freedom to continue exploring possibilities, and that it would interfere with others recognizing their own contributions to the work. They wrote:

> There is another reason to resist such naming. With regard to ideas and practices, we do not believe that we are in any one place for very long ... one of the aspects associated with this work that is of central importance to us is the spirit of adventure. We aim to preserve this spirit, and know that if we accomplish this our work will continue to evolve in ways that are enriching to our lives, and to the lives of those persons who seek our help.
>
> (White & Epston, 1992, p. 9)

They did eventually name the work narrative therapy[1] because they decided that was preferrable to its being called by their names.

The ways of working that White and Epston developed continued to evolve through the contributions of many people in many contexts. From the beginning, they recognized that as two White men, with the privilege that entails, they should attend to the importance of cultural differences and power relations. They carefully avoided treating the practices they created as universally applicable. Rather, they looked to partner with people of various cultures so that they could learn with and from them how to adapt their practices to fit the values, traditions, and customs of those who had sought consultation. Cheryl White and others suggested feminist readings that brought an important strand of ideas to further shape narrative practice (White & Epston, 1990). In Australia, from the early days, they engaged in partnership with Aboriginal people including Barbara Wingard and Tim Agius (White, 2003; Wingard et al., 2015; Wingard & Lester, 2001). In

DOI: 10.4324/9781003369097-12

New Zealand, the work of the Just Therapy Team (Waldegrave et al., 2003), which was made up of Maori, Pacific Islanders, and Pakeha (Anglo) people had a huge and lasting influence.

Epston has continued to develop new ideas and practices to this day (see, for example, his online publication *Journal of Contemporary Narrative Therapy*) and White constantly added nuance and complexity by creating, teaching, and writing about new theory and practice right up until his death in 2008 (see e.g., White, 2011 and https://dulwichcentre.com.au/michael-white-archive/writings-by-michael-white).

By the mid-1980s, therapists in countries around the world were becoming familiar with White and Epston's ideas and adapting them to fit their own cultural contexts (e.g., Kalisa et al., 2022). Various teams also developed ideas for narrative community work (e.g., Ncube, 2006; Denborough, 2008).

White's early publications (e.g., 1986) draw from the work of Gregory Bateson (1972, 1979), and show some theoretical overlap with strategic and cybernetic approaches. Epston, who had been reading widely in the then-current anthropology and cultural psychology literature, brought in the narrative metaphor from the work of Jerome Bruner (1986, 1990, 1991). Readings in philosophy (Derrida, 1988; Foucault, 1965, 1975, 1977, 1980), sociology (Goffman, 1961), and anthropology (Geertz, 1983, 1986; Myerhoff, 1986) contributed to the work. Foucault's writings on discourse and Myerhoff's ideas about definitional ceremonies were especially influential.

Although the specific implementation has changed over time and from place to place, with contributions from different therapists, narrative practice has consistently avoided focusing on pathology. Narrative practitioners focus on relationships rather than on individuals, and they seek to help through situation-and-context-specific approaches rather than universal one-size-fits-all solutions. Basic ideas include the following:

1 *Problems are separate from people.* This idea is often stated as "The person is not the problem. The problem is the problem."
2 *Problems are located in sociocultural discourses.* In couples therapy we particularly attend to gender discourses, to power relations that support inequity, and to the ways in which idealized images of what constitutes a good partner or a good relationship make people feel that they or their relationships don't measure up.
3 *Identity is multi-storied and is constructed through time by the choices we make and by our relationships with others.* This way of thinking about identity can be very important in working with couples because the way they know themselves through each other's eyes can be very significant. Exploring whether and how the relationship supports each in becoming the person they want to be is often a part of this. Culture, language, and discourse contribute to people's conception of their identities, so we explore all these aspects of experience.
4 *People are the experts on, and the privileged authors of, their own lives.* This idea makes us favor a collaborative therapeutic relationship. We think of the therapist as accompanying couples, rather than directing them.
5 *People organize their lives through stories of their experience.* We refer to this idea as the narrative metaphor. It is a central organizing principle of narrative therapy.
6 *People are not passive recipients of experience.* They are always responding, even in the midst of extreme hardship.

The Narrative Metaphor

In therapy organized by the **narrative metaphor**, we work with people to find new meaning in their lives by experiencing, telling, and retelling stories of as-yet-unstoried aspects of their lives.

Imagine that each of the dots below (Figure 12.1) represents a life experience.

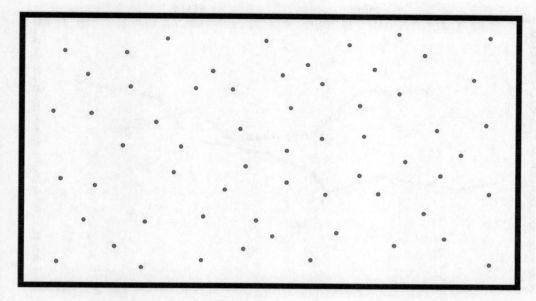

Figure 12.1 People have many life experiences.

When couples consult with a therapist, they are usually caught up in rather thin stories that focus on only a few of their many life experiences. Although the stories may share some events, often each member of a couple describes different incidents that they believe illustrate the problem. For example, although Steve and Carissa might both name arguments as the problem, Carissa might give examples to illustrate her disappointment in not experiencing Steve's commitment to become a parent. Steve might talk about Carissa complaining about many things, such as his spending too much time with friends and not doing his share around the house.

As therapists, our first job is to listen to these stories, and to orient to them as a few of many possible stories (see Figure 12.2). Listening with that attitude helps us notice when people make implicit or explicit reference to events that wouldn't be predicted by the plots of the problematic stories. The circled dot (Figure 12.3) represents such an event. An example might be that although Carissa might suggest that Steve is not very interested in becoming a parent, we learn that he has participated in going to fertility doctors and supported trying in-vitro fertilization. That participation would not be predicted by Carissa's description of the problem and provides a different picture of Steve's commitment.

We can then ask questions that invite people to step into those events, and to tell us (and themselves) about the meaning of the events, developing them into memorable and vivid stories (Figure 12.4). The initial part of this process is to linger with the event, asking questions that invite details, setting, other people, etc. If we were to inquire about Steve's participation in consultation about fertility, we might learn that although becoming a parent is not as important to him as it is to Carissa, he has thought positively about being a father. We might hear some of the images and possibilities that he has entertained about that. Additionally, we might ask questions that would facilitate Steve talking about wanting to support Carissa's dreams and his worry that continuing fertility treatment would put them in a very difficult place financially and might only lead to more disappointment.

Then we ask about related events through time, developing a new plot line (Figure 12.5) that runs through their lives and through their relationship.

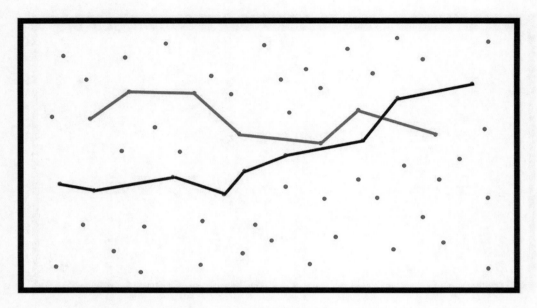

Figure 12.2 People story only a few of their many life experiences.

Over time, this process leads to the development of multiple storylines with rich and complex meanings that speak of multiple possibilities for people's lives and relationships. This process does not take away problematic stories, but problematic stories often have a different meaning when they are only strands of multi-stranded stories (Figure 12.6).

Post-structuralism

Narrative ideas are based in **post-structuralist philosophy** (Foucault, 1988; White, 1997) which focuses on contextualized meaning-making, rather than on generalizations or universal truths. Post-structuralism grew out of structuralism. Structuralism seeks to categorize and name all the entities in the universe. Structuralist scholars sought to develop categories and rules that applied everywhere in all situations. As some structuralist scholars tried to categorize, classify, and name finer and finer levels of complex systems, they encountered ambiguities and paradoxes. For instance, anthropology students sent to study "primitive" peoples found wisdom and wondrous events that they could not fit neatly into the structural categories they were learning in school. Their experience was that no system of universal categories could capture people's lives in all their complexity. These scholars became more interested in local, specific stories than in universally applicable generalizations. At some point people with such interests began to describe themselves as *post*-structuralists.

Post-structuralists believe that it is useful to focus on contextualized meaning-making, rather than on universal truths or an all-encompassing reality. In this meaning-focused approach, culture, language, and discourse are explored in terms of how they contribute to the experience and identity of people in their specific cultural contexts. Proponents of post-structuralism seek details of people's experience. Lives are valued in terms of how they embody exceptions or uniqueness, rather than how they fit into general categories.

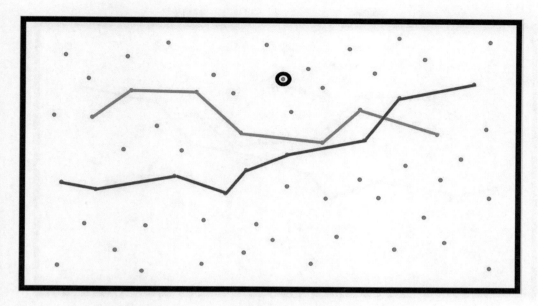

Figure 12.3 Some events fall outside of the plots of people's problematic stories.

Guided by the narrative metaphor, narrative practitioners assume that people's experiences of problems are shaped by stories (which are constructions). But these are not the constructions of individuals. In any social group, small or large, we are participants in each other's stories. We each shape, and are shaped by, the beliefs, intentions, and actions of others. Collectively, we participate in discourses. Rachel Hare-Mustin (1994, pp. 19–20) defines discourse as "a system of statements, practices, and institutional structures that share common values… ." She goes on to say "discourses bring certain phenomena into sight and obscure other phenomena. The ways most people in a society hold, talk about, and act on a common, shared viewpoint are part of and sustain the prevailing discourses."

The norms and expectations of a culture are communicated through discourses, and they are largely taken for granted. Unless we look, listen, and feel for them, they are invisible. For example, gender discourses still often shape the partners in a heterosexual couple to believe that the man should earn more money than the woman. If the woman earns more, both partners in the couple may think there must be something wrong with their relationship. This discourse-based comparison is in the background, shaping their relationship and contributing to the sense that it is problematic.

Post-structuralist therapists assume that since we are all part of culture, we can all be caught up by discourses, and we can all too easily reproduce unhelpful discourses in the therapy room without recognizing what we are doing (Hare-Mustin, 1994). For post-structuralists, no one is in a position to be an objective expert on someone else's experience. Further, we recognize that the power relations of the political context influence our lives both in and out of the therapy room. Knowing this, narrative therapists strive to facilitate awareness of discourses and power differentials that support problems. We work from a position of collaboration, recognizing clients as the privileged authors of their own stories. This reflects a movement in the social sciences known as "**the interpretive turn**" (Bruner, 1986; Geertz, 1983), which is a shift in who is doing the interpreting. Specifically, it denotes a shift away from experts making interpretations about other people's

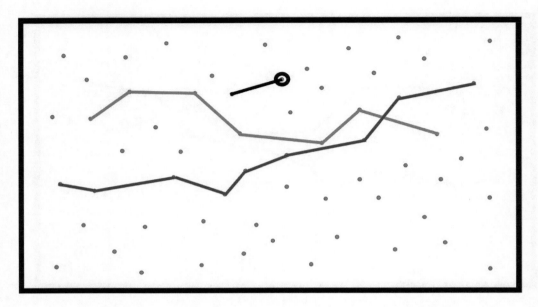

Figure 12.4 Narrative therapists help people to thicken the description of a unique outcome event.

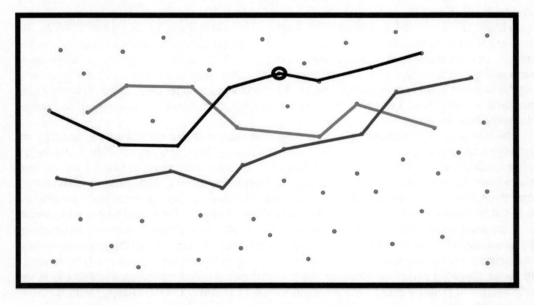

Figure 12.5 A new plot line is developed that connects events that weren't previously acknowledged.

lives, and toward people making interpretations and meaning of their own lives. The interpretive turn favors local, personal, contextualized knowledge rather than universal, generalized expert knowledge. This does not completely change the power relations in the therapy room, but it does encourage us to find ways of collaborating, rather than imposing our values and opinions.

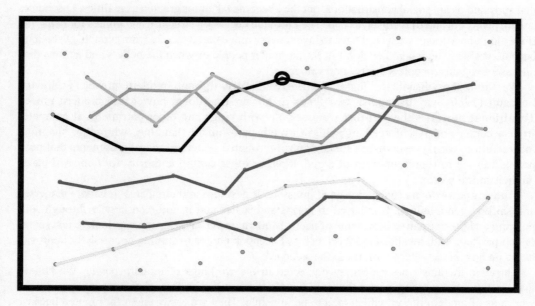

Figure 12.6 People have multiple storylines that offer a multitude of possibilities for their lives.

Conceptualization of Problem Formation

As we have already noted, narrative therapy has come to be known for the statement "The person is not the problem. The problem is the problem." Narrative therapists assume that problems are separate from people. This is in opposition to the structuralist notion that people's actions are a manifestation of essential internal characteristics. Rather than thinking of people as problematic, we think about problems as entities that are outside of and acting on people.

Members of couples often locate problems in each other. They often enter therapy hoping that the therapist will help them fix their deficient partner. In our work, we **externalize** problems; we think about problems as separate from either partner, and work to define and understand the problems that come between couple members. We do not work to create a shared problem. We accept that each partner has different desires and a different experience of the relationship. We can, and often do, work with more than one problem. Whether it is a single agreed-upon problem or separate problems, we ask questions to facilitate **experience-near descriptions** of what's problematic. As therapy progresses and situations change, problem descriptions and names usually shift. We try to flow with these shifts.

Because we want to help partners understand each other's experience of problems, we ask questions to facilitate that understanding, with the hope that each person will get a new perspective. We work to bring forth a detailed understanding of the landscape in which each problem exists. We ask about the effects of problems in the life and relationships of each member of the couple. We ask where problems show up and where they don't. We want to know whether and how different problems work together. When a person identifies an effect of a problem, we ask them to evaluate it. Is it useful or not? Do they think the effect is good or bad? Etc. Then we ask them to explain their evaluation—why they find it useful or not (White, 2007). Throughout these explorations, we treat problems as entities that are influencing the relationship and its members.

We believe that problems are shaped and supported by clouds of **discourse**—discourses that dictate norms, expectations, standards of behavior, markers of success, and the like. The discourses that surround us are social constructions, but they become taken for granted as realities. Discourses are not always in and of themselves bad. They provide necessary structure and guides for behavior. If we didn't have them, we would have to invent every move that we make from scratch. Discourses become problematic when they don't fit for particular people or when the beliefs and actions they propose go against people's desires and values.

We think that discourses make themselves known through modern power. Following Foucault (1980), we distinguish two types of power: traditional power and modern power. **Traditional power** is the sort that we associate with kings and other patriarchs. It emanates from a center and is enforced in public through punishment (hanging, whipping, shaming, incarceration, etc.). It establishes social control through a system of moral judgments that push people to look to representatives of a god, king, or other central authority for approval based on their moral worth.

Modern power is more insidious and invisible. It develops and circulates in widely dispersed and shifting communities. It is based in norms and scales and is enforced largely through self-policing and the normative judgments of peers. Modern power invites people to look to test scores or comparisons with idealized models (such as Facebook photos of smiling couples) for approval, based on how closely they conform to the standard.

Narrative therapists are especially interested in the workings of modern power. We believe that the thin, unsatisfying stories that lead people to consult with therapists are supported by the workings of modern power, which tend to be invisible. They are easily taken for granted because of the way they hide in the norms, standards, and scales that we so willingly use to measure ourselves and each other.

We see modern power as carried in the stories we tell each other about what is worth pursuing and what is not worth pursuing, what constitutes success or failure, who is "in" and who is "out," and where we measure ourselves to be on this or that continuum of normality. The looks that Carissa and Steve get in the South may well be the work of modern power. The desire to have biological children is also supported by modern power.

Although Steve and Carissa have much in common, as a Black woman who grew up in a small town, Carissa would likely have different cultural assumptions than Steve who grew up in a considerably bigger city as a White male. The discourses that would shape their evaluations of themselves and each other would be different, which would lead each of them to focus on different moments in their experience as problematic. They would probably also identify some of the same experiences as problematic. Because he is White and a man, race and gender discourses that are still prevalent would place Steve in a more powerful position than Carissa. Our responsibility as therapists is to be aware of power inequities like these and to consider how they might shape the problems that bring couples to therapy.

There are also discourse-level ideas about the difficulties of being an inter-racial couple. Steve's father predicted that the relationship wouldn't last because of these difficulties. Other people's views of inter-racial relationships could create problems for Steve and Carissa or could create an unsupportive context. We would not want to assume that we knew how they experience these discourses, but we would want to be alert as to how Carissa and Steve experience their effects.

Our speculation in the above paragraphs about the norms and expectations supporting this couple's problems could be completely off-target. If we were seeing Carissa and Steve, we would unpack and investigate evidence of discourses in their relationship, carefully checking our understanding, and only cautiously exploring the possible norms and standards that those discourses implied.

All our study of the workings of modern power is in the service of developing awareness of the many discourses that can feed people's problems. Exploring the discursive cloud that surrounds a given couple makes it possible for us to interact in ways that invite partners to see each other in the light of different stories. In that light, they can imagine, experience, and live out previously unseen possibilities for satisfying life stories.

Conceptualizing Diversity

Even though we are focusing on work with couples, as narrative practitioners, we want to be clear that there are many ways to lead satisfying lives and many kinds of relationships besides couple relationships.

From very early in the development of what came to be known as narrative therapy, there has been an openness and responsiveness to critiques. Some of these critiques came from the feminist movement; others came from indigenous people in various locations. Michael White, particularly, stressed that it is not possible to leave the sociocultural context outside of the therapy room. The awareness of both cultural differences and power relations has always figured in the work.

Many models of therapy are exported to different places as exactly as possible in their original form. Narrative therapists have always adapted and changed their practices to fit with the particularities of local cultures. For example, narrative therapy in Rwanda includes local song, local proverbs in local language, games, and, at times, gardening and farming (Kalisa et al., 2022). As narrative ideas have spread across the world, narrative practitioners take pains to fit their actions and rhythms to the local culture.

Wherever it is practiced, narrative therapy locates problems in discourses that support standards in that culture of what is desirable. Problems may arise on the basis of discourses that focus on class, wealth, gender, race, beauty, academic achievement, athletic ability, psychological functioning, or some local norm we haven't yet encountered. These discourses support and privilege some people while marginalizing others. Narrative practitioners endeavor to support people in having different relationships with these standards—to claim meaningful lives even when they do not fit them and at times to celebrate nonstandard lives (Olinger, 2010; White, 2002).

Additionally, we are alert to power relations—both those between therapists and people coming for help, and between members of families or couples or other kinds of relationships. This ethic has us resist neutrality and locate our position as striving to support **social justice** (Reynolds & Hammoud-Beckett, 2018). We endeavor to be aware of power relations and other forms of injustice and shape our responses to expose these forms of injustice and make room for other possibilities. The therapist's position is important in accomplishing this.

The Role of the Therapist

A narrative therapist's position is **decentered but influential** (White, 1997). We want to place the couple coming for consultation at the center of the conversation. We privilege the stories couple members tell, their experience of what is problematic, and their evaluation of what is useful and not useful. We work hard to rid ourselves of preconceived ideas about what a healthy couple looks like or how a successful couple organizes itself. We try to support the ideas and values that members of the couple put forward. If our context allows it, we ask people at the end of each conversation if they would like to meet again, and if they would, when they would like to meet again. Rather than following a prescribed way of doing things, this invites couple members to decide for themselves. We also want couples to decide when to end therapy. Sometimes, even though we note that the problem which brought them is no longer at play, some couples find it valuable to keep telling and retelling preferred stories in a therapy context for some time. Others prefer to keep these conversations to a minimum.

Although we work to stay decentered (to keep the people who have come for help in the spotlight), we also endeavor to be influential. That is, we don't simply reflect back what members of a couple say. We intentionally shape the conversation in ways that we hope will facilitate people thinking about things they haven't thought about before. We take responsibility for helping them entertain new possibilities. The balance between staying decentered and exerting influence varies from situation to situation and from therapist to therapist, but our desire is that people be the principal authors of their own lives.

We hope to facilitate a collaborative relationship in which we are joining people or working alongside them or accompanying them. But despite our vision of therapy relationships, members of a couple often orient to us as though we are judges or expert teachers. They may hope that we take their side rather than their partner's or they look to us to offer guidance about how they should be as a couple. In order to avoid both of these roles, we often speak to one partner at a time, referring to the other in the third person. Our purpose is to create a **witnessing** position from which each couple member, in turn, can understand the other's experience (Freedman, 2014). We are not hoping for negotiation or agreement, but for understanding.

Epston (1999) thinks about therapy as **co-research**. This supports collaboration and discovery, treating everyone—therapist and couple members—as a research team. Therapy shifts based on reflections offered on the ongoing process. Insider knowledge from those who have consulted us informs our work with others.

The main way that narrative practitioners communicate with couples is through questions. Posing a question is a very powerful move. Questions propose the domain of the answer and are very influential. But the person answering chooses how to answer, which is also very important. We think of questions as a way of staying decentered but influential. We endeavor to ask real questions that we do not know the answers to; not ones that are constructed to point people in directions we favor.

We are not blank slates; we hope to be skilled practitioners taking sides with people's preferred stories and with positions that favor social justice. We see our main task as one of facilitating the telling, retelling—and thereby experiencing—of preferred stories, and that means that we want to be influential in listening for openings to preferred stories and asking questions about them. As new, favored, stories come forth, we often make documents that record and continue these retellings (Fox, 2003). Narrative documents featuring the words of the people we work with offer the opportunity to re-engage with preferred stories between our meetings.

Another part of our role is to recognize power relationships and help make visible the way they affect members of a couple. As we recognize power relationships and examine their effects, we can ask partners if those effects are what they want in their relationship. Knowing that we are often in positions of power over those we work with, we endeavor to keep our focus near to their experiential worlds so that we can keep their skills, abilities, and knowledge, rather than our own, in the spotlight.

We avoid giving expert advice, and we strive for transparency in our relating. We situate what we say by acknowledging our values and lived experience, so that people know how to take our contributions. We also engage in **taking it back practices** (White, 1997), acknowledging that our relationships are not one-way—that we learn from and are moved by our relationships with people who consult us. We share with people how their words and stories make a difference to us.

Conceptualization of Problem Resolution

In narrative therapy, we do not aim for problem resolution. We think people and relationships are multi-storied, and we don't subscribe to the idea that couple members must always negotiate or agree. We do think that it is helpful for people to understand what is problematic for their partners. We are interested in engaging members of couples in the telling and retelling of preferred stories and in understanding (not necessarily agreeing with, but understanding) each other's stories. Sometimes when people are immersed in preferred stories, they are in touch with ways of resolving problems. At other times, the problem stories simply become a much smaller part of the overall picture—a single thread in a rich and varied tapestry—and are no longer a matter of great concern. Of course, at times, agreement *is* important. Sometimes it is necessary to make a choice or take an action as a couple. When people understand each other's stories, it is easier for them to reach this kind of agreement.

Rather than focusing on resolving problems, narrative therapists invite people to explore experiences that lie outside of or do not fit with the problematic stories. We facilitate people telling, and through their telling, experiencing stories that include memories, present events, and possibilities that they prefer. We start by using **double listening**—listening to understand problematic stories, and at the same time listening to hear openings to other possibilities. As members of a couple listen to understand their partner's stories, we are also listening, striving to understand the specifics of their struggles. And, simultaneously, we take on an additional task—listening to hear possible openings to other stories. This double listening takes practice, and there are several things that we have found useful to practice listening for:

1 Unique outcomes

A **unique outcome** is an event that would not be predicted by the plot line of the problematic story. It may be an exception to the problem, but it is not limited to an exception. It could also be anything that does not fit with any aspect of the plot of the problematic story. For example, Carissa may name Steve choosing to spend weekends with his friends instead of her as a problem. As we ask externalizing questions, she may name the problem "lack of closeness." One of the effects of the lack of closeness is that Carissa has lost interest in caring for the house plants the couple used to enjoy together. In a later conversation, we hear that Carissa bought a new house plant. The lack of closeness is still there, but when the new plant caught her eye, she remembered the pleasure she used to take from watering and pruning the now-neglected plants at home. The problem has not changed, but buying a new house plant does not fit with the problem story, so it is a unique outcome—a decision where the problem did not dominate Carissa's experience and may provide an opening to an alternative story.

2 Initiatives

An **initiative** is anything a person does which shows that they have agency—that they can initiate actions that may have some role in shaping their lives. An initiative need not be related to the problem. For Steve and Carissa, simply making a therapy appointment and attending therapy could be viewed as an initiative. Or we might discover other steps they have taken to put themselves in charge of their lives and relationships. Perhaps they have recently re-financed their home. This could be an initiative showing how they are taking charge of their financial life. Questions about how they decided to do this and followed through with it could bring out awareness of skills and abilities that support a different story about their relationship.

3 Possible discourses

Unpacking a problem story—examining details and developing a more complex understanding of it and exposing the discourses that support it—can yield gaps that let us perceive events or experiences that create openings to construct stories of other possibilities. **Externalizing conversations** deconstruct the idea that a person or a relationship is problematic. They open possibilities for constructing stories that feature non-problematic selves or relationships. A conversation which exposes a discourse that is influencing members of a couple could put them in the position to make decisions about whether the discourse fits for them. For example, Carissa's displeasure with Steve for spending weekends with his friends instead of with her could have to do with the discourse that members of a couple should be everything to each other. If this idea is found to be at play, and if the therapist can help Carissa examine its effects, then she can have some choice about how to relate to the discourse. She won't be spellbound by the discourse's invisible power.

4 *Cues to the absent but implicit*

The **absent but implicit** rests on the idea that for someone to discern that something is problematic, they must be comparing it to something important that is missing or betrayed. For example, disappointment is evidence that something has been expected and eagerly awaited but it hasn't come. When we talk about the absent but implicit, the conversation moves from talk of a problem to consideration of a treasured value. If Steve and Carissa name the problem as "arguing and tension," we might wonder what this says about what they long for. Our conversation may reveal that they long for excitement about their future, rather than arguments about the present. We can then ask questions to develop vivid stories of exciting future possibilities.

5 *Responses to problems*

We believe that people are always responding (Wade, 1997, 2002; Yuen, 2009). They are not passive recipients of the events in their lives. Not all responses are successful or even memorable, but any response can be the basis of a useful story. This idea would have us asking about ways—these could be quite small—that Carissa and Steve have already responded to what they have named as problematic. Maybe after one of their arguments, Steve has imagined a calmer future together. Carissa may not have known anything about this, but when she hears Steve mention it in the therapy conversation, she may begin to wonder about and entertain the possibility of a calmer future. We could then ask questions to bring forth experience of a story that conveys what a calmer future might be like. We could ask questions that invite both partners to connect the calmer future to past times when they have enjoyed calmness together.

In our conversations with couples, we often talk with one member of the couple at a time, while the other is in a listening or **witnessing position**. It is important for each member of a couple to understand what the other finds problematic, and to appreciate the steps the other has taken to respond and move toward more satisfying experiences. When we turn to ask the witnessing member questions, we want to invite them to show understanding, perhaps to appreciate their partner, and, when possible, to develop and extend the preferred story.

Let's imagine that Steve names "arguing" as the problem. In our conversation with him, we find that one of the effects of this arguing is that he has stopped initiating things that he and Carissa can do together. Instead, he is spending more time with friends, and when the two of them are home, they watch more and more television. However, in a later conversation, we hear that an old friend of Steve's came into town and Steve could have arranged to have lunch or drinks just with him, but instead arranged a dinner including Carissa. We interview Steve about this while Carissa listens. She may start to interrupt to make an alternative meaning, perhaps suggesting that Steve just didn't want to reveal the problems in their relationship. Our role is to help Carissa focus her attention on Steve's telling and then ask questions that invite her to join the story. We might ask, "Are you surprised to hear that although Steve has said that arguing has made him reluctant to initiate doing things together, he wanted to include you in his friend's visit? Can you see how to me this could be an example of continuing to try to build the relationship, instead of letting arguing stop him? … If I'm right about this, why do you think it might be important to Steve? … What does it mean to you to consider the dinner invitation in this light?"

All the practices we are describing come to life in conversations where we ask questions and attend carefully to people's responses. We are interested in asking about the not-yet-said. In inviting exploration of new expressions, we use questions to *generate experience*, rather than to gather information. We don't want the therapy conversation to be simply a retelling of the problematic story. Instead, we work to facilitate not only the telling of an alternative story, but the *experiencing* of it (Freedman & Combs, 1993). We believe that a story will only have memorable meaning and useful effects if people relive it as they retell it. To help stories be experientially "thick" and vivid, we ask about many things:

- Details that will enhance experiential involvement, such as sensory experience.
- Time, including the steps leading up to the event being storied, past experiences that relate to the event in some way, and steps in the near future that the developing story could facilitate.
- People—both others present for events in the story and people who support the direction of the story or who have shown through their life that these kinds of events are possible.
- Other viewpoints—what this new story would mean to the younger Carissa and Steve if they could have looked ahead and seen it, or how a friend might describe the alternative story they are developing.
- Knowledge, skills, and abilities that members of the couple are drawing on to create a preferred story. We can also ask what new skills and knowledge they are developing through imagining how the new story might play out.
- Meaning, which includes things like hopes and intentions the story illustrates or implies, values that are important in the story, what the story suggests about what is important to members of the couple, or what the story shows is significant about the relationship.

We think about two different landscapes (Bruner, 1990) as we compose our questions: the **landscape of action** in which people relate what happened (a sequence of events over time); and the **landscape of meaning or identity** in which people reflect on the meaning of what happened and relate that to what they give value to and what that implies about their identities. We weave between these two landscapes, asking about events and then inviting reflection on their meaning.

The way we think about identity (Combs & Freedman, 2016) can play a significant role in working with couples. We think about "self," or identity, not as a noun referring to a container filled with resources and deficits, but as a verb referring to a project we are pursuing in active, ongoing relationship with other people across a wide variety of contexts. We view identity as relational, distributed, performed, and fluid.

We think of identity as relational because our identities are shaped by our experience with others and our perceptions of how they perceive us. Our relationship to culture and context also shapes our sense of self.

By describing our identity as distributed we mean that we inhabit different roles in different places, and we experience ourselves differently in those different roles or contexts. Our identity is different at work than it is at home. It is different in front of a large group than when we are alone. Thinking about identity as distributed reminds us to invite different aspects of identity into different contexts in ways that may support preferred stories.

Our description of identity as performed has to do with the idea that what we actually do contributes to our identity. We become who we enact. We are all performers in each other's ongoing dramas, and we are literally making each other up moment-by-moment as we go through life.

Taken together, the descriptions of identity as relational, distributed, and performed imply that our identities are fluid. Identity is a process, not a possession. Because we are always stepping into new identities, change is impossible to avoid. The question is, "How are we changing, and according to what values, ethics, and intentions?"

Carissa and Steve's perceptions of how the other perceives them seem to have changed over time and under the influence of the problems they now face. Being able to reclaim the ways they used to know themselves through their partner's eyes may be very significant. It also might be important to explore how cultural differences have shaped their identities and for each of them to have an understanding about this from the other's perspective. If they decide to continue to pursue becoming parents, we might wonder if ways that they know themselves differently in different contexts (distributed identity) may be useful in dealing with fertility problems in a different way. And if they become parents, this will certainly impact their identities and may be something they would like to prepare for in therapy.

Another way we engage in the retelling of developing stories is through the creation of documents (e.g., Fox, 2003). The following include some types of documents and their purposes:

- THERAPY NOTES that document preferred directions in life
- LETTERS summarizing therapy conversations, extending or thickening emerging ideas and stories, and at times including people who did not attend a session
- CERTIFICATES of membership, completion, special achievements, statements of position, etc.
- LISTS (especially for children) of accomplishments, knowledge, important people or relationships, etc.
- ARTISTIC RESPONSES of all kinds, including drawings and paintings, poetry, and songs featuring words from the therapy conversation
- COLLABORATIVE DOCUMENTS sharing insider knowledge and giving people the opportunity to make contributions to others.

Case Transcript

In making up a case transcript, it is helpful to think about the therapist's social location. It is often not realistic to attempt to find a therapist who matches the location of people coming for therapy, but it does make a difference if the therapist shares certain aspects of their identity with one partner and not another. It is important to keep this in mind, and for the therapist to consider getting supervision from someone whose social location is more similar to the other partner. For example, in this transcript, the therapist is White, so it may be helpful for her to seek out a Black supervisor. It is also important that the therapist offers the possibility of a conversation about the differences, and is prepared to respond to how these differences are important to members of the couple. In this example, the therapist is a cisgender White, heterosexual woman.

Therapist: Hello! It's lovely to meet you… Is it okay if we start out by talking about some things that probably have nothing to do with why you are here?

We don't want the problem to take over the way we see members of the couple, so we want from the beginning to hear about things outside the problem. We also want to convey to couple members that we know that they are more than the problems they bring.

          (*Steve and Carissa nod*)
Therapist: I'm wondering if we could start by each of you telling me what you appreciate about each other?

Sometimes we start by simply asking each couple member questions about their lives and what they are involved in doing. If we sense great tension between couple members, we do not start by asking for appreciation of each other, but with Steve and Carissa, the therapist is hoping these questions may set a supportive tone (Marsten et al., 2016).

Steve: Okay… Carissa is a good person. She is honest and loyal. She is friendly. Everyone loves her and I know she can be fun. Also, she is responsible. She works hard.
Therapist: Carissa, what was it like hearing Steve's description of you?

The therapist is introducing the idea of each partner witnessing what the other says and is inviting Carissa to draw meaning from it.

Carissa: I wasn't expecting that. It felt good.

This is a useful response. The conversation has already entered the realm of the not-yet-said, or at least not-said-in-a-while.

Therapist: And Carissa, what do you appreciate about Steve?
Carissa: Well, I appreciate that he can surprise me, like he just did. He is also honest. He is a caring person. He never speaks badly of people behind their backs. I like him. And usually, he is flexible.
Therapist: Steve, could you say something about what it was like to hear Carissa's appreciations?
Steve: Good. I'm glad that's not all lost…
Therapist: That's got me wanting to ask why you are glad, but I think I'm going to go ahead with a question that might be a little bit harder… What do you appreciate about the relationship … Carissa?
Carissa: Well, it hasn't been so great lately. But appreciation… We have been able to keep it going even when we were apart for long periods of time. I guess it has been pretty stable. And… We are good together. We cook well together. Every couple can't say that.
Steve: And we dance well together. And in a day-to-day way, we are really compatible.
Carissa: Yeah, but it's like that seems to be falling apart. We are more talking about how it used to be.

Narrative therapists are interested, at times, in introducing other perspectives. Things may look different to the relationship than to its members.

Therapist: Okay, I am curious about the cooking and dancing, but it sounds to me like you might be wanting to talk about what brought you here. Is it okay if we do one other thing before we get to that?
             (*Steve and Carissa nod*)
Therapist: Are there any questions you would like to ask me?

This question is meant to contribute to a collaborative two-way relationship.

Carissa: What do you mean?
Steve: I don't know what we're supposed to ask.
Therapist: Well, you are deciding whether to open your life to me. There may be some things it's important to know about me as you do that.
Carissa: You came well recommended.
Therapist: Okay, but as we talk, if you have questions—even questions about why I'm asking a particular question—please feel free to ask me… And with another couple I saw recently, it was a heterosexual couple, the man wondered if he would feel ganged up on with two women in the conversation. He wanted to know how I would handle that. I don't know if questions like that would be in play for you, Carissa, with two White people being in the conversation.
Carissa: I'm used to being in a context with more White people, but I appreciate your bringing it up. It sort of gives me room to talk about race if it seems important at some point. Usually, I'm the one who has to bring it up.

Therapist: Yes, please do talk about race or about anything that makes a difference in how your relationship or our conversations are going.
Carissa: I will.

This last interchange may seem out of balance, but it is more about responding to a context that is already out of balance in our culture, with White people having built-in power and advantages simply because they are White.

Therapist: I spoke with you a little bit on the phone, Carissa, so I'll start with you, Steve. Can you tell me a little bit about what brought you here?

Narrative therapists don't have a set idea of who should speak first, but we want both members of the couple to feel connected with us, so we keep that in mind in directing questions. It is a difficult choice with a heterosexual couple because we don't want to go along with the dominant idea that the woman is in charge of maintaining the relationship, nor reinforce the dominant power relationship that gives the man more say. If we hadn't already briefly talked about possible racial dominance we may have begun with Carissa, rather than Steve.

Steve: I don't know exactly. It seems like Carissa is jumping all over me for any little thing these days. She is turning into an angry person.
Carissa: That's not fair!
Therapist: (*Turning to Carissa*) Is it okay if I talk with one of you at a time and the other listens? Then I'll ask whoever is listening about what you heard.
Carissa: But he isn't telling the whole story!
Therapist: I know that you each would describe what happens differently and that you probably think that different things are important, and Carissa, I'm going to ask Steve to listen to you just the way I'm asking you to listen to him. Is that okay?
Carissa: I guess so.

To create a witnessing position, sometimes we speak about it explicitly. It is also important to watch the witnessing partner for cues about whether they are listening, and to catch it early if they are tracking disagreements or rehearsing their next argument, rather than listening to understand.

Therapist: Can you give me an example of what you were talking about, Steve?
Steve: Well, she just criticizes everything lately—my going out with friends, chores around the house, what I'm wearing … like she's unhappy about everything.

The therapist is listening for details that might help externalize the problem, rather than locate it in Carissa. The word "lately" stands out. This cues the therapist to shift from naming the problem to asking about the absent but implicit.

Therapist: When you say "lately," does that mean it was different before?
(*Steve nods*)
Therapist: Is there something about the way it was different that you long for now?

This is an absent but implicit question which may help make clear what Steve has given value to in the past that he is missing as he compares his current relationship to what he remembers.

Steve: Yeah… absolutely. I'd say it was a fun, loving relationship. I miss that.

Therapist: This might seem like a funny question, but why do you miss that?

Steve: It was easy. It was fun. We could count on each other. We, I don't know. I felt love. Like, this is the person I want to spend my life with. But now, I sometimes feel like I don't know her and she's always mad, like I was explaining.

Therapist: Okay, I know that it's different now, but can we just stay a while with what you long for?

Steve: I guess.

Therapist: You said it was fun. You could count on each other. You wanted to spend your life together. I think you said something about love… Carissa, what is it like to hear what Steve longs for?

We are hoping that from the witnessing position Carissa will understand Steve's story and maybe even contribute to it.

Carissa: I don't know. It makes me sad that it's not that way now.

Therapist: Does the sadness speak to something you long for too?

This time the absent but implicit question is for Carissa. Often in working with couples, asking about the absent but implicit early in the therapy sets a tone that has to do with what partners value, rather than focusing on disappointment and blame.

Carissa: Well really, pretty much the same thing. But we have had some big disappointments… Maybe it's more like I have been disappointed with Steve.

Therapist: Okay, I'm hearing that the two of you are in touch with the anger and disappointments you have been experiencing recently. There will be room to talk about that, but I think it would be useful to stay with what you have said you long for before we do. Is that okay with you?

Carissa: Okay.
       (*Steve nods*)

Therapist: Can each of you say what it is like to hear that your partner longs for the same kind of relationship that you long for? Carissa?

Carissa: It's good. It is a little hard to sink into that, but it is good to hear.

Therapist: Steve?

Steve: Yeah, hopeful.

Therapist: Okay, Steve, can you hold on to that hope and that shared vision of what you long for while I talk to Carissa?

Steve: Yes, but I'm still thinking about Carissa talking about being disappointed in me and I'm wondering if that's what she's so mad about.

Therapist: Okay, if you think it would be more important to talk about the anger and disappointment than the shared longing, we can do that. Would it be important to have that conversation first?

Steve: I don't know… I guess we can go with the shared vision.

Therapist: Is there something that would help you hold on to hope while I talk with Carissa?

Steve: No, I like the idea of holding on to hope.

We now have a position not only of listening, but also of hope.

Therapist: Okay, I understand that you have had a relationship that has really given both of you fun and love and being able to count on each other. And Carissa, you have mentioned disappointments. Is it important to talk about that or is it okay if I ask you about the shared longing?

Carissa: Well, even when it was good, there have been some disappointments. That's really what I think we should talk about. Like, Steve spends weekends doing sports with his friends. I let him know that I wanted some of that weekend time. It seemed like he agreed, but it didn't change anything. I could live with that, but I guess that whole relationship we were talking about, for me, was the foundation for a family. And I know that was always more important to me than him, but it seems like he has just given up.

Therapist: Okay, so would you say that disappointment about not creating the future you were imagining is the problem here?

Carissa: Yeah, I think that is fair to say.

This marks the beginning of an externalizing conversation in which disappointment about not creating a future, rather than Steve, is the problem. The therapist had been hoping to talk with Carissa about the absent but implicit longing. This would have been a way of beginning to develop a preferred story that Steve would have witnessed and perhaps joined. But since this is a collaborative relationship, after attempting to influence the focus of the conversation, the therapist honors Carissa's preference and the focus turns to disappointment. However, disappointment is being externalized, rather than located in Steve.

Therapist: Would it be okay to talk about what some of the effects of the disappointment are? I think I heard that one is anger.

*The therapist is interested in hearing about effects of the problem, in understanding its workings in the relationship. Questions about effects are the first part of **relative influence questioning** (White, 1986) in which the effects the problem has on the person and the effects the person has on the problem are both made visible.*

Carissa: Yes. And worry too about the uncertainty of the future and whether we can make it work.

Therapist: Okay, disappointment leads to worry and uncertainty about the future. Would you say that it also lets blame into the picture?

Carissa: Yeah, I guess so.

Therapist: How do you think that works? Where does blame come from?

*This is the beginning of a **deconstruction conversation** that continues over the next several exchanges. The intent is to unpack the problem, showing how it was constructed. This holds the possibility of making discourses that contribute to the problem visible.*

Carissa: I'm not really sure.

Therapist: Well, you have talked about the future, and the foundation of a family. Where do you think your vision of that comes from?

Carissa: I've always seen myself as a mother and having a family.

Therapist: I'm not saying that's not a wonderful role to have in the world, but I'm curious about where that vision comes from for you.

Carissa: Of course, that's the usual path of life … and so many of our friends are having children now.

Therapist: So, would you say that comparisons feed the problem?

Carissa: I'm not exactly sure what you are saying.

Therapist: Well … if you weren't around friends having children and families, do you think the disappointment would be less?

In beginning to expose a discourse that includes the idea of children, the therapist is not intending to change Carissa's mind about having children. The intent is to invite a position from which Carissa can decide on the kind of relationship she wants to have with the discourse, rather than taking it for granted as the only way.

Carissa: It's funny to think about it that way, but yes, I do think it would be less… But I do want to have children.

Therapist: Yeah, I'm focusing on the experience of disappointment, not whether to have children. And I'm just wondering what the disappointment keeps you from appreciating about your relationship or about Steve.

After a brief glimpse of a discourse that may be at play, the therapist is continuing to ask about the effects of the problem.

Carissa: Hmmm. Well, even though Steve would be okay not having children, he has gone to infertility treatment for a couple of years and been right there with me through it until recently. It's hard to stay in touch with that since he has stopped wanting to do it.

The therapist hears what may be a unique outcome, "he has gone to infertility treatment for a couple of years and been right there with me through it…"

Therapist: So, he has been right there with you through it! What does that say about him?

As the possible unique outcome may be an opening to a preferred story, the therapist asks more about it in the landscape of identity or meaning.

Carissa: He's loyal. He's strong. He cares about me.

Carissa is now in touch with these aspects of Steve's identity.

Therapist: Can you tell me about a time, maybe one that didn't have anything to do with trying to have children, that showed Steve's loyalty, strength, and care about you?

This question invites Carissa to expand the story that is developing through time by connecting it with a past event. It also holds the possibility of helping her step into and re-experience that past event.

Carissa: Well, when Steve graduated, he was offered quite a good job, but it was in Charlotte. He took a job in Orlando because it was only about two hours away from Gainesville, where I was going to school. He drove to see me almost every weekend. There were times I could see that he was tired and times he had to work on the weekend, and times I could see that if he stayed and socialized with the guys at his company, he might get ahead. Instead, he spent almost every weekend with me. And he was so obviously happy when he arrived in Gainesville, and he stretched the time to the very last minute… I knew I could count on him and that he loved me.

Therapist: What was it about that year that told you that you could count on Steve and that he loved you?

This question invites Carissa to become further experientially involved in the retelling.

Carissa: Well, just that he did it … but also the way he looked at me when he arrived, and when he didn't want to leave.
Therapist: How did he look at you?
Carissa: Oh, it's hard to describe, but I could just feel that he really wanted to be right there with me.
Therapist: Right there with you… How did all this time together happen when you were living in different places? Did you plan it together?

These questions facilitate thickening the story.

Carissa: When Steve got the job offer in Charlotte, he told me about it, and he said that he didn't want to be that far away from me. And I didn't want him to be that far away either. So when he took the job in Orlando that was not as good a job, that meant a lot to me… And he told me that he was taking it to be near me, so I knew we would see each other—but I didn't know that it would be almost every weekend. It became clear that we both wanted to see each other as often as we could.
Therapist: How did it become clear?
Carissa: (*Chuckles*) We both hinted about it, and then one evening early on in that year we had been to this little Italian restaurant, and we were sharing a dessert; seeing each other by candlelight, and Steve said, "This is good." I knew he meant me, not the tiramisu, and I was feeling so moved I couldn't speak, so I reached my hand across the table, and we sat looking into each other's eyes.

There is a stillness in the room. Carissa is re-experiencing this important moment. The therapist has been watching Steve and thinks that he may have been too. Now the therapist would like to offer the possibility for Steve to more actively join in this preferred story.

Therapist: That started out as a story about Steve but ended up being about both of you. Is it okay if I talk to Steve about that?
(*Carissa nods*)
Therapist: Steve, what was it like to hear Carissa talk about how you were loyal and strong and that she could count on you?
Steve: (*A little teary*) It was pretty wonderful.
Therapist: Did you know that she saw you this way?
Steve: Not exactly, and definitely not recently.
Therapist: What is it like to see yourself through her eyes, the way she saw you that she was just describing?
Steve: Pretty wonderful, yeah.
Therapist: If you had to put a name to the relationship in that moment that Carissa was describing, what would you call it?
Steve: Love and persistence.
Therapist: Love and persistence… And what would you say Carissa contributed to that?
Steve: I'm sort of surprised about what comes to mind… Carissa has a great family… They are really close, and they've been wonderful to me. My family is more fractured, you could say. Especially my father; he hasn't been welcoming at all. Even my mom… She's been

accepting, but not like Carissa's parents who have made me feel like part of the family. But Carissa … she has always been up for seeing my family and being positive around them and not saying anything negative about them. I think that's love and persistence.

Therapist: What has it meant to you that Carissa is always positive and willing to see your family?

This is another question in the landscape of meaning. It provides an opportunity for Carissa to hear what meaning Steve attributes to her actions.

Steve: That we are a team; that she gets it that my family isn't what I'd wish for, but they're my family. That I can count on her.

Therapist: Carissa…

Carissa: You've never said that to me.

Therapist: (*To Carissa*) What is it like hearing Steve describe this now for the first time?

Carissa: Wow! I'm glad he feels that way… I've really tried with his family, and hearing this makes it worthwhile. And maybe I'm more interested in children because of my family, and he's less interested because of his…

Steve: It's just that it has been messing us up financially, and personally too.

Therapist: Okay… Clearly there have been disappointments between you and misunderstandings, and it may be important to talk about them more. I can hear that right now you are both seeing some of the problems in a different light, and I would guess that is important. We don't have a lot of time left today. Would it be okay if we stay with the conversation about the relationship that you long for?
(*Both nod*)

Therapist: I'm wondering what stands out for you. Carissa?

Carissa: That Steve has appreciated how I've been with his family. That he knew it wasn't easy. And that he sees us as a team… And, also … that year when we lived two hours apart but saw each other almost every weekend … and the night over candlelight in the restaurant.

Therapist: And what about for you, Steve?

Steve: This conversation didn't go like I expected it to at all! I was afraid to talk about my family, but it made things better, not worse! I guess what stands out to me is our history. We have a pretty amazing history.

Therapist: Was this conversation helpful?
(*Talking at the same time*) Yes, it was.

Therapist: Would you like to come again?

Carissa: Yes.

Steve: Yes.

Therapist: Okay, when would you like to come back?

Carissa: Isn't this a once-a-week thing?

Therapist: I've found that sometimes as time is up, we are in the middle of talking about something, and it would be helpful to come back really soon to continue the conversation. Other times when something significant has come from the conversation people want to sit with it for a while before talking again. Some couples are involved in so many things that if we schedule once a week, they may have hardly seen each other. So, of course, if your schedules require it, we can find a regular time, but if we can, I like to ask each time when it would be good to talk again.

Steve: Well, I think we are in a different place, but we still have some big decisions, so I think soon.

Carissa: Yeah, soon.

Setting appointments this way fits with a decentered position.

Therapist: I would like to send you a letter that I hope captures some of what we talked about today. Would that be okay?
Carissa: Great!
            (*Steve nods*)

The therapist sends the following letter:

Dear Carissa and Steve,

It was lovely to meet you and hear about your lives and relationships. I am sending you some notes of my impressions. If I get anything wrong, please let me know when we talk again. And I'd also be curious about your answers to any of my questions.

My understanding is that some arguing and disappointments have recently entered your life. Even though these problems have begun to take over your relationship, it became clear that you both have a longing for the way you have experienced each other and your relationship in the past. How does it make a difference to know that you both have this longing?

Steve, you said that it was a fun, loving relationship and you knew that you wanted to spend your life together. You said that you were a team. You appreciated how Carissa is willing to spend time with your family and how she is always positive when she does.

Carissa, you agreed that you have had a fun, loving relationship. You spoke about Steve's loyalty, strength, and caring about you.

Do you think it would be helpful to claim these descriptions and hold on to them even when there are disagreements about the future that could lead to anger or disappointment?

You have spoken about being good together—cooking and dancing. I'm curious about the skills that go into being good together in these ways. Maybe we can talk about that next time.

Looking forward to seeing you again,

Your Therapist

The therapist is using this letter to offer another retelling of the developing story, being careful to let the couple be in charge (tell me if I get anything wrong) and wanting to offer the possibility of extending the stories already told through additional questions.

Note

1 Susan Munro, White and Epston's editor at W.W. Norton for *Narrative Means to Therapeutic Ends* and other works has suggested that this naming was a response to the book title. (personal communication)

References

Bateson, G. (1972). *Steps to an ecology of mind*. Ballantine.
Bateson, G. (1979). *Mind and nature: A necessary unity*. Dutton.
Bruner, J. (1986). *Actual minds/possible worlds*. Harvard University Press.
Bruner, J. (1990). *Acts of meaning*. Harvard University Press.
Bruner, J. (1991). The narrative construction of reality. *Critical Inquiry, 18*(1), 1–21.
Combs, G., & Freedman, J. (2016). Narrative therapy's relational understanding of identity. *Family Process, 55*(2), 211–224.
Denborough, D. (2008). *Collective narrative practice: Responding to individuals, groups, and communities who have experienced trauma*. Dulwich Centre Publications.
Derrida, J. (1988). *Limited, inc*. University of Illinois Press.

Epston, D. (1999). Co-research: The making of an alternative knowledge. In P. Moss (Ed.), *Narrative therapy and community work: A conference collection* (pp. 137–157). Dulwich Centre Publications.

Foucault, M. (1965). *Madness and civilization: A history of insanity in the age of reason* (R. Howard, Trans.). Random House.

Foucault, M. (1975). *The birth of the clinic: An archeology of medical perception* (A. M. Sheridan Smith, Trans.). Random House.

Foucault, M. (1977). *Discipline and punish: The birth of the prison* (A. Sheridan, Trans.). Pantheon Books.

Foucault, M. (1980). *Power/knowledge: Selected interviews and other writings, 1972–1977*. Pantheon Books.

Foucault, M. (1988). The political technology of individuals. In L. Martin, H. Gutman & P. P. Hutton (Eds.), *Technologies of the self* (pp. 14–162). University of Massachusetts Press.

Fox, H. (2003). Using therapeutic documents: A review. *International Journal of Narrative Therapy and Community Work, 4*, 25–35.

Freedman, J. (2014). Witnessing and positioning: Structuring narrative therapy with families and couples. *Australian and New Zealand Journal of Family Therapy, 35,* 20–30.

Freedman, J., & Combs, G. (1993). Invitations to new stories: Using questions to explore alternative possibilities. In S. Gilligan & R. Price (Eds.), *Therapeutic conversations* (pp. 291–303). Norton.

Geertz, C. (1983). *Local knowledge: Further essays in interpretive anthropology*. Basic Books.

Geertz, C. (1986). Making experiences, authoring selves. In V. W. Turner & E.M. Bruner (Eds.), *The anthropology of experience* (pp. 373–380). University of Illinois Press.

Goffman, E. (1961). *Asylums: Essays on the social situation of mental patients and other inmates*. Doubleday.

Hare-Mustin, R. (1994). Discourses in the mirrored room: A postmodern analysis of therapy. *Family Process, 33,* 19–35.

Kalisa, J., Mukarusanga, B., & Nyirinkwaya, S. (Eds.). (2022). *Land of a thousand stories: Rwandan narrative therapy and community work.* Dulwich Centre Foundation.

Marsten, D., Epston, D., & Markham, L. (2016). *Narrative therapy in wonderland: Connecting with children's imaginative know-how.* Norton.

Myerhoff, B. (1986). "Life not death in Venice": Its second life. In V. W. Turner & E. M. Bruner (Eds.), *The anthropology of experience* (pp. 261–286). University of Illinois Press.

Ncube, N. (2006). The Tree of Life Project: Using narrative ideas in work with vulnerable children in Southern Africa. *International Journal of Narrative Therapy and Community Work, 1,* 3–16.

Olinger, C. (2010). Privileging insider-knowledges in the world of autism. *International Journal of Narrative Therapy and Community Work, 2,* 37–50.

Reynolds, V., & Hammoud-Beckett, S. (2018). Social justice activism and therapy: Tensions, points of connection, and hopeful skepticism. In C. Audet & D. Pare (Eds.), *Social justice and counseling: Discourses in practice* (pp. 3–15). Routledge.

Wade, A. (1997). Small acts of living: Everyday resistance to violence and other forms of oppression. *Contemporary Family Therapy, 19*(1), 23–39. (Also appears in French in *Thérapie familiale*, Genève, 1999, Vol. 20, No. 4, pp. 425–438.)

Wade, A. (2002). From a language of effects to responses: Honouring our clients' resistance to violence. *New Therapist*, September/October, 14–17.

Waldegrave, C., Tamasese, K., Tuhaka, F., & Campbell, W. (Eds.). (2003). *Just therapy—A journey: A collection of papers from the Just Therapy Team*. Dulwich Centre Publications.

White, C. (2016). *A memory book for the field of narrative practice.* Dulwich Centre PTY LTD.

White, M. (1986). Negative explanation, restraint and double description: A template for family therapy. *Family Process, 25*(2), 169–184.

White, M. (1997). *Narratives of therapists' lives*. Dulwich Centre Publications.

White, M. (2002). Addressing personal failure. *The International Journal of Narrative Therapy and Community Work, 3,* 33–76.

White, M. (2003). Narrative practice and community assignments. *The International Journal of Narrative Therapy and Community Work, 2,* 17–55.

White, M. (2007). *Maps of narrative practice*. W. W. Norton.

White, M. (2011). *Narrative practice. Continuing the conversations*. (D. Denborough, Ed.) W. W. Norton.

White, M., & Epston, D. (1990). *Narrative means to therapeutic ends.* Norton.

White, M., & Epston, D. (1992). *Experience, contradiction, narrative & imagination: Selected papers of David Epston & Michael White, 1989–1991.* Dulwich Centre Publications.

Wingard, B, Johnson, C., & Drahm-Butler, T. (2015). *Aboriginal narrative practice: Honouring storylines of pride, strength and creativity.* Dulwich Centre Publications.

Wingard, B., & Lester, J. (Eds.). (2001). *Telling our stories in ways that make us stronger.* Dulwich Centre Publications.

Yuen, A. (2009). Less pain, more gain: Exploration of responses versus effects when working with the consequences of trauma. *Explorations: An E-Journal of Narrative Practice, 1,* 6–16.

13 Choice Theory and Reality Therapy Couples Counseling

Patricia A. Robey

"Dr. Glasser's therapy is based on inescapable truths: Meaningful relationships are central to the good life, the choice we make will determine their quality, and we can create them only if we take responsibility for ourselves without controlling other people" (Breggin, in Foreword, Glasser, 2000, p. xiii.).

History of the Model

William Glasser, M.D., was a psychiatrist who was trained to work with clients from a psychoanalytic perspective. However, in response to his experiences in practice, including work in a correctional institute for young women and with patients in a mental hospital, Glasser concluded that a different understanding of what causes psychological problems was needed. Essentially, Glasser proposed that individuals have needs that are unmet, and their problems are based on their inability to get their needs met in ways that do not deprive others of their ability to meet their own needs.

In his book *Reality Therapy: A New Approach to Psychiatry*, Glasser (1965) explained the reality therapy process as having three interwoven procedures, beginning with involvement, then working with clients to face reality and see how their current behavior is unrealistic, and finally, teaching clients to find more effective ways to fulfill their needs. Involvement requires the use of counseling skills to create an environment in which clients feel safe and confident that the therapist is working from a collaborative perspective. As part of this process, the therapist helps clients understand that they have basic needs and that their behavior is motivated and put into action as their best attempts to get their needs met. Therapists take on a non-judgmental stance, in which they help clients accept responsibility for their behavior without feeling criticized by the therapist. Although therapists using reality therapy recognize the significance of past experiences, the process is generally oriented to the present, which is where clients have the opportunity to make changes that will help them meet their needs in more responsible ways. Within this caring environment, clients can meet their need for connection to others which also leads to the development of self-worth.

In 1985, based on William Powers' (1973) explanation of internal control and Glasser's understanding of human behavior, Glasser published his book *Control Theory: A New Explanation of How We Control Our Lives* (1985). Powers' book provided an explanation of control theory, which was based on cybernetic theory (Wiener, 1948). Powers hypothesized that human behavior originates within a person rather than being caused by external events. Glasser elaborated on Powers' work, specifically in Glasser's explanation that our behavior is determined by our perception of events and how we act in response to our perceptions. For example, the statement, "Rainy days are depressing," gives power to the rainy day as if it could create depression. If rainy days really had this power, everyone would feel depressed on a rainy day. Instead, the statement, "It's a rainy day and I feel depressed," links the reality of the day as being rainy to the internal perception that the individual associates with it and the feeling that the individual assumes on that day.

DOI: 10.4324/9781003369097-13

As Glasser continued to focus more sharply on behavior as a choice that is based on meeting five human needs, he changed the name of his theory from control theory to choice theory and introduced his book *Choice Theory: A New Psychology of Personal Freedom* (1998). Choice theory became the guiding theory that supported the reality therapy process. Building on the framework of reality therapy, choice theory explained Glasser's view of human nature and explained human behavior and motivation. The integration of choice theory in counseling has now become part of the reality therapy process, as explained in Glasser's book *Counseling with Choice Theory: The New Reality Therapy* (2000).

Concepts of Choice Theory

Basic Human Needs

Glasser (1998) proposed that human beings are motivated by five genetic and universal basic needs. Unlike a hierarchy of needs, Glasser's theory proposes that the significance and importance we attach to these basic needs is innate and unique to everyone, and how we define the meaning we attach to them is also unique. For example, the basic need for **survival** can be described as the motivation to continue living through activation of bodily functions, but can also be described in the context of interpersonal and social implications. In this sense, it can be described as including sexual activity, safety, and security. Other needs include: **love and belonging**, experienced as the need for connection with others and self; **power**, which is often felt as a need for achievement, inner control, personal significance, or self-worth; **freedom**, the desire for independence, autonomy, and the ability to make choices; and **fun**, a sense of enjoyment, playfulness, or learning.

Quality World

We meet our needs through very specific people, places, things, values, and beliefs. Over our lives, we develop these ideals and store them in our memory in what Glasser (1998) referred to as our **Quality World**. In any moment, we are trying to get our needs met through the attainment of the quality world picture that is most significant at that time. It is important to note that quality world pictures are ideals; they may be unattainable or unrealistic, but we still want them. For example, in relationships, we often have an idealized "perfect" picture of the person we want to spend our lives with. It is unlikely that one person could meet all the criteria of perfection. In these cases, it is important to remember that these pictures meet basic needs, so we can accept a "less than perfect" partner and still get our needs met in other ways.

Quality world pictures may also conflict with one another. For example, you might want to go to Europe on a vacation (fun and freedom), but you also want to buy a new car (survival or power). You don't have money for both. In this case, you can identify what need(s) you are trying to meet in either case and find a way to negotiate a win-win solution; for example, you might buy a used car and go on a weekend trip to a spa.

Quality world pictures are developed over time and through experiences that make a person, place, thing, value, or belief significant and need-satisfying. The criteria for significance are that the picture satisfies one or more of the basic needs, and there is usually a level of emotion attached to the attainment of the want that the picture represents. Because of this attachment, it is not easy to change our own pictures. This is significant when considering our interactions with others and how the idealized images of the perfect relationship influence our success in relationships. It's important to realize that, although we are reluctant and unlikely to change an idealized picture, we can make the choice to add a related picture that is more reasonable and attainable. We also must accept that we cannot change anyone other than ourselves, so to be successful in getting our needs met in relationships we need to utilize negotiation and compromise with our partners.

Perceived World

Not everything we experience is significant enough to become a picture in our quality world. Most often what we experience is stored as a perception in what Glasser (1998) referred to as our **perceived world**. In any given moment, we compare our perception of what we think is happening in the "real world" with what we want (our quality world picture in that moment). As a result of the comparison of what we want versus what we perceive we have, we are motivated to take action for change or to maintain what we have through our choice of behavior.

Total Behavior

Choice theory proposes a unique view of behavior. Glasser (1998) explained behavior as **total behavior**, which consists of four components that are all in play at one time: *acting*, *thinking*, *feeling*, and *physiology*. For example, if I am feeling depressed, I am thinking depressed, acting depressed, and my physiology is depressed. We often are most aware of our feelings and physiology, which provide information and alert us to evaluate if we are doing well or if something needs attention. However, we have the most control over our acting and thinking, so these are the components of total behavior we must recognize as associated with the feelings and physiology that are calling for attention. We need to address our acting and thinking to change feelings and physiology.

Glasser (1998) discussed total behavior as a system that includes creativity and reorganization. Over time, we develop behaviors that we use repeatedly and that may be more or less successful in their application. For example, if you've ever lost your keys, you look for where you usually find them, and if they aren't there you look elsewhere, but you may continue to look for them where they should be with the possibility that you might have missed them the first time you looked. Sometimes this works! This is what Glasser would define as organized behavior. Creative behavior can be described as something that you have not previously put into action, but you now choose as a way of doing something different to solve the problem. For example, you might look for your keys in the refrigerator! Creative and reorganized behavior is our system's attempt to take information and behaviors that we already know and have found useful and combine them into new behaviors that could be used as needed to regain control over our lives. For example, if you found the keys in the refrigerator, you are likely to look for the keys there again the next time you lose them.

All Behavior Has Purpose

The concepts of basic needs, quality world, perceived world, and total behavior work together to provide a systemic picture of human behavior and motivation. We are constantly motivated to get what we want (our quality world pictures) to meet one or more of our basic needs (love and belonging, power, freedom, fun, survival). We consistently compare our perceptions of what we believe we have to what we want, and our behavior is motivated to maintain what we are doing if our needs are being satisfied, or to make new behavioral choices if our needs are not being met. In summary, *all behavior is purposeful—to act on the world, to get what we want, which satisfies one or more of our basic needs.*

The 10 Axioms of Choice Theory

1   The only person whose behavior we can control is our own.
2   All we can give or get from other people is information. How we deal with that information is our or their choice.

3   All long-lasting psychological problems are relationship problems.
4   The problem relationship is always part of our present lives.
5   What happened in the past that was painful has a great deal to do with what we are today, but revisiting this painful past can contribute little or nothing to what we need to do now: improve an important, present relationship.
6   We are driven by five genetic needs: survival, love and belonging, power, freedom, and fun.
7   We can satisfy these needs only by satisfying a picture or pictures in our quality worlds. Of all we know, what we choose to put into our quality worlds is the most important.
8   All we can do from birth to death is behave. All behavior is total behavior and is made up of four inseparable components: acting, thinking, feeling, and physiology.
9   All total behavior is designated by verbs, usually infinitives and gerunds, and named by the component that is most recognizable. For example, I am choosing to depress or I am depressing instead of I am suffering from depression or I am depressed.
10   All behavior is chosen, but we have direct control over only the acting and thinking components. We can, however, control our feelings and physiology indirectly through how we choose to act and think.

(Glasser, 1998, pp. 332–336)

Conceptualization of Problem Formation

In his book *Choice Theory* (1998), Glasser explained that the difficulty we have with relationships is that we are trying to control others in an effort to get what we want. Based on a worldwide belief in the efficacy of external control, we have learned to focus on trying to change people through reward and punishment when dealing with problems, instead of thinking how we can change the systems that support this behavior.

Glasser defined four variations of external controlling behaviors that are common in relationships:

1   You are trying to force someone to do what you want them to do regardless of whether they want to do it;
2   Someone else is trying to force you to do something you don't want to do;
3   Both you and someone else are trying to make each other do what neither of you want to do;
4   You are trying to force yourself to do something you found painful or even impossible to do.

(Glasser, 1998, pp. 13–14)

Another reason relationships fail is because the pictures in the partners' quality worlds are incompatible. When counseling with choice theory, we understand that all people have basic needs and are motivated to meet these needs through very specific people, places, things, values, and beliefs that are represented by mental pictures and memories stored in their quality worlds. Our behavior is chosen in an effort to get our wants, which in turn, satisfies one or more of our basic needs.

Life might be easier, but maybe less interesting, if we all shared the same pictures of what we want, and all had the same needs profile. However, that's not usually the case. In fact, it seems that we often choose partners whom we believe will fill a gap in our lives that we can't fill on our own. For example, consider the case of Steve and Carissa. Both showed high needs for love and belonging, and connection with others, as evidenced by their close family attachments, and their early behavior in the courting period of their relationship. While Carissa was in school, however, the couple's primary focus changed from intimacy with one another to developing friendships outside of their relationship. Carissa developed friendships at school and Steve made friends at work. As a result of this behavior, the disconnect in their pictures of a quality relationship became obvious when Carissa graduated. Once Carissa no longer had schoolwork and friends at school to occupy her weekends, her picture of a quality relationship shifted back to the kind of relationship she valued with Steve, which was high in behaviors that represented love and belonging. To Carissa, this meant spending more time with him, cooking and eating together, exercising, and watching shows together like they had in the past. In contrast, Steve's picture of a quality relationship appeared to minimize intimacy and, instead, reflected his need for freedom and fun. On the weekends, Steve engaged in activities with his friends instead of making the time for Carissa that she wanted.

The contrast in their pictures of what makes a quality relationship was heightened by the issue of having children. Carissa's need for love and belonging included children and she was highly motivated to meet that need. Steve supported Carissa in this goal, even though his picture of a quality family relationship did not have a strong focus on children. Eventually, Carissa's inability to become pregnant and the pressure that this put on the marriage took a toll on the relationship. Steve, who had a higher need for safety and security than Carissa had, began to push back on the fertility treatments because his focus was on maintaining a secure financial position.

As they each tried to get their needs met in the relationship, Carissa and Steve both began to use disconnecting behaviors in an effort to control one another. They developed values and beliefs about what the relationship should look like and how to manage problems from what they observed from their parents and the conclusions they drew about what makes a good relationship.

We develop our quality world pictures regarding relationships through our experiences in life. Sometimes our ideal relationship pictures are created in opposition to what we observed that we never wanted for ourselves. For example, Steve observed the discord between his parents, who argued in front of the children as well as behind closed doors. This discord eventually resulted in his parents' divorce when he was 10 years old. After the divorce, he didn't see his father often as his father had moved an hour away from where they lived. We might hypothesize that Steve has a picture in his quality world of a good relationship as having no conflict and no arguing. He may believe that if he had that type of relationship, he would feel loved, safe, and comfortable. When he experiences conflict in his relationship with Carissa, after engaging in arguments again and again, he chooses to withdraw in times of trouble and spends time with his friends rather than dealing with Carissa to solve the conflict.

Carissa's picture of a quality relationship was developed differently. Although Carissa was 10 years old when her father moved out of the house for two weeks, she didn't know that there was a problem until years later when she learned that he had cheated on her mother. Her experience was that after the two-week separation, which she did not perceive as a troubling event, her parents were together again, and they are currently still married. Here, we could hypothesize that Carissa's picture of a good relationship is one in which partners can have problems but are able to work them out, as evidenced by what she saw with her parents. However, instead of behaving in the way that was modeled by her parents, because Steve is withdrawing instead of negotiating to solve the problem, Carissa has tapped into her creative system and is trying new behaviors. Unfortunately, the behaviors she is currently putting into action in her relationship with Steve reflect her effort to control the situation through arguing, which has resulted in an escalation of the problem.

What we see in Steve and Carissa's relationship is their attempt to control the situation and one another through disconnecting behaviors that people often use in an effort to get what they want. Glasser (1998) identified some of these disconnecting behaviors as criticizing, blaming, complaining, nagging, threatening, punishing, and bribing or rewarding in an attempt to control. We tend to use these behaviors because this is what we've experienced in our own lives. They often seem to work, as evidenced by changes we have made in response to them, and as evidenced by changes we observe in the person on whom we have used the behaviors. However, anyone who has been on the receiving end of these behaviors is likely to agree that, although they may make some changes in response to these behaviors, in the long run, they do not tend to improve their relationship with the person who is using the behavior.

In the case of Steve and Carissa, the coercive behavior they admit to using is to argue with one another in an effort to get what they want in the relationship. They admit that it hasn't worked but they continue to do it, as evidenced by the fact that the arguing has been steadily increasing over the last two years. They continue to use this behavior because they don't have a clear idea of what to do instead. They are each trying to control and change the other through ongoing arguments in which they continue to maintain their differing perspectives.

The use of external control and coercive behaviors has escalated as Carissa has been unable to become pregnant and Steve is at the point where he wants them to stop trying. The tension around this situation has intensified and they now find that they snipe at each other more often about what seem like inconsequential items.

From a choice theory perspective, we know that couples often request therapy because they are unable to satisfy their need for love and connection in their relationship. Regardless of the specifics of the problem, the therapist begins by creating an environment that is nurturing and explores their current interactions to get a clear picture of how they treat one another. The therapist models behavior that is conducive to helping clients get their need for connection in the therapeutic relationship. This provides an example of how the couple can use behaviors that will result in less coercion and more effective communication. Among these effective behaviors are listening, supporting, encouraging, respecting, accepting, and negotiating differences (Glasser, 1998).

It is likely that a couple who is not experiencing love and belonging in their relationship is also not getting their other needs met. For example, it is not unusual for the therapist to notice that couples often feel powerless or insignificant in their relationship and are trying to meet this need by attempting to control their partner. This power struggle is often at the source of relationship conflicts. Their sense of freedom and autonomy and opportunities for fun are hampered by attempts to control one another, which often is perceived by the receiver as feeling trapped and victimized. All of this has impact on basic survival needs, which may be reflected in total behavior that includes acting, thinking, and feeling sadness, loneliness, hopelessness, and the accompanying physiological symptoms associated with those segments of total behavior.

A needs assessment is often an effective technique that serves the purpose of identifying areas of compatibility or concern in a couple's relationship. It also provides an opportunity to initiate a conversation about each person's specific pictures of how they want to get their needs met. The therapist explains the concept that we all have needs for love and belonging, power, freedom, fun, and survival, and then asks clients to rate the importance of those needs in their lives, on a scale of one to five, with five being high importance, three being average importance, and one being low importance. In the case of Steve and Carissa, for example, we might anticipate the needs assessment to look like Table 13.1.

After each partner privately rates their perception of their need bases, the therapist explains that the difference in their ratings doesn't mean that their relationship is at risk. The purpose of this assessment is to open a conversation about how each person is motivated and to provide a starting place to negotiate any differences.

Table 13.1 Choice Theory needs assessment for Steve and Carissa

Need	Love & belonging	Power	Freedom	Fun	Survival
Carissa	5	4	2	3	4
Steve	3	2	4	4	4

In the case of Carissa and Steve, we can see that they differ in most areas, most significantly in their rating of love and belonging. Carissa is highly motivated for connection with Steve and others in her life. We see this in the intensity of her relationships with her family, her desire to spend a lot of time with Steve, and her wish for children. Steve rates himself as having an average need for love and belonging, which is influenced by his higher need for freedom and fun. This is evidenced by his desire to spend time with Carissa, but also to be free to spend time outside the relationship with his friends and engage in activities like sports. Carissa, on the other hand, has a lower-than-average need for freedom and an average need for fun. Her above-average need for power is evidenced by her pursuit of her education and her important work as an accountant. Because she has a lower need for freedom and fun in her life, she can focus on meeting her higher needs for power and belonging.

When looking at the challenges this couple might face, it's also interesting to note the difference between the need for power in the couple. In this case, Carissa, with the higher power need, is likely to want to control Steve and be sure everything in their relationship is in order. Steve, with his high needs for freedom and fun, is likely to resist Carissa's control.

It is notable that Carissa and Steve both scored above average at a level four for survival. At first glance, this looks compatible, but when discussing this need, it becomes evident that the quality world pictures—what it means to each person to satisfy this need—are different, which can result in conflict. For example, Carissa describes survival as being healthy and having children to carry on her family legacy. Steve describes survival as having financial security, safety, and comfort, knowing that he has shelter and can feel confident that he will never lack for food or the necessities in life.

The therapist uses the assessment to point out the areas of difference in their needs and how this has influenced their relationship and their behavior. In their attempt to meet their individual needs, Steve and Carissa have been choosing ineffective behaviors in an effort to control one another and get what they want. Of the behaviors Glasser (1998) identified as disconnecting (i.e., criticizing, blaming, complaining, nagging, threatening, punishing, and bribing or rewarding in an attempt to control), we see that Carissa has been *complaining* that Steve is away from home too much, *nagging* him to help with the chores at home, *criticizing* his behavior with his friends, *blaming* him for the tension in their relationship that has influenced her ability to get pregnant, *criticizing* him for his inability to provide financially for fertility treatments, and *threatening* divorce. Steve has been *complaining* about Carissa's nagging, *punishing* her by leaving her to be with his friends, and *blaming* her for creating an environment in which he can't feel relaxed and important. It is evident that these behaviors are not helping them resolve their problems, and, in fact, they are growing further apart as evidenced by the fact that they have not yet had an open conversation about their growing tension. Neither understands how the other is feeling and thinking, and both think their position is the right one.

Carissa is wondering whether she made a mistake in marrying Steve. She has contemplated divorce, thinking that it would be easier to do it now before they have a child. Steve thinks he is being a good husband and that the only problem they have is that Carissa is becoming more out of control. Finally, after an intense argument, they both agreed that they would give couples therapy a try since neither was happy with how things currently are in their relationship. Ironically, they finally reached an area of agreement for addressing their concerns. They both agreed they were unhappy and they both wanted to go to therapy.

Conceptualizing Diversity

Reality therapy is an established form of therapy that initially began as a practice used primarily in the United States but is now being taught globally, along with choice theory, to therapists and other professionals and to individuals interested in personal growth. In 2013, William Glasser

International (WGI) was formed and included an international board that represented many of the countries in which choice theory and reality therapy have been taught and put into practice. Training in Glasser's work has been offered in 35 countries around the world (www.wglasserintern ational.org/wgi/who-we-are/).

The commitment to diversity and multiculturalism is evident in the WGI mission statement, which includes the words, "We operate through Member Organizations around the world offering culturally respectful training & innovative initiatives." WGI also states that "We accept and uphold Choice Theory psychology as an explanation of human behavior, mental health, happiness, and personal wellbeing. WGI is international in nature, representing the Choice Theory psychology movements around the world," and "We accept and uphold the United Nations Universal Declaration of Human Rights" (www.wglasserinternational.org/wgi/who-we-are/).

The process of therapy with choice theory and reality therapy is useful across cultures because it does not impose values and beliefs on clients. Choice theory is Glasser's attempt to understand human behavior and motivation through the concepts of basic needs, quality world pictures, and total behavior, but those needs, pictures, and behaviors are understood to be unique to everyone. The relational focus of this approach allows for all participants to engage in a process that promotes mutual understanding and appreciation for another's point of view. For example, the respectful exploration of the quality world allows clients to share their unique worldviews through their own cultural lenses. Therapists recognize that clients are the experts on their own quality worlds and how they meet their basic needs in relationship to their cultural values and beliefs is respected by the therapist.

Wubbolding (2017) noted that through the facilitation of self-evaluation, clients determine the effectiveness of their behavior and their readiness to make change. The relevance of self-evaluation to diversity and multiculturalism is its acknowledgement that motivation is internal and behavior is chosen in an effort to meet needs and wants with consideration for cultural norms and ideals. As part of the self-evaluation process, therapists encourage clients to compare the effectiveness of their behavior with the values and beliefs of the culture in which they live.

Clients can be taught the ideas of choice theory and can implement them in only a few sessions, which can be useful in settings in which resources, culture, economic status, location, time, and other situational factors may limit clients' access to therapy (Wubbolding, 2000, 2011, 2019). Culturally competent therapists modify their work with their clients as required to meet the needs required from diverse populations (Arredondo et al., 1996; Haskins & Appling, 2017; Wubbolding, 2000).

Choice theory is the underlying theoretical construct that supports the reality therapy process (Glasser, 2000). Notably, choice theory does not ignore the influence of external events over which people have little or no control. Through exploration of their client's quality world, therapists embrace differences, listen without judgment, and accept the reality of the client's experience. Therapists understand that a client's underlying problems lie in difficulty in their relationships (Glasser, 1998). Therefore, when working with couples, therapists recognize that each person's behavior is motivated to get their needs met in a way to deal with external situations that are out of their control (Glasser, 2000; Haskins & Appling, 2017; Wubbolding, 2000.) Therapists empathize with clients as they deal with the circumstances that limit their choices, and then work to empower clients to manage their responses to environmental constraints (Wubbolding, 2000, 2011; Wubbolding & Brickell, 2015).

Negotiating Diversity Differences in a Couple Relationship (The Case of Steve and Carissa Hogarth)

According to Glasser's model of Choice Theory (1998), we are motivated to get our needs met through the specific people, places, things, values, and beliefs that are important to us, which he referred to as *quality world* pictures. We develop these pictures through our interactions with significant people and events in our lives which provide information that we evaluate as important or unimportant. Included in these are ideas relevant to cultural values and beliefs. Relationships struggle when one or both persons in a relationship attempt to control the other or when the pictures in their quality worlds are incompatible (Wubbolding & Robey, 2012).

Steve and Carissa came to their relationship with quality world pictures that each had developed over time, based on family, community, and external information that shaped their views. Among these were cultural values related to what it meant to be a White cisgender male and what it meant to be a Black cisgender female in the South, and, what it meant to be a bi-racial couple. Judgments, challenges, disapproval, and conflicts can come from family, friends, and the community (Bustamante et al., 2011). In this case, both Steve and Carissa were concerned about the reaction of their families to their relationship.

Steve's Family History

A review of Steve's history shows the development of some family cultural values that shaped his view of what a relationship should look like. Among them were values passed down from Steve's father, Ethan, who emphasized the importance of living up to expectations and demonstrated the guilt and shame he felt when he was unable to live up to the expectations of his family. This shame was exacerbated by Ethan's perception that he couldn't make enough money to support his family, as evidenced by the fact that Steve's mother, Melanie, continued to teach after her first child was born because the income was needed to pay the bills.

Steve's parents modeled communication patterns that were likely to influence Steve's perception of how conflict was managed in a marriage. Ethan didn't discuss with Melanie his feelings of guilt, shame, and inadequacy regarding his inability to support his family. If he had done so, he may have discovered that Melanie enjoyed working in the classroom, so Ethan's feelings about her work were unwarranted. Among other problems, tension developed in the relationship because of two miscarriages. Even though the couple eventually had two more children, Steve and Patrick, the tension maintained itself and was exacerbated when Ethan had a vasectomy without consulting Melanie. The pattern of behavior that the couple used in their relationship proved to be so disconnecting that Ethan and Melanie eventually divorced.

As a result of these early family cultural experiences, it is likely that Steve put pictures in his quality world of doing well in school, staying out of trouble and being a good person, and that family members should always get along with one another. From his experiences outside of his family he also developed pictures of the importance of social interaction and connections.

Carissa's Family History

Carissa was the second daughter born to Earl and Natalie, who bonded in high school because they were among a few Black students in a school in a small town in Florida that was primarily White. After graduating from high school, neither attended college. They both found local employment and were married at age 20. At that time, they were able to buy a small house and one year later, Carissa's sister Lori was born.

Family cultural values seemed to rest on the importance of hard work and finding ways to navigate problems in the family by focusing on maintaining relationships. This is evidenced by the close relationship Carissa had with her sister, Lori, mother Natalie, and grandmother, as well as by the model set by Earl and Natalie, who were able to reconcile after Earl had cheated on Natalie.

Family values regarding education included an expectation that the girls would do well in their schoolwork, but Earl and Natalie did not push them to go further. Carissa and Lori continued to maintain their relationship with one another while they pursued their advanced education. Carissa received scholarships and worked to pay for her tuition, but also was able to enjoy time at the university and made many friends before graduating with a degree in accounting.

As a result of Carissa's early experiences, we can hypothesize that she developed quality world pictures of family values that placed importance on maintaining relationships even through times of stress. Challenges to the marital relationship can be overcome. However, Carissa did not see *how* Earl and Natalie navigated the process of negotiating differences. Carissa developed the concept in her quality world that working through relationship challenges was valued, but the actual process of negotiating differences was never modeled for her.

Steve and Carissa—Culture in the Context of the Relationship

> We live in a highly interconnected world in which more and more individuals, in different parts of the globe, are seeking democratic relationships based on companionship, partnership, and love. However, in my view, it is crucial for the therapist to keep in mind that these expectations are happening in different ways and at different paces as they are integrated with values and priorities of specific cultures and subcultures.
>
> (Scheinkman, 2019, p. 553)

Steve and Carissa's values and beliefs were shaped by their family culture and also by their experiences growing up in the South. These social and cultural expectations influenced how they saw their roles in their relationship and the community. The diversity of values, beliefs, and attitudes makes it likely that couples will face challenges in their relationships (Hsu, 2001). It's to be expected that in any couple relationship, each person brings their own distinct cultural values that are shaped by variables such as ethnicity, race, religion, economic status, education, etc. For example, the perspective of individualist countries supports rights and privacy before the needs of a group effort. On the other hand, people in a collectivist society tend to focus on, and value, the contributions they can make to the group (Brooks, 2008). Because of the vastly different information we have regarding expectations and what is important, it's no wonder that couples struggle with negotiating differences as they attempt to form a relationship. Accepting diversity requires partners to make a conscious effort to engage in communication with a goal of understanding the other's cultural perspective (Waldman & Rubalcava, 2018). Tension develops when partners in a relationship take the position that they are "right," and the other person is "wrong." Growth occurs when couples respond with curiosity and a desire for understanding the other's position (Olver, 2011, 2012).

The Role of the Therapist

Reality therapy originated in the early 1960s as a method for providing mental health services through a practical approach that was easy to understand, but required practice to use the process creatively and with intention. Intention is now based on the integration of choice theory into therapeutic practice. Therapists utilizing reality therapy understand that choice theory is the psychological foundation for understanding human behavior and motivation. Theory informs how therapists understand what is happening with clients; therapy is the process of putting theory into action in work with clients. The integration of choice theory and reality therapy in couples therapy provides an explanation for what needs to occur in therapy to improve human relationships. When using choice theory as a general foundation for understanding Steve and Carissa, the therapist knows that they each have unique quality world pictures of what a relationship looks like, and their behavior is their attempt to meet the needs that these pictures represent. However, the therapist does not make assumptions about what these pictures are or should be. The therapist is an explorer in their quality worlds and makes discoveries by facilitating questions and using therapeutic skills that draw the relationship story from Steve and Carissa (Wubbolding & Robey, 2012).

The role of the therapist is to facilitate a process that provides a road map for understanding human behavior and to educate the couple to use specific tools that will enhance their relationship. This intervention includes teaching the couple about choice theory, which will provide the foundation for understanding themselves and one another. A relationship that is built on these ideas will initiate behavioral changes in the couple with the goal of creating a mutually satisfying relationship that leads each person to experience a sense of connection, personal control and significance, freedom, enjoyment, and increased satisfaction (Glasser, 2000; Wubbolding & Robey, 2012).

The therapeutic relationship with Steve and Carissa begins with creating a caring, supportive environment in which they feel confident that the therapist is working with their best interest in mind. The general goals of therapy are to help Steve and Carissa recognize that there are three entities in the therapy room; that is, the couple and the relationship between them. The therapist helps them to explore the strengths of their relationship and assess whether there is any agreement regarding the potential for the relationship. When this agreement is made, the therapist facilitates a process that will help Steve and Carissa to change their perceptions of one another, make behavioral changes that will include opportunities for quality time together, and find commonalities in quality world pictures, expectations for behavior, and shared perceptions that will bring them closer together (Wubbolding & Robey, 2012).

Specific behaviors utilized by therapists in this process include using ethical behavior that demonstrates empathy and communicates a sense of hope for the relationship. Therapists use creativity and innovative ways to connect with clients and to facilitate connection between the clients. Interactions include reframing negatives into positives, using the past tense to discuss problems and the present or future tense to discuss solutions, and acknowledging feelings without overly focusing on them (Wubbolding, 2011; Wubbolding & Robey, 2012). Therapeutic procedures specific to counseling with choice theory and reality therapy include exploring Steve and Carissa's quality world pictures regarding the relationship, discussing their perception of how much control they have over what they want in their lives, and sharing their perceptions about who they are as individuals and as partners in their relationship. The therapist helps Steve and Carissa identify goals and develop specific behavioral plans about how to work toward goal attainment. Steve and Carissa will be guided to identify and self-evaluate the effectiveness of the current behaviors they are using in an attempt to get what they want in the relationship. This self-evaluation includes an assessment of the outcomes of their actions, how they are thinking about the relationship and their own and their partner's behavior, and how those actions and thinking influence how they feel and even how they physically experience the relationship (Wubbolding & Robey, 2012).

Conceptualization of Problem Resolution

The therapeutic process begins by establishing a relationship with clients in which they feel safe and confident that the therapist is acting in their best interest, without judgment. Therapists employ caring relationship habits of listening, supporting, encouraging, respecting, accepting, and negotiating differences (Glasser, 2000), which are useful in building a collaborative relationship, and avoid habits that blame or criticize clients for the outcomes of their behavior (Wubbolding & Brickell, 2015). Relationship failure tends to occur when one or both partners attempt to control the other in a way that is unacceptable to that person.

The goal of therapy is initially to help clients collapse the conflict through mutually agreeing that they both want to improve the relationship. Glasser (2000) created a model of **structured reality therapy**, in which the first question asked is "Do you want to improve the relationship?" If both answer yes, the therapy moves forward. If not, the therapist asks what the clients are looking for from therapy and will determine whether therapy is appropriate for what they hope to accomplish.

The structured reality therapy process in the first session emphasizes that the relationship is a partnership in which there are actually three entities—the two people in the relationship and the relationship itself. The therapist works with the couple to focus on what is good for the *relationship*, not what is good for each person within the relationship. Glasser (2000) explained that this process limits the potential for the therapist to take sides or to determine that one person is more responsible for the problems in the relationship than the other.

After spending some time getting acquainted with the couple, the therapist using this process will explain what the expectations will be for the initial line of inquiry. The therapist informs the couple that they will be presented with five questions which each person will answer for themselves, without interruption from the other. After each person agrees that they want to improve the relationship, the second question is, "Whose behavior can you control?" This question is based on the belief that we can only control our own behavior, which leads the couple to take ownership of what they are doing in the relationship and to evaluate the effectiveness of their own behavior on the relationship.

When the partners in the couple agree that they can only control their own behavior, in the third step in the process, the therapist gives each person an opportunity to talk about what they see as being wrong in the relationship and to express their feelings. This is where it is important for the therapist to listen without taking sides. Once each person has shared their perception of what is wrong with the relationship, the therapist empathizes with what they have shared and assures them that the purpose of this process is to help them with their relationship, which is what they agreed that they want from therapy. This leads to the fourth question, which asks the couple to each take the opportunity to explain what is good about their relationship. It's interesting to note that Dr. Glasser included a warning with this question, and that was, "If either one of you believes that there is nothing good about your [relationship], then the counseling is over" (Glasser, 2000, p. 43). Paradoxically, this step is important to shift the focus from the problem to recognizing why the relationship is worth saving. After both individuals have had a chance to respond, the final question leads to an initial change of behavior that is likely to have an immediate positive impact on the relationship.

> Each of you tell me what's one thing that you [individually] could do all this coming week that you think will make your [relationship] better? Assuming that each of you can come up with something, then you'll go home and do it for a week. If you don't do it, or if it doesn't help the [relationship], then I don't see any sense in you coming back. But let's not worry about that right now. Let's see what you come up with.
>
> (Glasser, 2000, p. 45)

The purpose of this last statement is to make sure that the couple understands the importance of this question and that the success of the therapy depends on their ability to commit to making changes that will positively affect the relationship.

In the second session, the couple will be asked to report on what happened because of the actions they took during the time since the first session. If the couple didn't follow up with their plan, the therapist can ask the couple if they want to repeat the process from the first week, or if they are ready to give up on the relationship. If they did follow through on their commitment, the therapist will acknowledge their success and will explain that there is still a lot of work to do, but they are off to a good start. The therapist will teach the couple to think about their relationship as an entity that envelops them both and that the good of the relationship is more important than the individuals within the relationship. The therapist will present the process of working for the good of the relationship as working within the **solving circle**. When the individuals are in conflict, rather than escalate the conflict, they can agree to have a conversation within the circle, where they use the caring relationship habits to negotiate differences and make plans for the good of the relationship (Glasser, 2000).

As therapy continues, the therapist works with the couple to discuss their quality world pictures of their expectations for the relationship, themselves, and one another. The purpose of this process is to help each understand the motivation for their behavior and to share this with their partner in an attempt to develop a mutual understanding of what each finds important and where they agree and disagree about values, beliefs, and goals. The therapist teaches clients choice theory to help them understand the ultimate purpose of their behavior (to meet needs) and to recognize that they can only control themselves. Therefore, when using the solving circle concept, the couple can use the caring habits to explore what is happening and to make plans for what behaviors they can use to support the relationship.

Case Transcript

As in any therapeutic approach, practitioners have differing approaches to initiating the relationships with clients in the first session. However, for the purpose of demonstrating the model Glasser suggested for the first session, this first session "transcript" is based on Glasser's structured reality therapy process, which he explains in Chapter 4 of his book *Counseling with Choice Theory: The New Reality Therapy* (2000).

Therapist: (*After greeting the clients and inviting them to make themselves comfortable in the office*) Let me tell you a little about how I work and what my expectations will be regarding our time together in counseling. In any relationship, there are always differences in perception about what or who is right or wrong, but I don't get deeply involved in the issues that have brought you to therapy or in finding fault with either one of you. Instead, my goal is to work together with you by focusing on what you can do from here forward that will be best for your marriage. To begin, I want to do a simple assessment of your commitment to saving the relationship. I will ask you each to answer five questions. Please do not interrupt or talk over your partner when they are answering the question. You will each have an opportunity to answer in your own way. This may seem a bit abrupt to you, but I want to assure you that I want to do the best I can to help you meet your goals regarding your relationship if you want to work on saving it. Are you ready to begin?

The therapist informs the couple of what they can expect from the session and provides the rationale for the therapist's behavior. When counseling with choice theory and reality therapy, the process is transparent. The expectation is that the therapist and clients will work together for the sake of the other entity in the room, and that is the relationship itself. The purpose of the first question is to assess the commitment to the process.

Carissa: I'm ready, I guess.
Steve: Same here.
Therapist: OK, good. So, my first question for both of you is—Are you here because you want to get help for your relationship?

The purpose of this question is to assess the level of commitment the clients are bringing to the therapy, and to get their buy-in to the process. If the clients are not in agreement that they want to get help for the relationship, the therapist may discuss options for a separation and referral to another source for assistance.

Steve: Yes, we need help! It seems like nothing I do is right, though, so I'm not sure if therapy will be successful.

Therapist: I appreciate your concerns, Steve, but I want to be sure that I have a concrete answer to my question. Are you here because you want help for your relationship?

Steve: Yes, that's why I'm here.

Therapist: Thank you. Carissa, same question. Are you here because you want help for your relationship?

Carissa: Yes.

Therapist: OK, it's good that you both agree about that. My goal is to work with you with the good of your relationship always at the center of what we do together in sessions. So— next question: Whose behavior can you control?

Carissa: Well, I can control the people who work for me most of the time, and sometimes I can control Steve if I give him something he wants that makes him feel nicer toward me.

Therapist: I hear you saying you can control people most of the time, or when you try to gain control with bribing, but it sounds like you are negotiating with them rather than having the ability to control them. My guess is that even your employees are only choosing to do what you want them to do because it is less trouble than resisting you or they don't want to lose their jobs. Note that I say they are making that choice. So, let me ask you the question again. Whose behavior can you actually control?

Carissa: Well, when you put it that way, I guess the only person I can always control is myself. But it really seems that I'm able to control others sometimes.

Therapist: Yes, it seems that way sometimes, but would you agree that ultimately if a person doesn't want to do what you want them to do, that means you can't really control them?

Carissa: I guess that's true. I just don't like the idea of not being in control.

Therapist: I understand. It might be nice if we could get what we want by controlling others around us, but that's not the way things work, is it? So, let me ask you one more time. Who can you control?

Carissa   (*Sighing*) Only myself.

Therapist: Thank you! Steve, now it's your turn to answer the question. Who can you control?

Steve: Well, after listening to that conversation, I know the correct answer is I can only control myself.

Therapist: Do you believe that?

Steve: Yeah, I see your point and I agree with you.

The purpose of this question is to help each person to understand that they can only control their own behavior. This is an important first step to helping them realize that if they want to make a change in the relationship, they are each responsible for their own behavior. If it is true that each person can only control their own behavior, they begin to realize that they don't have to be victims of the other's behavior. How they respond is under their own control. This helps to limit blaming. However, it is important that each person has a chance to tell their story so they feel heard, which leads to question three.

Therapist: OK, good, so you agree regarding two things. One, that you are here to help the relationship, and two, that you each can only control your own behavior. So now is what you have probably been waiting for—your chance to express your feelings about your current relationship. At this point I want each of you to tell me what you think is wrong with your relationship right now. Who would like to go first?

The therapist wants to be sure the couple realizes that they already are agreeing to two important questions, which sets the stage for collaboration. If the couple begins to argue, the therapist can always remind them of what they said is their goal for therapy—to help the relationship—which will help put an end to arguing and shift the focus to creating behaviors that will bring them closer together.

Steve: I will go first this time. When we got together everything seemed to be so great. We had a lot of fun together and it seemed like we were always on the same wavelength. I was perfectly happy with how we were, but then Carissa said she wanted to have a baby, which seems to have thrown everything out of whack. I don't particularly care if we have kids or not, but it's a big deal for her, so fine. But now, she can't get pregnant, and our sex life seems to be built around a calendar and a clock, so I have to be ready to perform when it's the right time. I feel like it's all we ever talk about and I'm getting tired of it. I'm working myself to death trying to get enough money to cover fertility specialists with no results. The only relief I get is when I go out golfing with my friends, but then Carissa nags at me for not being at home, and when I'm home she nags and complains about everything I do. There is no pleasing her.

Therapist: OK, I think I have a pretty good picture of your concerns. Is there anything else you want to add?

Steve: I think that's enough for now.

Therapist: Carissa, you have a chance to speak now. What do you believe is wrong with the relationship?

Carissa: Well, you heard it, didn't you? Only it's not fair that Steve is blaming me for all of this. He knew before we got married that I wanted to have children, and he never said he didn't. So now he's being a real jerk about the fertility process, and he isn't supportive at all. He is absolutely cruel in response to my feelings about this. When he's home, he just tunes me out, and he's not home that much anymore. He's always out with his friends, and he leaves all the chores at home for me to do. For example, he won't clean up the kitty litter, which is really an issue for me because there are chemicals in the litter that are not good for me to inhale. I've been talking to my mother about all this, and she says I should try to work it out with Steve, but I'm at the point where I'm not sure how to even get started to deal with all the problems we have.

At this point, the clients are feeling angry, and each of them feels justified in complaining that the problem lies in the behavior of their partner. They attempt to escalate their complaints, but the therapist just acknowledges how difficult the situation is and moves the process forward to the next question. The therapist is careful not to take sides or to challenge the couple's perception of their problems. The point of this intervention is that each can feel their concerns are heard, and for the therapist to get a baseline idea of what the problems are. As they begin to see improvement in the relationship it can be measured in comparison to what the problems were when they started counseling.

Therapist: OK, I appreciate hearing your perspectives regarding the problems in your relationship. I want to remind you that you both agreed that you are here because you want to help the relationship, so I want to shift the focus of our assessment a bit with question four. That is—what do you think is good in your relationship right now? Take your time in answering this. If one or both of you think there is nothing good about your relationship, then we will discontinue therapy and I will refer you to someone who can advise you about other steps you might take.

This is a paradoxical approach which is designed to catch the clients off guard as they contemplate how serious this question is and the potential outcome if they can't come up with any good points in their relationship. Steve and Carissa complain a bit as they try to shift their focus from their problems to what is working in the relationship. The therapist gives them some space for the process and then reminds them that they must answer the question so they can move forward in the session.

Steve: Well, one of the things I always appreciated about Carissa is how smart she is. She really keeps us on track financially because she has a degree in accounting. I always liked hanging out with her, watching old movies, and just relaxing after work. She's a great cook, too! We used to enjoy barbecuing on the patio and cleaning up together afterward. We used to experiment with recipes. Some of them were great, but we also had some real disasters that made us laugh. I miss those times.

Carissa: (*Tearfully*) Wow, I didn't know you really appreciated all those things, Steve. It seems we've been fighting so much that I can't remember the last time we laughed together. I miss it too. Since we are talking about what's good about our relationship now, I guess I would have to say that we are still trying to pull it together so there must be something still there to fight for. I do appreciate how hard you work so we can have a nice home and cars and some money in the bank. You've always made sure that I had everything I need to live in a nice environment. I appreciate that.

The tone in the therapist's office has changed as the clients have shifted from the focus on the problem to a recognition of what is good about their relationship. The therapist now wants to capitalize on this shift through use of the last question, which will guide the couple in making an action plan for the next week. The goal is to help them move in the direction of helping the relationship instead of focusing on the problem.

Therapist: Thank you for your answers. You both seemed sincere in what you said, and I am feeling optimistic about your chances for success in repairing your relationship. So now we will move forward to taking action with that in mind. The last question for each of you is—what is one thing that you each can do in the next week that you think will help improve your relationship? You must come up with something you can commit to and actually do it for a week. If you can't, or if it doesn't help the relationship, then you can let me know and we can discontinue therapy. But I feel confident that you will take some positive action and that you will come back next week with good news to report on how it went.

Carissa: OK, well, I will try to stop nagging about Steve going golfing with his friends so often.

Therapist: That's a good thought, but let me provide a little more guidance on this assignment. You need to commit to something you can do, not something you will not do. So, for example, Carissa, instead of stopping the nagging, how can you communicate with Steve in a way that would bring you closer together and reignite some of those moments you just referred to?

Carissa: I see. Um, I guess if Steve is on board, I can plan a nice dinner and we can spend time watching a funny movie together after we clean up from dinner.

Steve: I would like that. We can decide what night that will be. I can take a day and do some of those chores that have been waiting for my attention instead of going golfing on Sunday. I know you will feel happy if that happens!

Therapist: So, do you both agree that if you did those things, it would help your relationship?

Carissa: Yes!

Steve: Yes, I think so.

The therapist spends time creating a SMART plan with the couple. To be successful, plans must be very Specific about time, place, and behavior, and Measurable—how will they know the plan is accomplished? Plans need to be Attainable—can they actually do this? What might get in the way and how would they address this? Are the plans Realistic and Relevant to the goal of helping the relationship? The plan needs to be Timely, so the couple will know what to expect. Finally, the couple needs to make a commitment to putting the plan into action.

Case Transcript Discussion and Second Session Follow-Up

This first session transcript is a brief hypothetical account of what a session might look like when using Glasser's (2000) model of structured reality therapy in couples therapy. Of course, in an actual session, the therapist should expect that clients are likely to be a bit more resistant to the process and to spend more time elaborating on their complaints. However, the process has been shown to be effective in many applications, as evidenced by case studies presented in Robey et al.'s book *Contemporary Issues in Couples Counseling: A Choice Theory and Reality Approach* (2012).

Assuming the couple puts their plan into action, and it helps their relationship, the expectation is that they will return for a second session. In this session, the therapist will check in to see what happened with the plan. Using Glasser's (2000) model, the second session will include a discussion of the solving circle process. The couple is taught that the needs of the relationship are more important than the needs of each individual. In times of trouble, the couple agrees to enter the imaginary solving circle in which problems are considered by how they are affecting the relationship, and the solution comes from what is best for the relationship, not necessarily for the individuals in the relationship.

In the second and ongoing sessions, the therapist will teach the clients about choice theory, including the impact of external control behaviors on the relationship, and will help them create new options for behaviors that are likely to bring the partners closer together. When partners understand how they are motivated by basic needs and quality world pictures, and understand the purpose of behavior, they can reconsider how they understand the dynamics of their relationship and make choices that serve the individuals and the relationship itself. The goal is win-win-win as much as possible.

The ultimate relationship question that should drive behavior in a relationship is, "Is what I'm about to do or say going to bring us closer together or push us further apart?" If the answer is further apart, this is a signal to take a time out and re-evaluate what is going on and make plans for different behavior that will support the relationship.

References

Arredondo, P., Toporek, R., Brown, S. P., Jones, J., Locke, D., & Sanchez, J., et al. (1996). Operationalization of the multicultural counseling competencies. *Journal of Multicultural Counselling & Development, 24,* 42–78. https://doi.org/10.1002/j.2161-1912.1996.tb00288.x

Brooks, D. (2008). Harmony and the dream. *The New York Times.* Retrieved from www.nytimes.com/2008/08/12/opinion/12iht-edbrooks.1.15207937.html

Bustamante, R. M., Nelson, J. A., Henriksen, R. C., Jr. & Monakes, S. (2011). Intercultural couples: Coping with culture-related stressors. *Family Journal, 19*(2), 154–164. doi: 10.1177/10664807113997233

Glasser, W. (1965). *Reality therapy: A new approach to psychiatry.* Harper & Rowe.

Glasser, W. (1985). *Control theory: A new explanation of how we control our lives.* HarperCollins.

Glasser, W. (1998). *Choice theory: A new psychology of personal freedom.* HarperCollins.

Glasser, W. (2000). *Counseling with choice theory: The new reality therapy.* HarperCollins.

Haskins, N., & Appling, B. (2017). Relational-cultural theory and reality therapy: A culturally responsive integrated framework. *Journal of Counseling and Development, 95*(1), 87–99. doi:10.1002/jcad.12120

Hsu, J. (2001). Marital therapy for intercultural couples. In W.W. Tseng & J. Streltzer (Eds.), *Culture and psychotherapy: A guide to clinical practice* (pp. 225–242). American Psychiatric Press.

Olver, K. (2011). *Secrets of happy couples: Loving yourself, your partner, and your life.* Inside Out Press.

Olver, K. (2012). Multicultural couples: Seeing the world through different lenses. In P. A. Robey, R. E. Wubbolding & J. D. Carlson (Eds.), *Contemporary issues in couples counseling* (pp. 33–58). Routledge.

Powers, W. T. (1973). *Behavior: The control of perception.* Aldine de Gruyter.

Robey, P. A., Wubbolding, R. E., & Carlson, J. D. (2012). *Contemporary issues* in *couples counseling.* Routledge.

Scheinkman, M. (2019). Intimacies: An integrative multicultural framework for couple therapy. *Family Process, 58*(3), 550–568. doi:10.1111/famp.12444

Waldman, K., & Rubalcava, L. (2018). Psychotherapy with intercultural couples: A contemporary psychodynamic approach. *The American Journal of Psychotherapy, 59*(3), 227–245. https://doi.org/10.1176/appi.psychotherapy.2005.59.3.227

Wiener, N. (1948). *Cybernetics.* John Wiley & Sons.

William Glasser International. www.wglasserinternational.org/wgi/who-we-are/ Accessed December 16, 2023

Wubbolding, R. E. (2000). *Reality therapy for the 21st century.* Brunner Routledge.

Wubbolding, R. E. (2011). *Reality therapy: Theories of psychotherapy series.* American Psychological Association.

Wubbolding, R. E. (2017). *Reality therapy and self-evaluation: The key to client change.* American Counseling Association.

Wubbolding, R. E. (2019). The relationship between professional diversity/multicultural guidelines and choice theory/reality therapy. *International Journal of Choice Theory and Reality Therapy, 38*(2), 36–42.

Wubbolding, R. E., & Brickell, J. (2015). *Counselling with reality therapy* (2nd ed.). Speechmark Publishing.

Wubbolding, R. E., & Robey, P. A. (2012). Introduction to choice theory and reality therapy. In P. A. Robey, R. E. Wubbolding & J. D. Carlson, (Eds), *Contemporary issues* in *couples counseling* (pp. 3–20). Routledge.

14　Context Areas of Couple Therapy

Kayleigh Sabo and Michael D. Reiter

This book has introduced 11 distinct therapy models commonly employed in couple therapy. In this final chapter, we pivot slightly to discuss several broader contextual domains that couples might bring into therapy. These domains are crucial to consider when therapists construct their case conceptualization. It's important to note that this chapter doesn't delve into the therapeutic approaches for working with couples; that's the focus of the preceding 11 chapters. Our intention here is to detail the various contextual factors that couple therapists might encounter. Regardless of which of these factors are relevant to the couple in the therapy room, any of the models detailed in this book can still be applied, including those not covered due to space constraints. The contextual factors we will discuss include same-sex couples, interracial couples, intimate partner violence, financial issues, in-laws, infidelity, consensual nonmonogamy, and kinks.

Same-Sex Couples

In June of 2015, the United States Supreme Court voted 5-4 in favor of partners who are part of a **same-sex couple** (SSC) being able to marry regardless of state, marking a significant milestone in the legalization of same-sex marriage. This decision brought about a transformation in the legitimacy and opportunities available to thousands of SSCs. Media coverage of this event often framed it in political/legal, religious/morality, or civil rights/equality terms (Colistra & Johnson, 2021). The framing of the legalization of same-sex marriage as a civil rights and equality issue had a more positive tone, while framing it as a conflict between religion and morality resulted in a more negative tone. How SSCs are portrayed in the media has a profound impact on how they are perceived and ultimately treated by others and how they view themselves as members of an SSC. Knowing this, therapists can be more open to the possibility that the SSC may have experienced both positive and negative messages and reactions from individuals and social structures.

The experiences of SSCs have undergone significant changes in recent decades. While SSCs tend to exhibit more egalitarian relationships than heterosexual couples, there has been a slight divergence in trends (Gotta et al., 2011). Heterosexual couples are moving toward greater equality, while SSCs are experiencing a slight decrease in egalitarianism. Within SSCs, female couples divide household labor more equally than male couples (van der Vleuten et al., 2021). As van der Vleuten et al. (2021) pointed out, "Even though same-sex couples challenge traditional gender norms within the partnership, they still exhibit behavior that aligns with their gender roles as a couple" (p. 162). Thus, gender role socialization influences both same-sex and different-sex couples (DSCs).

The experiences of SSCs also vary depending on their relationship status. Once married, same-sex partners often report a stronger bond with each other, possibly due to a sense of legitimacy and security in their relationship (Kennedy & Dalla, 2020). However, marriage may not hold the same significance for same-sex couples as it does for mixed-sex couples (Bosley-Smith & Reczek,

DOI: 10.4324/9781003369097-14

2018). This disparity may be due to society's hesitation in legalizing same-sex marriage or embracing alternative lifestyle choices. For example, males in same-sex couples, compared to individuals in other relationship pairings, are less likely to view their relationship as sexually exclusive (Joyner et al., 2019). Thus, therapists might explore with the couple their choices in how they want their relationship to be, not expecting that any couple wants or should be moving toward marriage.

While we often discuss same-sex couples as a distinct group and DSCs as another, it is important to acknowledge that there are both universal factors that apply to all couples and specific factors that pertain to SSCs. Additionally, there is diversity within both groups (Pentel & Baucom, 2022). Just as not all DSCs are the same, not all SSCs are identical. Same-sex and different-sex couples share many similarities in terms of core relationship processes and outcomes as both SSCs and DSCs experience similar levels of satisfaction, commitment, and emotional intimacy with their partners (Joyner et al., 2019).

However, they differ in terms of relational dynamics, such as the level of egalitarianism as well as the challenges they face from larger social processes, such as discrimination (Scott et al., 2019). For instance, individuals in SSCs tend to be more accepting of others and are more likely to enter interracial relationships compared to DSCs (Jones et al., 2021). Moreover, according to Gottman et al. (2020), SSCs generally are happier in their relationship when they seek therapy compared to DSCs. Like all couples, LGBTQ+ (lesbian, gay, bisexual, transgender, queer/questioning+) relationships thrive when partners engage in relationship maintenance behaviors that contribute to positive relational quality, commitment, satisfaction, and closeness (Haas & Lannutti, 2022). Assurances between partners play a crucial role in this regard, so this is something for therapists who work with such couples to keep in mind.

Main Challenges for SSCs

Individuals in same-sex relationships face **interpersonal stigma** from individuals and **structural stigma** from institutions (Petruzzella et al., 2019). **Homophobia** poses a significant social obstacle for SSCs, as members of these couples may internalize societal prejudices, leading to intrapsychic and interpersonal distress (Pepping et al., 2019; Totenhagen et al., 2018a). **Internalized homophobia** stems from society's negative attitudes toward sexual minorities, which LGBTQ+ individuals may internalize. Despite originating externally, these feelings become internalized and can persist as a vulnerability for the individual. For instance, higher levels of internalized homophobia are associated with increased daily stress, greater conflict with a partner, and lower relationship quality (Totenhagen et al., 2018a). **Concealment practices**, often used as a coping mechanism for internalized homophobia, are linked to lower relationship satisfaction (Pepping et al., 2019).

These experiences of one's sexuality and who knows about it have significant impact for the individual and the couple. Differences in "outness" within a same-sex relationship can lead to discord. Totenhagen et al. (2018a) found that individuals who were less open about their sexual orientation and had a partner experiencing stress reported lower commitment levels. Conversely, those who experience affirmation of their LGBTQ+ identity tend to have higher levels of relationship satisfaction (Pepping et al., 2019). Therapists working with SSCs might explore early in the therapy each person's outness as well as the overall outness that they have as a couple.

SSCs are more likely than DSCs to experience relationship dissolution. In a study by Allen and Price (2020), 25.1% of SSCs and 15.2% of DSCs studied ended their relationships. The disparity is even more pronounced for SSCs with children, with 46.7% of such couples ending their relationships compared to 14.9% of DSCs. Thus, SSCs with children may face a three-fold higher risk of relationship dissolution. Female same-gender couples tend to have higher dissolution rates than male same-gender or mixed-gender couples. Reasons for breakup among females in same-gender relationships include frequent arguments, conflicts, concerns about a partner's mental health, infidelity, and a lack of sexual satisfaction (Scott et al., 2022). When working with an SSC who is presenting with relationship issues, therapists should be aware of these challenges specific to SSCs to have a more comprehensive understanding of their presenting concerns.

Wider Social Networks

SSCs face unique challenges as a minority group. They encounter **minority stress** in the form of prejudice and discrimination, which can have negative effects on the individuals and the dynamics of their relationships (Feinstein et al., 2018; Stewart et al., 2019). Partners who experience higher levels of general stress, suffer internalized stigma, encounter microaggressions, and are not fully open about their sexual orientation tend to have more negative interactions within their relationships (Feinstein et al., 2018). While SSCs in the United States and over 30 other countries now have the legal right to marry, not all choose to do so. As with heterosexual couples, the decision to marry or not depends on various factors. When SSCs opt not to marry, they often experience less support from their social networks, possibly due to perceptions of lower commitment (Lannutti, 2018). Family support plays a significant role in the well-being of SSCs, and concealing their relationship from others has negative impacts on relationship commitment and satisfaction (Haas & Lannutti, 2022).

Therapists working with SSCs should consider both the universal factors that apply to all couples and the unique experiences and challenges faced by SSCs in a society that is still adapting to the visibility and acceptance of LGBTQ+ relationships. Creating an open and safe space for same-sex couples to discuss their experiences is crucial, as they often navigate external systems and factors that influence their relationship.

Interracial Couples

In 1967, the landmark Supreme Court case *Loving* v. *Virginia* struck down anti-miscegenation laws that prohibited interracial marriages. At that time, 13 states had such laws, making this ruling a significant moment in American history. In 1958, only 4% of Americans approved of interracial couples, but recently that number has risen to 94% (Pew Research Center, 2017). This change in approval is reflected in the growing number of married interracial couples, which has increased from 3% in 1967 to 20% today. Thus, therapists should be prepared to see an increasing number of interracial couples in their therapy office as these couples continue to date, be in committed relationships, and possibly marry.

Despite the increase in interracial couples, **homogamy**, or marriage between people of similar backgrounds, remains the prevailing norm. Homogamy is supported by underlying racism and classism, which contribute to the separation and segregation of individuals based on their group affiliations (Killian, 2001a, 2001b). The images we often see of couples in popular culture tend to depict couples of the same race, ethnic background, religion, age, and social standing.

Foeman and Nance (1999) propose that interracial couples go through their own unique stages of development in addition to the typical stages of relationship formation. These stages include racial awareness, coping with social definitions of race, identity emergence, and maintenance. **Racial awareness** involves partners developing an understanding of their own racial perspectives, their partner's perspectives, and the perspectives of their respective racial groups. **Coping with social definitions of race** requires navigating a society that can be racist and prejudiced, and the partners must reconcile their own views with those of their larger social groups. **Identity emergence** occurs when partners take ownership of their individual and collective racial identities. **Maintenance** involves developing effective strategies and perspectives for maintaining the relationship. Couples may cycle through these stages multiple times over the course of their relationship. Therapists can be curious as to the couple's current stage of development and the impact of that stage on their relational dynamics.

While interracial couples go through the typical stages of relationship formation, they often find unique aspects of their partner to connect with. Interracial daters tend to rate their partner more positively in terms of attractiveness and intellectual attributes, and they believe their partners view them positively in these areas as well (Wu et al., 2015). Notably, independent raters consider inter-racial daters to have more desirable attributes compared to intraracial daters, particularly in terms of physical attractiveness.

Nguyen et al. (2016) explain that interracial couples have both visible and invisible differences and similarities. To help couples address these aspects of their relationship, clinicians may use a **visible–invisible grid** as a tool to enhance their awareness and facilitate open discussions. This grid highlights the visible differences and similarities that members of a couple have along with the invisible differences and similarities. Nguyen et al. (2016) explain the useful-ness for couples in using a tool such as this, "The continuum of invisible and visible helps the couple recognize the salience of perspective when it comes to what people define as difference and similarity, which is ultimately constructed by individuals and society" (p. 219). Bringing these dynamics to the forefront of the couple's conversations helps each of them to better understand themself, the other person, and them as a couple. Seshardri and Knudson-Martin (2013) suggest that therapists initially assist interracial couples in identifying the relationship structures influenced by their cultural backgrounds, as this can provide insight into their current relationship patterns.

Interracial relationships tend to form earlier in life rather than later, and individuals entering remarriages are less likely to cross racial boundaries (Choi & Tienda, 2017). Racial and ethnic sorting is more prominent in remarriages, leading individuals to avoid interracial relationships. This trend is especially pronounced for White–Black relationships compared to White–Hispanic, White–Asian, or other pairings. People in interracial relationships evaluate their commitment to the couple based on the quality of alternatives and satisfaction with their interracial relationships rather than solely on investments (Brooks et al., 2018). Overall, individuals in interracial relationships exhibit both secure and insecure attachment styles, suggesting a socio-emotional intimacy within these couples (Gaines et al., 1999).

Relationship Satisfaction

Relationship satisfaction in interracial marriages has both similarities and differences compared to homogamous marriages. Women in interracial marriages report higher levels of gender inequity than men, and perceived unfairness in the relationship is associated with poorer marital quality (Forry et al., 2007). African Americans also tend to have higher levels of ambivalence toward their relationships compared to White partners. While interracial couples tend to report higher relation-ship satisfaction overall, they do not differ significantly from homogamous couples in terms of relationship quality, conflict patterns, or attachment style (Troy et al., 2006). However, initially, women in interracial relationships tend to report lower relationship quality compared to women in intraracial relationships (Brown et al., 2018).

On the one hand, certain types of interracial couples—such as White men with Asian biracial children, Black women with White biracial children, and Asian women with White biracial children—are more likely to maintain their marriages (Kuroki, 2017). On the other hand, White female–Black male and White female–Asian male marriages face a higher risk of divorce compared to White–White couples (Bratter & King, 2008). Racial identity, particularly for African American–White couples, emerges as a significant predictor of marital quality (Leslie & Letiecq, 2004). Partners who demonstrate pride in their own racial identity while also accepting those of other races tend to have higher marital quality. While interracial and intraracial couples generally follow similar trajectories of relationship quality, Black–Hispanic interracial couples have a higher likelihood of separation (Brown et al., 2018). As with all couples, most couple therapy is about increasing relationship satisfaction. Understanding the unique impact that being in an interracial relationship has on the couple can bring this topic to the forefront so that it can be more overtly addressed.

Perceived Prejudice

Interracial couples face unique challenges related to societal disapproval and the effects of racial privilege in addition to the common relationship issues experienced by all couples, such as communication, finances, intimacy, and gender roles (Leslie & Young, 2015). Friends and family members in the psychological networks of interracial couples often align with dominant discourses of homogamy, attempting to prevent these couples from forming. Consequently, partners in interracial relationships must make strategic decisions regarding when and how to disclose their relationship status, as dating or marrying interracially can have serious social and psychological implications for their relationships with friends and family (Killian, 2001a). Interracial couples may downplay the significance of race in their relationships as they navigate the intersection of global relationship issues and the implications of race, discrimination, and societal expectations (Leslie & Young, 2015).

Prejudice and discrimination against interracial couples manifest in various ways, including stares, disapproving expressions, vocal disapproval, and harassment (Killian, 2001a, 2001b). White individuals tend to perceive interracial couples as less compatible, particularly when the non-White partner is African American rather than Asian American (Lewandowski & Jackson, 2001). Interracial couples may feel socially isolated, especially in areas such as leisure, family, and work, due primarily to race and racism (Hibbler & Shinew, 2002). Consequently, they are less likely to engage in public displays of affection due to potential negative social reactions. The lack of social support and societal discrimination against one or both partners may also contribute to higher rates of migration (Böhm & Shapley, 2013). Interracial couples experience **racist nativism** (prejudice against them based on being perceived as an immigrant) differently based on the gender and race of their partners, with Latina women facing more microaggressions and Latino men experiencing more macroaggressions (Schueths, 2014).

Therapists will likely work with interracial couples at some point in their career. Therapists can adopt strategies such as **broaching**, which involves openly discussing race-related differences within the couple and between the couple and the therapist. This approach can help reduce the stigma experienced by interracial couples and foster acceptance and support. Relationship stigma has been found to negatively impact relationship satisfaction, although religious and spiritual wellbeing may partially mediate this effect (Vazques et al., 2019). Interracial couples actively navigate and confront racism, often through educational efforts, with Black partners educating their White partners on effectively handling racial conflicts (Bell & Hastings, 2011).

Intimate Partner Violence

Intimate partner violence (IPV) is a potential presenting problem that a couple (or an individual client who is in a relationship) may present with when coming to therapy. While it seems that the terms domestic violence and IPV are at times both used to represent a use of harmful physical, sexual, and/or mental behaviors between romantic partners, Patra et al. (2018) state that domestic violence involves such behaviors between any family members while IPV is strictly between intimate partners. Since we are focusing on the dynamics between couples in this book, we will use the term IPV (although some of the literature we cite references these dynamics in terms of domestic violence).

What Is IPV?

There are several features of IPV that therapists should be aware of before working with a couple or an individual presenting with IPV. First, there are different ways in which IPV can manifest in a relationship. Ali et al. (2016) discuss these elements of IPV in depth. There are three overarching classifications of IPV: physical, sexual, and psychological. **Physical violence** (utilized to enforce pain and suffering) may present in a plethora of ways, including beating, slapping, pushing, injuring with weapons, and kicking. **Sexual violence** includes both forced sexual acts and forced attempts to engage in sexual acts against the victim's will. **Psychological IPV** involves verbal abuse (e.g., name-calling), threats (e.g., threatening to harm the victim or the victim's children), and the control over factors in the victim's life (e.g., prohibiting the victim from seeing their family or having educational access). Behaviors from each of these major categories may be present in a relationship.

Second, Ali et al. (2016) note that there are often controlling and coercive elements in the perpetration of IPV (i.e., attempts to make a partner dependent on the perpetrator and efforts to harm or scare the victim, respectively). **Controlling behaviors** may include preventing the victim from engaging with others, utilizing the victim's resources, and governing the victim's daily schedule and activities. **Coercive behaviors** may consist of threats to and intimidation of the victim. At the same time, there is also what Johnson and Ferraro (2000) reference as **common couple violence**, which lacks the element of control and is less likely to involve severe or escalating violence. This scenario involves couples where intense situations, such as arguments, may lead to violent outbursts due to challenges with emotional regulation by one or both partners.

In addition to being aware of the common defining features of IPV, it is vital for therapists to have knowledge of the common presenting traits that can aid in the identification of IPV. There are, of course, the physical signs of IPV, as victims may likely have bruises, cuts, and other visual markings from physical abuse. As with child abuse, it is especially noteworthy if a client continuously has fresh bruises or cuts (as this would indicate that continued harm is happening rather than a one-time accident having occurred). Threatening, jealous, and aggressive behavior by the potential perpetrator is noteworthy as well, along with frequent missed or canceled appointments (Cronholm et al., 2011).

IPV in the Therapy Room

With the dynamics of IPV in mind, it is also helpful for therapists to be cognizant of how they might come across IPV in the therapy room. While this book focuses on couples, and IPV is certainly a couple's dynamic that both partners may present with in therapy, it may also just be one partner in a relationship coming in for therapy. The overtness of IPV may also vary: Some couples or individuals come in with this as a clear presenting problem whereas other clients enter therapy for something else but divulge the presence of IPV during the process of therapy. It is necessary to reflect on these factors—along with the actual manifestation/types of IPV—when determining how to work with such cases. For example, Karakurt et al. (2013) emphasize that it is "important to understand distinctions between various types of violence when discerning the appropriateness and safety of working with both partners in a relationship" (p. 3). Some partners may be entering therapy with the perpetrator having acknowledged the abuse with a desire to change. However, other partners may enter for other concerns, and it is unsafe for the victim to express any occurrences of IPV. It is thus essential for therapists to be aware of the signs of IPV and the dynamics of each couple and/

or individual that present in therapy to determine (a) if IPV is present and (b) how to handle this information depending on the dynamics of the relationship.

Practical Considerations of IPV

So far, we have discussed the overarching definitions, manifestations, and dynamics of IPV. Now, we want to note a few practical considerations for therapists to keep in mind when they work with clients presenting with IPV. First, there is the safety of both the clients and the therapist in the therapy room. Most couples experiencing IPV will not bring the physical dynamics from home into sessions. However, it is still appropriate for therapists to be aware of and plan for their own safety as well as their clients' if any conversations lead to physical altercations. Some considerations may include making sure that the arrangement of the office enables the therapist to be able to exit the room easily and talking with the couple about setting preventative ground rules for communication (e.g., using a talking stick).

Second, it is important to recognize the dominant discourses surrounding gender when talking about IPV. Much of the literature indicates that, in heterosexual relationships, women are victims of IPV more often than men (Ali et al., 2016; Cronholm et al., 2011) and women are more likely to be seriously injured or even killed as a result of IPV (Hornor, 2005; Patra et al., 2018). It is necessary to reflect on this information for two reasons. On the one hand, it alerts therapists to the potential physical severity that can accompany IPV, especially for women. On the other hand, it also becomes necessary to not assume that in every couple experiencing IPV, the man is the perpetrator and the woman is the victim. This assumption can potentially prevent therapists from attending to the dynamics of the couple in front of them, so staying curious and open concerning the roles and behaviors in each individual relationship is key for the safety of both partners.

IPV and Same-Sex Couples

As explained earlier, SSCs are similar to heterosexual couples on many levels. Unfortunately, experiencing IPV is one of these areas (Rollè et al., 2018). IPV has mainly been an event that is kept private within the household. This silence has been even more present in the LGBTQ+ community. However, the U.S. Supreme Court's 2015 decision in *Obergefell* v. *Hodges* made available more protections for individuals in SSCs who experience IPV (Durfee & Goodmark, 2020). As the legal recognition of same-sex marriages has increased, so has the rate of arrest in IPV cases for partners in SSCs (Addington, 2020).

Gerstenberger et al. (2019) found that male IPV perpetrators in same-sex relationships had lower assessed risk than their heterosexual counterparts. They were also less likely to be rearrested for a new offense. Conversely, female perpetrators in SSCs had a higher likelihood of reoffending. Males in SSCs are more likely to report their own IPV perpetration than victimization (Stephenson et al., 2019). This may be due to their adherence to ideas about masculinity. College students who are in SSCs are more likely to experience IPV resulting in physical injury (Graham et al., 2019).

Legal and Ethical Responsibilities

Because IPV brings an element of physical—and sometimes potentially life-threatening—harm to some clients, it is important to address the legal and ethical responsibilities of the therapist when working with clients experiencing IPV. These legal and ethical guidelines change depending on the state or country in which the therapist is licensed, so it is of the utmost importance that therapists purposefully understand and attend to all legal and ethical requirements set forth by their respective states. For example, Mascolo (2023) states that California's reporting law mandates that healthcare providers report visible or reasonably suspected domestic violence that resulted in bodily harm, and this source includes spousal abuse in the list of potential perpetrations. However, Johnson (2017) comments that marriage and family therapists do not fall under California's definition of a healthcare provider because they "do not provide medical services for physical conditions" ("Who Reports Domestic Violence?" section). Again, this further demonstrates the necessity for therapists to be aware of and follow their geographic location's laws regarding mandatory reporting for domestic violence.

Therapists also need to consider the legal and ethical responsibilities related to mandatory reporting when children are involved. Johnson (2017) addresses the considerations that a therapist needs to hold in mind when their clients experiencing IPV have children:

> The fact that a child's parent or guardian is a victim of domestic violence should not, in and of itself, be a sufficient basis for reporting suspected child abuse or neglect. Further, a child's exposure to a domestic violence incident, in and of itself, should not be a sufficient basis for reporting suspected abuse or neglect.
>
> (Johnson, 2017, "Abuse of Protected Classes" section)

First, this information suggests that therapists should not assume that an IPV situation indicates that there is also automatically child abuse going on as well. Second, however, this does mean that therapists need to listen for the presence of child abuse as they would in any other situation in order to make the necessary report. Again, similar to domestic violence reporting among adult partners, child abuse reporting laws may differ per locale. We cannot emphasize enough that therapists must be aware of the reporting laws in their area and take appropriate action based on those laws.

Financial Issues

It is widely known that finances are a common source of conflict and disagreement among couples (Crapo et al., 2021; Ford et al., 2020; Jeanfreau et al., 2020; Totenhagen et al., 2018b). However, despite the significance of financial issues in relationships, couples often prioritize discussions about sex and infidelity over conversations about money (Atwood, 2012).

Managing and controlling money within a couple involves power dynamics (Çineli, 2022). **Control of money** refers to who has the authority to make major financial decisions, while **managing money** pertains to the day-to-day financial choices in running a household. Over time, financial decisions have become more egalitarian, but this is influenced by income disparities. In heterosexual relationships, women with lower incomes tend to defer financial control to their male partners, whereas high-earning women adopt a more individualized approach to financial management (Hu, 2021).

As described, couples tend to talk more about sex and infidelity than finances since sexual infidelity is often a tipping point for people—whether they should maintain a relationship or not. But sexual infidelity is not the only arena where infidelity plays a significant role for a couple. Occasionally, one partner may engage in **financial infidelity**, which involves deceitfully keeping their use of the couple's finances a secret (Jeanfreau et al., 2020). This behavior often stems from a desire to avoid conflict. However, once the deception is discovered, issues of trust arise within the couple. It becomes a matter not only of undisclosed purchases, but also of the breach of trust caused by the deception.

While financial matters can cause distress in many couples, they do not have to be a source of conflict. Couples with strong relationships have learned how to effectively manage their finances through open communication and trust (Skogrand et al., 2011). These couples typically designate one person to handle day-to-day financial management while maintaining open communication. They also tend to have minimal or manageable debt and live within their means. Alignment in financial values contributes to better communication, relationship stability, and satisfaction (LeBaron-Black et al., 2022). Further, joint bank accounts and financial integration are associated with higher levels of relationship satisfaction, as increased financial integration leads to fewer financial conflicts (Addo & Sassler, 2010; Jeanfreau et al., 2020; Lim & Morgan, 2021).

Gender Differentials and Finances

Finances and gender play a role in how individuals perceive and manage money within relationships. Men often associate money with power and prefer shared finances with some level of control, while women often opt to keep some money separate due to concerns about potential financial loss in case of relationship dissolution.

The connection between finances and couple satisfaction is not straightforward. Higher finances do not necessarily guarantee higher satisfaction, and the impact of income varies depending on the earner's gender. As women's income increases, negative impacts such as increased housework and childcare issues, decreased couple stability, and higher likelihood of divorce may arise (Piao, 2021).

Couples with more gender-egalitarian beliefs tend to adopt individualized or joint money management systems instead of traditional "**breadwinner**" systems, resulting in higher relationship satisfaction and lower likelihood of relationship dissolution (Çineli, 2020; Gladstone et al., 2022). The perception of a partner's spending behavior also influences financial satisfaction, with individuals perceiving their partner as a saver reporting higher satisfaction, particularly among women (Grable et al., 2021).

Finances are both a reason for couples to stay together and decide to divorce (Bell et al., 2022). A divorce will likely negatively impact both members' finances. Thus, some people stay longer in a relationship because they fear the consequences of relationship dissolution. They might have to downsize their living arrangements, get a job, or potentially seek financial assistance from friends, family, or government sources.

Financial therapy can be beneficial for couples, as it addresses the impact of gender biases and helps facilitate open and healthy communication about finances and money management (Jeanfreau et al., 2020). Couples who jointly implement financial management practices experience improved communication and relationship quality (Zimmerman & Roberts, 2012). Engaging in financial therapy can increase couples' help-seeking behavior and lead to improved relationship outcomes (Ford et al., 2020). Although discussing finances may initially cause stress, it presents an opportunity for resilience and growth when approached with unity and a willingness to learn from one another's perspectives (Afifi et al., 2018). Therefore, finances may be a significant topic for therapists to explore in therapy when working with couples. The knowledge of these considerations we have discussed may help therapists to enter into these finance-related conversations with a better understanding of the impact that finances can have on couples.

In-Laws

When a couple comes together through marriage and/or a long-term committed relationship, their families of origin are also usually part of the equation. For some couples, the process of bridging one another's families is relatively smooth. In-laws can oftentimes be a huge source of support in a couple's life, including providing financial aid, emotional support, and childcare for grandchildren (Goetting, 1990). However, for other couples, relationships with in-laws can be strained and can cause significant stress in the couple's relationship. Because in-laws are likely involved in most couples' lives and the quality of these relationships can impact the couple's dynamics (Bryant et al., 2001), it is potentially a significant topic when a couple enters therapy.

Therapists need to understand where conflict with in-laws can stem from. Even though many families go through this process, merging two different families of origin is a tall order. Though one would hope that the couple is coming together because they feel connected to one another in many ways, their respective families and upbringings may be worlds apart. For example, one partner may have been raised with their parents enforcing strict table manners, such as being seated tall and using utensils properly, while the other partner was allowed to keep their elbows on the table and watch television during dinner. Perhaps one partner's religious upbringing was Christianity while their partner's was Islam. These smaller or larger differences in backgrounds (e.g., family rules, communication patterns, roles, family values, culture) can potentially be a foundation for conflict when families join and these distinctions emerge (Prentice, 2008). Additionally, navigating boundaries in the newly created family (i.e., the couple) and in the families of origin may be challenging, as in-laws and the couple themselves are trying to find their place in this new system. Partners may battle with feelings of disloyalty either to their partner or their family of origin. These components that are often a part of the family merging process can potentially be the basis for problems to surface.

The specific dynamics and nuances that unfold in every family are different; however, there are a few common themes concerning in-laws that are important to make note of as a therapist. While **in-laws**, by definition, are those who are relatives by marriage (Merriam-Webster, n.d.), we will use this term to refer to the parents brought together by a couple's relationship, whether the couple is married or not. This section, while not exhaustive, gives some perspective on these themes surrounding in-laws that therapists should keep on their radar when working with a couple.

Parental Approval

A frequent concern among couples is the approval from each partner's parents. Parental approval has been shown to impact the quality of a couple's relationship (e.g., Knobloch & Donovan-Kicken, 2006; Sprecher & Felmlee, 1992), so lack of parental approval may be a significant stressor for a couple coming into therapy. It is a common occurrence for partners to be nervous about meeting one another's parents for the first time. This goes both ways—a partner understandably wants their partner's parents' approval, and they also want their own parents to approve of their partner. One would hope that both sets of parents are accepting of the relationship and of the respective partners. However, when this is not the case, the stress in the couple's relationship can increase as they attempt to grapple with the disapproval from their families of origin.

There are myriad reasons that can be at the root of parental disapproval. Perhaps the parents simply don't like the personality of their child's partner. Maybe the ambitions, finances, and career goals that the partner has do not align with what the in-laws envisioned their child marrying into. Disapproval can also result from larger factors outside of the individual. For example, couples in interracial relationships face a whole other set of obstacles when one or both of the partners' parents do not approve of the relationship because of the difference in race (Bell & Hastings, 2015). Same-sex couples face similar challenges when parents do not approve of the relationship due to underlying issues with sexual orientation, which often puts more strain on the couple (Reczek, 2016). Therapists should not only recognize these reasons for disapproval, but also understand the meaning that the disapproval may have for the couple. Disapproval that arises from being against same-sex or interracial relationships, for instance, may make the couple (or an individual within the couple) feel like their personhood and identity are not being accepted or even challenged. Overall, it is crucial for therapists to understand that the reasons behind parental disapproval may vary and the meaning that accompanies this disapproval may significantly impact the couple—and each partner—in different ways.

Grandchildren and Time Spending

Fingerman (2004) states, "The relationship between a grandparent and a grandchild is a 'contingent' one, dependent on a middle generation rather than a direct path between two parties" (p. 1026). Here, Fingerman highlights the implicit role that parents have in the relationship between their parents/in-laws and their children. The welcoming of children can thus also potentially create discord between in-laws and the couple. This shift in the couple's role as parents and in the in-laws' role as grandparents may result in blurred boundaries (Daly & Perry, 2021). For example, one partner may believe that their partner's parents are overstepping their role as grandparents and are acting like the parents of the couple's child. In-laws may have their own viewpoint on how the child should be raised, and this can potentially result in criticism of one of the partners by their in-laws (Ward & Linn, 2020). The couple may also have different viewpoints on how involved their in-laws should be in their child's life. On the one hand, some couples may greatly appreciate their in-laws being involved with their children and actively rely on their in-laws to take care of the children at times (e.g., babysitting them, picking them up from school). On the other hand, one partner may believe that the grandparents shouldn't be this involved in taking care of their child or—conversely—believe that their partner's parents aren't involved enough in the child's life.

This leads to another possible factor concerning the involvement of in-laws that couples may disagree on: the amount of time the couple spends with their respective in-laws. One partner may want to visit with their parents frequently, whereas the other partner may have the expectation that they only see their in-laws for special occasions and holidays. These differing expectations may lead to arguments or conflict between the couple as they navigate these conversations that focus on their opposing wants and expectations.

Caring for In-Laws

Conflict may also result from taking care of in-laws. Sometimes, especially when partners' parents become older, a couple may be called upon to provide housing, financial support, assistance with daily tasks, medical care, and more to one (or sometimes both) of a partner's parents. This creates a shift in dynamics between the couple, and the family as a whole, which can sometimes result in issues between the couple. For instance, partners may disagree on what the right course of action should be regarding the caregiving for one of their parents. Perhaps one partner believes their mother should move in with them, but the other partner would prefer their mother-in-law to go to a nursing home. The emotional, physical, and mental effects that can accompany caregiving can also potentially bring stress to a couple's relationship (Strauss, 2013).

Stephens et al. (2001) mention that caregivers often experience conflict in other roles in their lives; they experience more depression and spend less time engaging in social and leisure activities. This is especially the case since the partner is usually caring for their parent around the same time they are caring for their own children. This has been called the **sandwich generation**, as the person's caretaking duties are vertically required in two directions, upward for their parent and downward for their child. The demands on time and attention that can be required when caregiving for an in-law can also present potential concerns. For example, if one partner is the primary caregiver for their parent, they may give more attention to them than to their partner (Stephens et al., 2001), leaving their partner feeling unsupported or undervalued. Additionally, the other partner may be leaned on more for support by the caregiving partner, potentially leading to the supporting partner feeling overwhelmed and burned out. These are just a few examples of what could arise from the caregiving of an in-law that therapists can be aware of.

Infidelity

Another common issue that couples present with—and that is perhaps one of the most daunting presenting problems for therapists to work with—is infidelity (Blow & Hartnett, 2005a). The literature boasts a range of definitions used to describe **infidelity**, which can include both physically related acts (e.g., kissing, sexual intercourse, pornography use) and emotionally related acts (e.g., flirting, texting others, falling in love with someone else) (Thornton & Nagurney, 2011). For example, Vowels et al. (2022) comment that infidelity "can broadly be defined as engaging in emotional or sexual relations outside of the agreed-upon bounds of the relationship" (p. 224). Similarly, Thornton and Nagurney (2011) suggest, "Ultimately, infidelity might be considered to be feelings or behaviors that go against a partner's expectations for the exclusivity of the relationship" (p. 52). It seems that many of the definitions of infidelity, although different in their exact wording, focus on the unexpected occurrence of a partner's behaviors that are outside the bounds of what was thought to be acceptable in the relationship. With the specifics of infidelity being multifaceted, there are several noteworthy elements of infidelity that might show up in the therapy room.

Gender and Infidelity

The differing definitions of infidelity in the literature are related to an essential aspect of infidelity between a couple for therapists to consider: Each individual within a partnership may have a different conceptualization of what infidelity looks like. As the therapist, it is thus crucial to understand how each partner defines infidelity. A typical issue therapists might encounter is when the individuals within the couple are not in agreement about the definition of infidelity. Thornton and Nagurney (2011) note that gender is a significant factor that can have an influence on these differing definitions, as women seem to consider emotional and physical involvement with another person as infidelity, whereas men are more likely to believe that physical intimacy rather than an emotional connection is an act of infidelity. These trends seem to be present in other research as well. In Tagler and Jeffers' (2013) study on attitude differences about infidelity between men and women, they found that, compared to women, men responded more negatively toward sexual cheating than emotional cheating.

Differences in the definition of infidelity may then lead to disagreements between the couple about whether one of the partners actually cheated, creating heightened conflict as a result. If the person who allegedly cheated is claiming that what they did does not constitute infidelity, the partner who believes they were cheated on may feel invalidated and angry when they perceive their partner's denial of the situation/refusal to take responsibility. Therapists must keep in the back of their minds the understanding that two partners may not always be on the same page about infidelity, in order to understand the couple's dynamics and concerns more effectively. Being aware that gender could play a role in these differing definitions may be beneficial for the therapist's understanding of any accompanying relational dynamics as well.

Culture and Infidelity

Culture, in addition to gender, is also commonly identified as a factor that can influence a couple's/each partner's conceptualization of infidelity. Needing to work within the couple's (and each individual's) cultural conceptualization of infidelity thus also applies, as cultural values, beliefs, and practices can potentially affect the perception of and reaction to infidelity in a relationship. Penn et al. (1997) state, "Infidelity has diverse meanings for people of different cultures and ethnicities" (p. 169).

For example, Blow and Hartnett (2005b) note that while many countries show disapproval of infidelity (specifically sexual relationships outside of the primary relationship) (e.g., the Netherlands), there are some countries that seem to be more open-minded about extramarital affairs (e.g., Russia, Denmark). Penn et al. (1997) also conduct an in-depth investigation of cultural differences with infidelity, specifically examining these differences among African Americans, Hispanic Americans, and Asian Americans. They acknowledge that the trends they identified are not present in every individual/couple within these cultural backgrounds. However, they found that—while all three groups identified infidelity as being more acceptable for males—it is tolerated (though not approved) for African Americans, frowned upon among Hispanic Americans, and is more likely to lead to blame of females for Asian Americans. Not only are there cultural differences in the disapproval/approval of and social factors related to infidelity, but there is also research that looks at the cultural differences in the accompanying emotional responses to infidelity. For instance, partners in the United States were more likely to identify sexual infidelity rather than emotional infidelity as more distressing compared to partners in Japan (Kato, 2021).

Emotional Experience of Infidelity

So far, we have discussed how it is beneficial for therapists to attend to each couple's (and each partner's) definition of infidelity, as it may change due to factors such as gender and culture. The emotional climate of a therapy session surrounding infidelity is also particularly noteworthy, as the discovery of infidelity often sends shockwaves of pain into a relationship. Though—as with the definition of infidelity—the specifics of the emotional experience of the couple and each individual partner may look different, it is safe to say that instances of infidelity oftentimes come with a shift in the emotional climate of the relationship.

The emotional reaction of the partner who was cheated on is often the first thing that people think of and is a dominant topic in the literature on infidelity. Feelings of betrayal often underlie the emotional experience of the partner who was cheated on (Rokach & Chan, 2023). This betrayal is commonly the result of unmet expectations between partners who enter into a committed relationship with one another with the expectation that they will remain faithful. Again, this is where the potential difference in the partners' definitions of cheating can become a foundation for unmet expectations. A range of related emotions also commonly accompanies the experience of infidelity. Shackelford et al. (2000) conducted a study specifically exploring emotional reactions as a result of infidelity. Common emotional themes that were present in the participant responses included jealousy, anxiety, sadness, hopelessness, shock, and helplessness. Warach and Josephs (2021) also comment on the "resulting traumatic reaction that infidelity can cause betrayed partners" (p. 68) which can consist of anxiety, flashbacks, obsessive thoughts, and other related trauma symptoms.

There seems to be less literature exploring the emotions of the partner who was the perpetrator of the infidelity. There is some research investigating the reasons behind a partner's engagement in infidelity (e.g., Hall & Fincham, 2009; Hunyady et al., 2008) and the perpetrator's perspective of the cheating narrative (e.g., Wilkinson & Dunlop, 2020), but there is scant literature on the emotional experience of the perpetrator after the cheating event and during the potential fallout with their romantic partner. Still, we can speculate what emotions might be present for this partner after the infidelity comes to light. Depending on the relationship as a whole and on the partners as individuals, the perpetrator may feel guilty or shamed because of their actions. In other circumstances, these individuals may feel angry and become defensive, perhaps because of being blamed by their partner for their actions. Like the victim, the perpetrator may also likely feel sadness and anxiety as they experience the rift that infidelity commonly causes in a relationship.

These are just some emotions that therapists may encounter from a couple that is dealing with infidelity. Infidelity can oftentimes be one of the most emotionally jarring incidents in a couple's relationship, so therapists should be aware beforehand that this particular presenting problem may come with intense emotional dynamics. Having an idea of the common emotional experiences of couples, while attending to the particular dynamics of each couple—and even each session—is beneficial. Therapists must be prepared, yet still meet each couple where they are at.

Infidelity versus Nonmonogamy

As we come to a close on the major themes of infidelity, there is one more item where we believe it is important to provide clarity: the difference between infidelity and nonmonogamy. When we addressed the various definitions of infidelity, we noted the common definitional component of the behaviors (whatever they specifically may be) being outside of what was expected/agreed upon for the relationship. **Nonmonogamy** refers to *consensual* non-exclusive sexual and/or romantic relationships (Mogilski et al., 2020).

Essentially, infidelity is the breach of what was expected for the relationship whereas nonmonogamy involves the consensual decision from all partners to be involved in outside relationships/behaviors in some form (Scoats & Campbell, 2022). This distinction is important to make because the two concepts are oftentimes confused. While nonmonogamy is often accompanied by negative connotations related to moral values (Mogilski et al., 2020), it is actually based on a consensual agreement, unlike infidelity. If a therapist finds out during the course of therapy that an individual with whom they are working has a partner who is sexually or romantically seeing another person, it should not automatically be assumed that it is the result of cheating. Once again, the therapist needs to be open and curious about the dynamics that the client is presenting with, in order to understand them accurately.

Consensual Nonmonogamy

Throughout this book, the term "couple" has been used to refer to people in a relationship. However, therapists might encounter multiple people—rather than just two individuals—that are involved romantically and/or sexually with one another. **Consensual nonmonogamy** (CNM) is the overarching term used to describe romantic and sexual relationships and practices that are consensual and involve multiple partners (Scoats & Campbell, 2022). There are several types of CNM relationships that can helpfully be defined and understood. While this list is not exhaustive, these are some of the common CNM relationships that a therapist may encounter—polyamory, swinging, open relationships (Scoats & Campbell, 2022), and polyfidelity (Levine et al., 2018).

The term polyamory first emerged in the 1990s and continues to have multiple uses and definitions in a variety of contexts (Cardoso et al., 2021). Hnatkovičová and Bianchi (2022) more recently defined **polyamory** as "a form of consensual non-monogamy (CNM) based on the belief that people can participate in and build multiple romantic and/or sexual relationships with the consent of all involved" (p. 184). A polyamorous relationship is thus comprised of more than two individuals—their genders, sexual orientations, sexual interactions with one another, shared children, and more differ depending on each individual relationship. Scoats and Campbell (2022) also note that there can be hierarchal or non-hierarchal polyamorous relationships. In a hierarchal relationship, partners can be identified as primary, secondary, and so on, and primary (or nesting) partners are commonly those who live together. In a non-hierarchal relationship, all individuals in the relationship have relations generally equal to one another.

Polyfidelity is similar to polyamory in that romantic relationships are with multiple partners (Levine et al., 2018). In contrast to polyamory, in which "individuals are open to the possibility of forming loving relationships with multiple partners" (Levine et al., 2018, p. 1140), polyfidelity consists of three or more people being in a romantic relationship with one another specifically.

Essentially, polyfidelity is a romantic relationship between several people within one group, where the romantic love is shared between all individuals within the relationship (Peterson, 2017).

Swinging involves couples (made up of two romantically involved people) engaging in sexual relations with other couples (Scoats & Campbell, 2022). Oftentimes, swinging happens at designated swinging events/clubs. The main point about swinging is that the romantic unit of the relationship remains between two people (the couple), but the consensual nonmonogamy comes in through the consensual sexual relations that the couple has with other couples (Vaillancourt & Few-Demo, 2014).

Similar to swinging, **open relationships** also involve a couple (two individuals who are involved romantically) having sexual relations outside of that dyad (Scoats & Campbell, 2022). However, open relationships differ from swinging in that couples in open relationships do not purposefully go to have sex with other couples at organized events or meetups. Rather, it is agreed upon in an open relationship that the two individuals in the romantic couple are free to explore other sexual relationships with whomever they choose. Thus, in swinging relationships, both partners are having sexual relations with the partners of another couple, usually at the same time (but perhaps not in the same room). In open relationships, the sexual encounter is likely not to involve another couple, but rather an individual that only one partner of the couple encounters.

We briefly want to take a moment and address a few other terms that are often associated with CNM, but do not seem to be a part of the umbrella of CNM in the literature. **Polygamy** is comparable to CNM in that the romantic relationship extends outside of just two people; however, Shaiful Bahari et al. (2021) explain that polygamy is different because it involves marital relationships between multiple individuals. There are three categories of relationships that fall within polygamous marriages: (1) **polygyny**—one male who is married to two or more females; (2) **polyandry**—one female who is married to two or more males; and (3) **polygynandry**—two or more females who are married to two or more males.

Client Conceptualizations of CNM

As with many labels, titles, or names for a concept, different people may have different conceptualizations of CNM (as indicated in our discussion on infidelity). This is one of the first things to be aware of—therapists may come across multiple clients who are in CNM relationships, but not all these clients will operate in their CNM relationships in the same way. Essentially, as with any other type of relationship, there is no "cookie cutter" CNM relationship. Each relationship will likely have different dynamics, roles, and expectations. Scoats and Campbell (2022) emphasize this notion as well: "These umbrella terms should be viewed with caution, at the individual level CNM is practiced in a variety of ways, producing a plethora of relationship configurations" ("Introduction" section, para. 3). It thus is crucial that therapists remain curious and non-assuming about these relational dynamics. They need to get to know the client's system and ways of functioning in that system, and allow them to provide the term that makes sense to them to define their relationship (if the client finds it important to do so). Again, this applies to all types of relationship. Therapists working with individuals in a CNM relationship should enter the worldview of their clients and see how they view their own relationship and the meanings that come with those viewpoints.

Stigmatization

Stigmatization could also potentially be a factor that influences a CNM relationship and resultantly be a factor that is present in the therapy room. Hnatkovičová and Bianchi (2022) acknowledge that there is still a stigma that surrounds polyamory (and most nonmonogamous relationships in general). This stigmatization can be found in the media and even in psychology-based research and literature, as much of it is littered with talk about romantic and/or sexual relationships in terms of a dyad and lacks equivalent attention to CNM relationships (Levine et al., 2018). Research that specifically explores individuals' attitudes to and perceptions of polyamory, for instance, indicates that negative beliefs are still pervasive. Séguin (2019) found that while there were some positive themes surrounding polyamory from the participants (e.g., valid, beneficial, and acceptable), the results also demonstrated adverse perceptions, such as polyamorous relationships being unsustainable, amoral, and deficient in true love. Barnett (2014) also notes the logistical and even legal repercussions of this stigmatization, such as not having the legal right to be married to more than one person (which comes with other concerns, including child custody and healthcare issues) or being directly criminalized if one went against these laws that ban polyamorous marriages in some states. Much of the stigmatization toward CNM stems from a pervasive Western ideal that sees serial monogamy as the hallmark of true romantic love (Moors et al., 2021).

If stigmatization is a significant experience for clients who are in a polyamorous relationship with one another, there are several considerations for therapists to keep in mind. First, it is important to recognize and validate that this stigmatization is present. Second, it is also key to remember that these negative beliefs may be coming from different contexts depending on the relationship. Perhaps the individuals in one relationship are from a city that legally recognizes CNM relationships and have family members who are supportive of this relationship as well. These clients might present differently than individuals who live in an area that has laws against CNM relationships or have family members whose beliefs strongly contrast with such a relationship. Even within one CNM relationship, the experience of each individual person may differ (e.g., one person's family may be supportive while the others' families are not). Overall, therapists need to (a) be aware of the general stigmatization of polyamory that is present in a variety of environments; and (b) still be curious about how this stigmatization may manifest differently in each relationship and in each individual within the relationship.

Mononormativity

It is also important to mention that just because a therapist might be sitting with a couple (i.e., two people in a relationship) in their therapy office, it does not mean that the entire relationship is necessarily comprised of only those two people. This brings up the concept of **mononormativity**, the assumption that a couple being committed to only each other is the healthy or normal standard for a sexual/romantic relationship (Ferrer, 2018). Just as it is necessary for therapists to work within the definition/dynamics of each CNM relationship, it is also crucial to remember that assuming a relationship solely consists of two people may be inaccurate. Because of the different dynamics that make up each CNM relationship, two people in that relationship may be presenting for therapy, while there still are other individuals in the relationship as a whole. It is important for therapists to ask questions that invite the dyad in the therapy room to be able to comfortably disclose these potential relationship dynamics.

Kinks

The definition of **kinks**, or kink behaviors, varies with its specificity in the literature. Rehor (2015) defines them as "unconventional sensual, erotic, and sexual behaviors" (p. 825). Similarly, Hughes and Hammack (2022) state that kinks are "consensual sexual, intimate or sensual activities that fall outside of typical social norms" (p. 360). Overall, the various descriptions of kinks seem to include three foundational elements: (a) they involve some sort of sexual, sensual, and/or intimate activity; (b) they are viewed as atypical/unconventional compared to "normal" sexual behaviors; and (c) the engagement in kink behaviors is consensual between all parties involved. Within this overarching concept of kinks are specific categories of kink behaviors. While we will not address all examples of kinks, there are a few common ones that we want to discuss to create a better understanding of these sexual practices.

BDSM—bondage and discipline (B/D), dominance and submission (D/S), sadism and masochism (S/M)—is one subset of kinks that is more commonly researched and well-known. Yates and Neuer-Colburn (2019) note that these three domains which make up the overlapping acronym of BDSM have different definitions/activities within themselves. **Bondage and discipline** involve the usage of both various physical and mental restraints. **Dominance and submission** center on the element of power, wherein one partner takes it while the other gives it up (again, this can be physical or mental). **Sadism and masochism**, often referred to as **sadomasochism**, focus on the experience of receiving and/or inflicting powerful stimuli and sensations. While BDSM is an overarching acronym that houses all three of these practices, each couple/individual who participates in BDSM may not partake in each one of these activities.

Fetishism involves sexual arousal and gratification from inanimate objects (Rees & Garcia, 2017; Ventriglio et al., 2019). Fetishes can include a range of inanimate objects (e.g., leather and rubber materials, clothing, shoes); however, a fetish can also be toward body parts, specific locations/situations, behaviors, or activities (Grimes, 2019; Ventriglio et al., 2019). In addition to fetishism being seen as a deviant sexual practice in general, specific stigmatization surrounding fetishism stems from the belief that the person is unable to see others as people, but rather as means for sexual gratification; these individuals thus direct their sexual energy toward non-living objects and have issues with finding and fostering sexual/romantic relationships with other people (Rees & Garcia, 2017).

Voyeurism and exhibitionism are often presented together in the literature, so we will discuss them together here as well. Thomas et al. (2021) define **voyeurism** as "arousal [that] comes from watching others undress or engage in sexual activities" (p. 2151) and **exhibitionism** as "arousal [that] comes from exposing oneself to strangers" (p. 2151). Much of the literature surrounding these two sexual behaviors is accompanied by a negative undertone, as the research seems to refer to voyeurism and exhibitionism just as instances of criminal behavior (e.g., Freund et al., 1988). While there are criminal cases involving these sexual practices, the word "consent" distinguishes these cases from other sexual activity. Pohtinen (2019) states that voyeurism and fetishism are subsets of kinky behaviors when consent and mutual agreement to engage in these practices are involved. However, there seems to be little research that talks about these two practices in a non-stigmatizing way.

Some forms of role-play, such as role-play related to age and gender, are also considered part of kinky behaviors (Pohtinen, 2019). Tiidenberg and Paasonen (2019) refer to age-related role-play and age-play. While **age-play** can be considered a part of BDSM in terms of its elements of dominance and submission, age-play brings in a more specific feature of the age of the roles that the partners take on during sexual activity. For example, the "older" roles may be mom/dad or schoolmaster, and the "younger" roles (often called Littles) may be a little boy/girl (Tiidenberg & Paasonen, 2019). Like age-play, **gender-play** encompasses the ability to experience stepping into different roles of different genders, regardless of one's gender identity or sexual orientation (Bauer, 2018). Bauer (2018) also notes that not only can this be a sexual experience, but it can also allow for "renegotiating what it means to be a mother, a father or other responsible adult, as well as non-biological reproductions of kinship" (p. 152). Overall, there seems to be less literature on age- and gender-play behaviors than other sexual practices under the kinky behaviors umbrella.

Pathology/Stigmatization

Like CNM relationships, kinks often come with stigmatization and are still frequently seen from a pathological viewpoint (Hughes & Hammack, 2022). This viewpoint stems from multiple realms, including religion, medicine, and psychiatry (Pohtinen, 2019). Practices such as sadism (especially in men) were originally believed to be sexual perversions and deviances from normal development by psychoanalysts such as Sigmund Freud and Richard von Krafft-Ebing (Rehor, 2015; Sabo, 2020). Trauma is also commonly seen and researched as the "root" of kinky preferences, giving kinky behaviors a negative connotation related to disturbing experiences from childhood (Hillier, 2019; Hughes & Hammack, 2022). Media portrayals of kink behaviors (often done in a violent, joking, or traumatic light) also contribute to kink practices' negative connotations (Pohtinen, 2019). Though the understanding of and the literature on kinks are beginning to change, this foundation of pathology still leads to stigmatization among individuals who practice kink behaviors (Hillier, 2019). It is necessary for therapists to keep in mind these stigmatizations and their associated effects on individuals within the kink community when working with clients who engage in kink behaviors to understand what kink practitioners' current experiences may be.

A significant area of life that can be impacted by the stigmatization of kinks is children. Much of the literature addresses the issue of bias in the legal system due to kink stigmatization that can result in custody issues, such as losing custody of children (Hillier, 2019; Pohtinen, 2019; Yates & Neuer-Colburn, 2019). An underlying experience of shame and anxiety also commonly accompanies those who practice kink behaviors, as these individuals often grapple with the decision of divulging these sexual preferences to others (Hillier, 2019). Dismissal from jobs and increased susceptibility to violence also might result from these stigmas (Pohtinen, 2019). In addition to kink practitioners facing discrimination in the healthcare system in general (Pohtinen, 2019), Hansen-Brown and Jefferson (2022) specifically point out that mental health professionals have been shown to experience more discomfort when working with the kink community compared to lesbian/gay clients or even clients who practice group sex. Again, though these experiences may not apply to every person participating in kink behaviors, knowing about these common experiences within this population may be helpful for therapists.

We want to end the conversation on pathology/stigmatization by highlighting a crux of kink behaviors—consent. Yates and Neuer-Colburn (2019) emphasize this notion as well, stating that the "practices of Kink community members hinge on one central construct: consent" (p. 16). Therapists must be cognizant of this consensual element of kink behaviors, as recognizing the importance of consent in the kink community helps to shift a lens of pathology off these practices. Yates and Neuer-Colburn (2019) also mention that this shift is evident in the fifth edition of the *Diagnostic and Statistical Manual of Mental Disorders* (APA, 2013), as paraphilic disorders included the criteria that (1) distress in the engagement of these behaviors needed to be present, (2) they cause problems with functioning, and (with certain diagnoses) (3) they include action against another person that was not consensual. This noteworthy clarification is analogous to our comments on consent separating infidelity from nonmonogamy as well.

The Kink Community

Much of the literature on kink behaviors references the kink community (e.g., Hughes & Hammack, 2022; Rehor, 2015; Yates & Neuer-Colburn, 2019). Rehor (2015) defines **kink practitioners** as individuals who participate in kinky practices and the kink community as the larger organizations that are made up of kink practitioners. Hughes and Hammack (2022) comment on the benefits of the kink community, such as the sense of identity and connection that the community brings to kink practitioners. Yates and Neuer-Colburn (2019) specifically address important components of the kink community that therapists need to understand to work more effectively with clients who identify with this population. Primarily, they note that while sexual practices are an important feature of the community, the community is a culture in and of itself that has values, customs, artwork/emblems, distinctive terminology, and more.

While the breadth and depth of the specific terms used in this community are beyond the scope of this discussion, we recommend that therapists become aware of these terms (but still work within the terminology presented by each individual client) to have a basic understanding of the kink community. Yates and Neuer-Colburn (2019) suggest utilizing a cultural lens when working with individuals in this community in order to create understanding and remove the stigma. While a client coming in for therapy may divulge that they engage in kink behaviors, these behaviors may not be related to the reason for seeking therapy; it is thus necessary for the therapist to remain focused on what the client is hoping for from therapy and not assume that kink behaviors are a problem. Overall, similar to our discussions on infidelity and CNM, we "encourage counselors to approach their sessions with curiosity and openness" (Yates & Neuer-Colburn, 2019, p. 20).

Summary

This chapter provided an overview of some of the primary contexts in which couples engage one another. Relational dynamics may depend on how the couple navigates each of these contexts, depending on their relevancy for the couple. Having a conceptualization of the case is based not only on one's primary theoretical model but also on the client's living situation. Therapists may need to adapt their conceptualization, even if using the same model, based on whether a couple is same-sex, interracial, or involved in an alternative lifestyle. We presented these various contexts here, understanding that this is just an introduction and that couples are housed within multiple contexts. A therapist's case conceptualization is always partial, but the more contexts that are layered into it, the closer a therapist can get to the client's experience.

References

Addington, L. A. (2020). Police response to same-sex intimate partner violence in the marriage equality era. *Criminal Justice Studies*, *33*(3), 213–230. https://doi.org/10.1080/1478601X.2020.1786277

Addo, F. R., & Sassler, S. (2010). Financial arrangements and relationship quality in low-income couples. *Family Relations*, *59*(4), 408–423. https://doi.org/10.1111/j.1741-3729.2010.00612.x

Afifi, T. D., Davis, S., Merrill, A. F., Coveleski, S., Denes, A., & Shahnazi, A. F. (2018). Couples' communication about financial uncertainty following the great recession and its association with stress, mental health and divorce proneness. *Journal of Family and Economic Issues*, *39*, 205–219. https://doi.org/10.1007/s10834-017-9560-5

Ali, P. A., McGarry, J., & Dhingra, K. (2016). Identifying signs of intimate partner violence. *Emergency Nurse*, *23*(9), 25–29. https://doi.org/10.7748/en.23.9.25.s25

Allen, D., & Price, J. (2020). Stability rates of same-sex couples: With and without children. *Marriage & Family Review*, *56*(1), 51–71. https://doi.org/10.1080/01494929.2019.1630048

American Psychiatric Association. (2013). *Diagnostic and statistical manual of mental disorders, fifth edition*. APA.

Atwood, J. D. (2012). Couples and money: The last taboo. *The American Journal of Family Therapy*, *40*(1), 1–19. https://doi.org/10.1080/01926187.2011.600674

Barnett, J. P. (2014). Polyamory and criminalization of plural conjugal unions in Canada: Competing narratives in the s.293 reference. *Sexual Research and Social Policy*, *11*, 63–75. https://doi.org/10.1007/s13178-013-0137-2

Bauer, R. (2018). Bois and grrrls meet their daddies and mommies on gender playgrounds: Gendered age play in the les-bi-trans-queer BDSM communities. *Sexualities*, *21*(1–2), 139–155. https://doi.org/10.1177/1363460716676987

Bell, G. C., & Hastings, S. O. (2011). Black and White interracial couples: Managing relational disapproval through facework. *Howard Journal of Communications*, *22*(3), 240–259. https://doi.org/10.1080/10646175.2011.590405

Bell, G. C., & Hastings, S. O. (2015). Exploring parental approval and disapproval for black and white interracial couples. *Journal of Social Issues*, *71*(4), 755–771. https://doi.org/10.1111/josi.12147

Bell, N. K., Harris, S. M., Guyette, E., Allen, S., & Roberts, K. M. (2022). Considering the roles of children and finances in the divorce decision-making process. *Journal of Divorce & Remarriage, 63*(7–8), 483–505. https://doi.org/10.1080/10502556.2022.2149031

Blow, A. J., & Hartnett, K. (2005a). Infidelity in committed relationships I: A methodological review. *Journal of Marital and Family Therapy, 31*(2), 183–216. https://doi.org/10.1111/j.1752-0606.2005.tb01555.x

Blow, A. J., & Hartnett, K. (2005b). Infidelity in committed relationships II: A substantive review. *Journal of Marital and Family Therapy, 31*(2), 217–233. https://doi.org/10.1111/j.1752-0606.2005.tb01555.x

Böhm, M., & Shapley, D. (2013). Interracial marriage trends and migration patterns: An analysis of LAFANS 2000. *Marriage & Family Review, 49*(3), 212–230. https://doi.org/10.1080/01494929.2012.762442

Bosley-Smith, E. R., & Reczek, C. (2018). Before and after 'I do': Marriage processes for mid-life gay and lesbian married couples. *Journal of Homosexuality, 65*(14), 1985–2004. https://doi.org/10.1080/00918369.2017.1423213

Bratter, J. L., & King, R. B., (2008). "But will it last?": Marital instability among interracial and same-race couples. *Family Relations, 57*(2), 160–171. https://doi.org/10.1111/j.1741-3729.2008.00491.x

Brooks, J. E., Ogolsky, B. G., & Monk, J. K. (2018). Commitment in interracial relationships: Dyadic and longitudinal tests of the investment model. *Journal of Family Issues, 39*(9), 2685–2708. https://doi.org/10.1177/0192513X18758343

Brown, C. C., Williams, Z., & Durtschi, J. A. (2018). Trajectories of interracial heterosexual couples: A longitudinal analysis of relationship quality and separation. *Journal of Marital and Family Therapy, 45*(4), 650–667. https://doi.org/10.1111/jmft.12363

Bryant, C. M., Conger, R. D., & Meehan, J. M. (2001). The influence of in-laws on change in marital success. *Journal of Marriage and Family Therapy, 63*(3), 614–626. https://doi.org/10.1111/j.1741-3737.2001.00614.x

Cardoso, D., Pascoal, P. M., & Maiochi, F. H. (2021). Defining polyamory: A thematic analysis of lay people's definitions. *Archives of Sexual Behavior, 50*, 1239–1252. https://doi.org/10.1007/s10508-021-02002-y

Choi, K. H., & Tienda, M. (2017). Boundary crossing in first marriage and remarriage. *Social Science Research, 62*, 305–316. https://doi.org/10.1016/j.ssresearch.2016.08.014

Çineli, B. (2020). Money management and gender equality: An analysis of dual-earner couples in Western Europe. *Family Relations, 69*(4), 803–819. https://doi.org/10.1111/fare.12465

Çineli, B. (2022). Who manages the money at home? Multilevel analysis of couples' money management across 34 countries. *Gender & Society, 36*(1), 32–62. https://doi.org/10.1177/08912432211057920

Colistra, R., & Johnson, C. B. (2021). Framing the legalization of marriage for same-sex couples: An examination of news coverage surrounding the U.S. Supreme Court's landmark decision. *Journal of Homosexuality, 68*(1), 88–111. https://doi.org/10.1080/00918369.2019.1627128

Crapo, J. S., Turner, J. J., Kopystynska, O., Bradford, K., & Higginbotham, B. J. (2021). Financial stress and perceptions of spousal behavior over time in remarriages. *Journal of Family and Economic Issues, 42*, 300–313. https://doi.org/10.1007/s10834-020-09697-6

Cronholm, P. F., Fogarty, C. T., Ambuel, B., & Harrison, S. L. (2011). Intimate partner violence. *American Family Physician, 83*(10), 1165–1172. www.aafp.org/dam/brand/aafp/pubs/afp/issues/2011/0515/p1165.pdf

Daly, M., & Perry, G. (2021). In-law relationships in evolutionary perspective: The good, the bad, and the ugly. *Frontiers in Sociology, 6*, Article 683501. https://doi.org/10.3389/fsoc.2021.683501

Durfee, A., & Goodmark, L. (2020). Domestic violence mandatory arrest policies and arrests for same-sex and opposite-sex intimate partner violence after legalization of same-sex marriage in the United States. *Criminal Justice Studies, 33*(3), 231–255. https://doi.org/10.1080/1478601X.2020.1786279.

Feinstein, B. A., McConnell, E., Dyar, C., Mustanski, B., & Newcomb, M. E. (2018). Minority stress and relationship functioning among young male same-sex couples: An examination of actor–partner interdependence models. *Journal of Consulting and Clinical Psychology, 86*(5), 416–426. http://dx.doi.org/10.1037/ccp0000296

Ferrer, J. N. (2018). Mononormativity, polypride, and the "mono–poly wars." *Sexuality & Culture, 22*, 817–836. https://doi.org/10.1007/s12119-017-9494-y

Fingerman, K. L. (2004). The role of offspring and in-laws in grandparents' ties to their grandchildren. *Journal of Family Issues, 25*(8), 1026–1049. https://doi.org/10.1177/0192513X04265941

Foeman, A. K., & Nance, T. (1999). From miscegenation to multiculturalism: Perceptions and stages of interracial relationship development. *Journal of Black Studies, 29*(4), 540–557. www.jstor.org/stable/2645869

Ford, M. R., Ross, D. B., Grable, J., & DeGraff, A. (2020). Examining the role of financial therapy on relationship outcomes and help-seeking behavior. *Contemporary Family Therapy*, *42*, 55–67. https://doi.org/10.1007/s10591-019-09511-y

Forry, N. D., Leslie, L. A., & Letiecq, B. L. (2007). Marital quality in interracial relationships: The role of sex role ideology and perceived fairness. *Journal of Family Issues*, *28*(12), 1538–1552. https://doi.org/10.1177/0192513X07304466

Freund, K., Watson, R., & Rienzo, D. (1988). The value of self-reports in the study of voyeurism and exhibitionism. *Annals of Sex Research*, *1*(2), 243–262. https://doi.org/10.1177/107906328800100205

Gaines Jr., S. O., Granrose, C. S., Rios, D. I., Garcia, B. F., Youn, M. S. P., Farris, K. R., & Bledsoe, K. L. (1999). Patterns of attachment and responses to accommodative dilemmas among interethnic/interracial couples. *Journal of Social and Personal Relationships*, *16*(2), 275–285. https://doi.org/10.1177/0265407599162009

Gerstenberger, C., Stansfield, R., & Williams, K. R. (2019). Intimate partner violence in same-sex relationships: An analysis of risk and rearrest. *Criminal Justice and Behavior*, *46*(11), 1515–1527. https://doi.org/10.1177/0093854819871984

Gladstone, J. J., Garbinsky, E. N., & Mogilner, C. (2022). Pooling finances and relationship satisfaction. *Journal of Personality and Social Psychology*, *123*(6), 1293–1314. https://doi.org/10.1037/pspi0000388

Goetting, A. (1990). Patterns of support among in-laws in the United States: A review of research. *Journal of Family Issues*, *11*(1), 67–90. https://doi.org/10.1177/019251390011001005

Gotta, G., Green, R.-J., Rothblum, E., Solomon, S., Balsam, K., & Schwartz, P. (2011). Heterosexual, lesbian, and gay male relationships: A comparison of couples in 1975 and 2000. *Family Process*, *50*(3), 353–376. https://doi.org/10.1111/j.1545-5300.2011.01365.x

Gottman, J. M., Gottman, J. S., Cole, C., & Preciado, M. (2020). Gay, lesbian, and heterosexual couples about to begin couples therapy: An online relationship assessment of 40,681 couples. *Journal of Marital and Family Therapy*, *46*(2), 218–239. https://doi.org/10.1111/jmft.12395

Grable, J. E., Kruger, M., Byram, J. L., & Kwak, E. J. (2021). Perceptions of a partner's spending and saving behavior and financial satisfaction. *Journal of Financial Therapy*, *12*(1), 31–50. https://doi.org/10.4148/1944-9771.1257

Graham, L. M., Jensen, T. M., Givens, A. D., Bowen, G. L., & Rizo, C. F. (2019). Intimate partner violence among same-sex couples in college: A propensity score analysis. *Journal of Interpersonal Violence*, *34*(8), 1583–1610. https://doi.org/10.1177/0886260516651628

Grimes, A. (2019). The science of fetishes. *Osmosis Magazine*, 1, Article 5. Retrieved from https://scholarship.richmond.edu/cgi/viewcontent.cgi?article=1014&context=osmosis

Haas, S. M., & Lannutti, P. J. (2022). Relationship maintenance behaviors, resilience, and relational quality in romantic relationships of LGBTQ+ people. *Couple and Family Psychology: Research and Practice*, *11*(2), 117–131. https://doi.org/10.1037/cfp0000186

Hall, J. H., & Fincham, F. D. (2009). Psychological distress: Precursor or consequence of dating infidelity? *Personality and Social Psychology Bulletin*, *35*(2), 143–159. https://doi.org/10.1177/0146167208327189

Hansen-Brown, A. A., & Jefferson, S. E. (2022). Perceptions of and stigma toward BDSM practitioners. *Current Psychology*. https://doi.org/10.1007/s12144-022-03112-z

Hibbler, D. K., & Shinew, K. J. (2002). Interracial couples' experience of leisure: A social network approach. *Journal of Leisure Research*, *34*(2), 135–156. https://doi.org/10.1080/00222216.2002.11949966

Hillier, K. (2019). The impact of childhood trauma and personality on kinkiness in adulthood [Doctoral dissertation, Walden University]. Walden University ScholarWorks. Retrieved from https://core.ac.uk/download/pdf/217233885.pdf

Hnatkovičová, D., & Bianchi, G. (2022). Model of motivations for engaging in polyamorous relationships. *Sexologies*, *31*(3), 184–194. https://doi.org/10.1016/j.sexol.2022.03.003

Hornor, G. (2005). Domestic violence and children. *Journal of Pediatric Health Care*, *19*(4), 206–212. https://doi.org/10.1016/j.pedhc.2005.02.002

Hu, Y. (2021). Divergent gender revolutions: Cohort changes in household financial management across income gradients. *Gender & Society*, *35*(5), 746–777. http://doi.org/10.1177/08912432211036912

Hughes, S. D., & Hammack, P. L. (2022). Narratives of the origins of kinky sexual desire held by users of a kink-oriented social networking website. *The Journal of Sex Research*, *59*(3), 360–371. https://doi.org/10.1080/00224499.2020.1840495

Hunyady, O., Josephs, L., & Jost, J. T. (2008). Priming the primal scene: Betrayal trauma, narcissism, and attitudes toward sexual infidelity. *Self and Identity*, *7*(3), 278–294. https://doi.org/10.1080/1529886070 1620227

Jeanfreau, M. M., Holden, C., & Brazeal, M. (2020). Our money, my secrets: Why married individuals commit financial infidelity. *Contemporary Family Therapy*, *42*, 46–54. https://doi.org/10.1007/s10591-019-09516-7

Johnson, A. (2017, February 1). *Domestic violence and the duty to make mandated reports*. CAMFT. Retrieved from www.camft.org/Resources/Legal-Articles/Chronological-Article-List/domestic-violence-and-the-duty-to-make-mandated-reports

Johnson, M. P., & Ferraro, K. J. (2000). Research on domestic violence in the 1990s: Making distinctions. *Journal of Marriage and the Family*, *62*(4), 948–963. https://doi.org/10.1111/j.1741-3737.2000.00948.x

Jones, N. E., Malone Jr., D. E., & Campbell, M. E. (2021). Same-sex and different-sex interracial couples: The importance of demographic and religious context. *Race and Social Problems*, *13*, 267–278. https://doi.org/10.1007/s12552-021-09340-5

Joyner, K., Manning, W., & Prince, B. (2019). The qualities of same-sex and different-sex couples in young adulthood. *Journal of Marriage and Family*, *81*(2), 487–505. https://doi.org/10.1111/jomf.12535

Karakurt, G., Dial, S., Korkow, H., Mansfield, T., & Banford, A. (2013). Experiences of marriage and family therapists working with intimate partner violence. *Journal of Family Psychotherapy*, *24*(1), 1–16. https://doi.org/10.1080/08975353.2013.762864

Kato, T. (2021). Gender differences in response to infidelity types and rival attractiveness. *Sexual and Relationship Therapy*, *36*(4), 368–384. https://doi.org/10.1080/14681994.2019.1639657

Kennedy, H. R., & Dalla, R. L. (2020). "It may be legal, but it is not treated equally": Marriage equality and well-being implications for same-sex couples. *Journal of Gay & Lesbian Social Services*, *32*(1), 67–98. https://doi.org/10.1080/10538720.2019.1681340

Killian, K. D. (2001a). Crossing borders: Race, gender and their intersections in interracial couples. *Journal of Feminist Family Therapy*, *13*(1), 1–31. https://doi.org/10.1300/J086v13n01_01

Killian, K. D. (2001b). Reconstituting racial histories and identities: The narratives of interracial couples. *Journal of Marital and Family Therapy*, *27*(1), 27–42. https://doi.org/10.1111/j.1752-0606.2001.tb01137.x

Killian, K. D. (2002). Dominant and marginalized discourses in interracial couples' narratives: Implications for family therapists. *Family Process*, *41*(4), 603–618. https://doi.org/10.1111/j.1545-5300.2002.00603.x

Knobloch, L. K., & Donovan-Kicken, E. (2006). Perceived involvement of network members in courtships: A test of the relational turbulence model. *Personal Relationships*, *13*(3), 281–302. https://doi.org/10.1111/j.1475-6811.2006.00118.x

Kuroki, M. (2017). Marital dissolution and formation for interracial couples: Evidence from parents of biracial children. *Race and Social Problems*, *9*, 255–261. https://doi.org/10.1007/s12552-017-9202-4

Lannutti, P. J. (2018). Committed, unmarried same-sex couples and their social networks in the United States: Relationships and discursive strategies. *Journal of Homosexuality*, *65*(9), 1232–1248. https://doi.org/10.1080/00918369.2017.1411690

LeBaron-Black, A. B., Saxey, M. T., Totenhagen, C. J., Wheeler, B. E., Archuleta, K. L., Yorgason, J. B., & James, S. (2022). Financial communication as a mediator between financial values and marital outcomes. *Family Relations*. https://doi.org/10.1111/fare.12786

Leslie, L. A., & Letiecq, B. L. (2004). Marital quality of African American and white partners in interracial couples. *Personal Relationships*, *11*(4), 559–574.

Leslie, L. A., & Young, J. L. (2015). Interracial couples in therapy: Common themes and issues. *Journal of Social Issues*, *71*(4), 788–803. https://doi.org/10.1111/josi.12149

Levine, E. C., Herbenick, D., Martinez, O., Fu, T.-C., & Dodge, B. (2018). Open relationships, nonconsensual nonmonogamy, and monogamy among U.S. adults: Findings from the 2012 National Survey of Sexual Health and Behavior. *Archives of Sexual Behavior*, *47*(5), 1439–1450. https://doi.org/10.1007/s10 508-018-1178-7

Lewandowski, D. A., & Jackson, L. A. (2001). Perceptions of interracial couples: Prejudice at the dyadic level. *Journal of Black Psychology*, *27*(3), 288–303. https://doi.org/10.1177/0095798401027003003

Lim, H., & Morgan, P. (2021). Financial integration and financial conflict: Does less financial integration relate to increased financial conflict between romantic partners? *Journal of Family and Economic Issues*, *42*, 273–281. https://doi.org/10.1007/s10834-020-09703-x

Mascolo, J. (2023). Mandatory reporting of domestic violence. *FindLaw*. Retrieved August 22, 2023, from www.findlaw.com/family/domestic-violence/mandatory-reporting-of-domestic-violence.html

Merriam-Webster. (n.d.). In-law. Retrieved September 19, 2022, from www.merriam-webster.com/dictionary/in-law

Mogilski, J. K., Mitchell, V. E., Reeve, S. D., Donaldson, S. H., Nicolas, S. C. A., & Welling, L. L. M. (2020). Life history and multi-partner mating: A novel explanation for moral stigma against consensual non-monogamy. *Frontiers in Psychology*, *10*, Article 3033. https://doi.org/10.3389/fpsyg.2019.03033

Moors, A. C., Gesselman, A. N., & Garcia, J. R. (2021). Desire, familiarity, and engagement in polyamory: Results from a national sample of single adults in the United States. *Frontiers in Psychology*, *12*, Article 619640. https://doi.org/10.3389/fpsyg.2021.619640

Nguyen, H. N., D'Aniello, C., & Hayes, B. (2016). Exploring visible and invisible differences and similarities in couple therapy. *Journal of Family Psychotherapy*, *27*(3), 215–220. https://doi.org/10.1080/08975353.2016.1199771

Patra, P., Prakash, J. Patra, B., & Khanna, P. (2018). Intimate partner violence: Wounds are deeper. *Indian Journal of Psychiatry*, *60*(4), 494–498. https://doi.org/10.4103/psychiatry.IndianJPsychiatry_74_17

Penn, C. D., HernÁndez, S. L., & Bermúdez, M. (1997). Using a cross-cultural perspective to understand infidelity in couples therapy. *American Journal of Family Therapy*, *25*(2), 169–185. https://doi.org/10.1080/01926189708251064

Pentel, K. Z., & Baucom, D. H. (2022). A clinical framework for sexual minority couple therapy. *Couple and Family Psychology: Research Practice*, *11*(2), 177–191. https://doi.org/10.1037/cfp0000187

Pepping, C. A., Cronin, T. J., Halford, W. K., & Lyons, A. (2019). Minority stress and same-sex relationship satisfaction: The role of concealment motivation. *Family Process*, *58*(2), 496–508. https://doi.org/10.1111/famp.12365

Peterson, J. R. (2017). Polyfidelity and the dynamics of group romantic relationships [Doctoral dissertation, Walden University]. Walden University ScholarWorks. Retrieved from https://scholarworks.waldenu.edu/cgi/viewcontent.cgi?article=4357&context=dissertations&httpsredir=1&referer=

Petruzzella, A., Feinstein, B. A., & Lavner, J. A. (2019). Sexual orientation-related stigma and relationship functioning among female same-sex couples. *Journal of Lesbian Studies*, *23*(4), 439–450. https://doi.org/10.1080/10894160.2019.1614861

Pew Research Center. (2017). *Intermarriage in the U.S. 50 years after Loving* v. *Virginia.*. Retrieved from www.pewresearch.org/social-trends/2017/05/18/intermarriage-in-the-u-s-50-years-after-loving-v-virginia/

Piao, X. (2021). Marriage stability and private versus shared expenditures within families: Evidence from Japanese families. *Social Indicators Research*, *153*, 533–559. https://doi.org/10.1007/s11205-020-02498-2

Pohtinen, J. (2019). From secrecy to pride negotiating the kink identity, normativity, and stigma. *Etnologia Fennica*, *46*, 84–108. https://doi.org/10.23991/ef.v46i0.74306

Prentice, C. M. (2008). The assimilation of in-laws: The impact of newcomers on the communication routines of families. *Journal of Applied Communication Research*, *36*(1), 74–97. https://doi.org/10.1080/00909880701799311

Reczek, C. (2016). Parental disapproval and gay and lesbian relationship quality. *Journal of Family Issues*, *37*(15), 2189–2212. https://doi.org/10.1177/0192513X14566638

Rees, G., & Garcia, J. R. (2017). An investigation into the solitary and interpersonal aspects of sexual object fetishism: A mixed-methods approach. *Psychology & Sexuality*, *8*(4), 252–267. https://doi.org/10.1080/19419899.2017.1383301

Rehor, J. E. (2015). Sensual, erotic, and sexual behaviors of women from the "kink" community. *Archives of Sexual Behavior*, *44*(4), 825–836. https://doi.org/10.1007/s10508-015-0524-2

Rokach, A., & Chan, S. H. (2023). Love and infidelity: Causes and consequences. *International Journal of Environmental Research and Public Health*, *20*(5), Article 3904. https://doi.org/10.3390/ijerph20053904

Rollè, L., Giardina, G., Caldarera, A. M., Gerino, E., & Brustia, P. (2018). When intimate partner violence meets same sex couples: A review of same sex intimate partner violence. *Frontiers in Psychology*, *9*, 1–13. https://doi.org/10.3389/fpsyg.2018.01506

Sabo, K. N. (2020). Sadomasochism: Appropriate, inappropriate, or somewhere in between? *Mako: NSU Undergraduate Student Journal*, Article 5. Retrieved from https://nsuworks.nova.edu/cgi/viewcontent.cgi?article=1016&context=mako

Schueths, A. M. (2014). 'It's almost like white supremacy': Interracial mixed-status couples facing racist nativism. *Ethnic and Racial Studies*, *37*(13), 2438–2456. https://doi.org/10.1080/01419870.2013.835058

Scoats, R., & Campbell, C. (2022). What do we know about consensual non-monogamy? *Current Opinion in Psychology*, *48*, Article 101468. https://doi.org/10.1016/j.copsyc.2022.101468

Scott, S. B., Garibay, B., & Do, Q. A. (2022). Reasons for relationship dissolution in female same-gender and queer couples. *Couple and Family Psychology: Research and Practice*, *11*(2), 132–140. https://doi.org/10.1037/cfp0000212

Scott, S. B., Whitton, S. W., & Buzzella, B. A. (2019). Providing relationship interventions to same-sex couples: Clinical considerations, program adaptations, and continuing education. *Cognitive and Behavioral Practice*, *26*(2), 270–284. https://doi.org/10.1016/j.cbpra.2018.03.004

Séguin, L. J. (2019). The good, the bad, and the ugly: Lay attitudes and perceptions of polyamory. *Sexualities*, *22*(4), 669–690. https://doi.org/10.1177/1363460717713382

Seshardri, G., & Knudson-Martin, C. (2013). How couples manage interracial and intercultural differences: Implications for clinical practice. *Journal of Marital and Family Therapy*, *39*(1), 43–58. https://doi.org/10.1111/j.1752-0606.2011.00262.x

Shackelford, T. K., LeBlanc, G. J., & Drass, E. (2000). Emotional reactions to infidelity. *Cognition and Emotion*, *14*(5), 643–659, https://doi.org/10.1080/02699930050117657

Shaiful Bahari, I., Norhayati, M. N., Nik Hazlina, N. H., Mohamad Shahirul Aiman, C. A. A., & Nik Muhammad Arif, N. A. (2021). Psychological impact of polygamous marriage on women and children: A systematic review and meta-analysis. *BMC Pregnancy Childbirth*, *21*, Article 823. https://doi.org/10.1186/s12884-021-04301-7

Skogrand, L., Johnson, A. C., Horrocks, A. M., & DeFrain, J. (2011). Financial management practices of couples with great marriages. *Journal of Family Economic Issues*, *32*, 27–35. http://doi.org/10.1007/s10834-010-9195-2

Sprecher, S., & Felmlee, D. (1992). The influence of parents and friends on the quality and stability of romantic relationships: A three-wave longitudinal investigation. *Journal of Marriage and Family Therapy*, *54*(4), 888–900. https://doi.org/10.2307/353170

Stephens, M. A. P., Townsend, A. L., Martire, L. M., & Druley, J. A. (2001). Balancing parent care with other roles: Interrole conflict of adult daughter caregivers. *Journal of Gerontology*, *56*(1), 24–34. https://doi.org/10.1093/geronb/56.1.p24

Stephenson, R., Sharma, A., Mimiaga, M. J., Garofalo, R., Brown, E., Bratcher, A., Wimbly, T., Hidalgo, M. A., Hoehnle, S., Thai, J., Sullivan, P. S., & Suarez, N. A. (2019). Concordance in the reporting of intimate partner violence among male-male couples. *Journal of Family Violence*, *34*, 677–686. https://doi.org/10.1007/s10896-019-00076-w

Stewart, S.-J. F., Frost, D. M., & LeBlanc, A. J. (2019). Understanding how emerging same-sex couples make meaning of minority stress: A narrative approach. *Journal of Family Psychology*, *33*(2), 183–193. http://dx.doi.org/10.1037/fam0000495

Strauss, J. R. (2013). Caregiving for parents and in-laws: Commonalities and differences. *Journal of Gerontological Social Work*, *56*(1), 49–66. https://doi.org/10.1080/01634372.2012.728185

Tagler, M. J., & Jeffers, H. M. (2013). Sex differences in attitudes toward partner infidelity. *Evolutionary Psychology*, *11*(4), 821–832. https://doi.org/10.1177/147470491301100407

Thomas, A. G., Stone, B., Bennett, P., Stewart-Williams, S., & Ottesen Kennair, L. E. (2021). Sex differences in voyeuristic and exhibitionistic interests: Exploring the mediating roles of sociosexuality and sexual compulsivity from an evolutionary perspective. *Archives of Sexual Behavior*, *50*, 2151–2162. https://doi.org/10.1007/s10508-021-01991-0

Thornton, V., & Nagurney, A. (2011). What is infidelity? Perceptions based on biological sex and personality. *Psychology Research and Behavior Management*, *4*, 51–58. https://doi.org/10.2147/PRBM.S16876

Tiidenberg, K., & Paasonen, S. (2019). Littles: Affects and aesthetics in sexual age-play. *Sexuality & Culture*, *23*(2), 375–393. https://doi.org/10.1007/s12119-018-09580-5

Totenhagen, C. J., Randall, A. K., & Lloyd, K. (2018a). Stress and relationship functioning in same-sex couples: The vulnerabilities of internalized homophobia and outness. *Family Relations*, *67*(3), 399–413. https://doi.org/10.1111/fare.12311

Totenhagen, C. J., Wilmarth, M. J., Serido, J., & Betancourt, A. E. (2018b). Do day-to-day finances play a role in relationship satisfaction? A dyadic investigation. *Journal of Family Psychology*, *32*(4), 528–537. http://dx.doi.org/10.1037/fam0000406

Troy, A. B., Lewis-Smith, J., & Laurenceau, J.-P. (2006). Interracial and intraracial romantic relationships: The search for differences in satisfaction, conflict, and attachment style. *Journal of Social and Personal Relationships*, *23*(1), 65–80. https://doi.org/10.1177/0265407506060178

Vaillancourt, K. T., & Few-Demo, A. L. (2014). Relational dynamics of swinging relationships: An exploratory study. *The Family Journal*, *22*(3), 311–320. https://doi.org/10.1177/1066480714529742

van der Vleuten, M., Jaspers, E., & van der Lippe, T. (2021). Same-sex couples' division of labor from a cross-national perspective. *Journal of GLBT Family Studies*, *17*(2), 150–167. https://doi.org/10.1080/1550428X.2020.1862012

Vazques, V., Otero, I., & Goodlow, J. (2019). Relationship stigma and Black-White interracial marital satisfaction: The mediating role of religious/spiritual well-being. *Mental Health, Religion & Culture*, *22*(3), 305–318. https://doi.org/10.1080/13674676.2019.1620189

Ventriglio, A., Bhat, P. S., Torales, J., & Bhugra, D. (2019). Sexuality in the 21st century: Leather or rubber? Fetishism explained. *Medical Journal Armed Forces India*, *75*(2), 121–124. https://doi.org/10.1016/j.mjafi.2018.09.009

Vowels, L. M., Vowels, M. J., & Mark, K. P. (2022). Is infidelity predictable? Using explainable machine learning to identify the most important predictors of infidelity. *Journal of Sex Research*, *59*(2), 224–237. https://doi.org/10.1080/00224499.2021.1967846

Warach, B., & Josephs, L. (2021). The aftershocks of infidelity: A review of infidelity-based attachment trauma. *Sexual and Relationship Therapy*, *36*(1), 68–90. https://doi.org/10.1080/14681994.2019.1577961

Ward, F., & Linn, R. (2020). The mother-in-law mystique: A tale of conflict, criticism and resistance. *Australian & New Zealand Journal of Family Therapy*, *41*(4), 381–392. https://doi.org/10.1002/anzf.1430

Wilkinson, D. E., & Dunlop, W. L. (2020). Both sides of the story: Narratives of romantic infidelity. *Personal Relationships*, *28*(1), 121–147. https://doi.org/10.1111/pere.12355

Wu, K., Chen, C., & Greenberger, E. (2015). The sweetness of forbidden fruit: Interracial daters are more attractive than intraracial daters. *Journal of Social and Personal Relationships*, *32*(5), 650–666. https://doi.org/10.1177/0265407514541074

Yates, S. M., & Neuer-Colburn, A. A. (2019). Counseling the kink community: What clinicians need to know. *Journal of Counseling Sexology & Sexual Wellness*, *1*(1), 14–22. https://doi.org/10.34296/01011007

Zimmerman, K. J., & Roberts, C. W. (2012). The influence of a financial management course on couples' relationship quality. *Journal of Financial Counseling and Planning*, *23*(2), 46–54.

Index

For Product Safety Concerns and Information please contact our
EU representative GPSR@taylorandfrancis.com Taylor & Francis
Verlag GmbH, Kaufingerstraße 24, 80331 München, Germany